Case Studies in Orthopedics

Case Studies in Orthopedics

Editor: Tom Dawson

AMERICAN
MEDICAL PUBLISHERS
www.americanmedicalpublishers.com

AMERICAN
MEDICAL PUBLISHERS
www.americanmedicalpublishers.com

Cataloging-in-Publication Data

Case studies in orthopedics / edited by Tom Dawson.
p. cm.
Includes bibliographical references and index.
ISBN 979-8-88740-613-8
1. Orthopedics. 2. Orthopedics--Diagnosis. 3. Orthopedics--Treatment.
I. Dawson, Tom.
RD731 .O78 2023
616.7--dc23

American Medical Publishers,
41 Flatbush Avenue,
1st Floor, New York,
NY 11217, USA

ISBN 979-8-88740-613-8 (Hardback)

Contents

Preface

This book was inspired by the evolution of our times; to answer the curiosity of inquisitive minds. Many developments have occurred across the globe in the recent past which has transformed the progress in the field.

Orthopedics refers to a medical specialty that focuses on the prevention, diagnosis and treatment of disorders and injuries related to the musculoskeletal system. The musculoskeletal system includes bones, joints, muscles, ligaments, tendons, and other connective tissues that provide structure, support and movement to the body. These include fractures, sprains, strains, dislocations, sports injuries, arthritis, spine disorders, deformities, and trauma-related injuries. Orthopedics utilizes both surgical and non-surgical methods to treat these conditions, depending on the specific needs of the patient. Prominent non-surgical treatments in orthopedics include physical therapy, medication management, immobilization with casts or braces, joint injections, and rehabilitation programs. Surgical interventions can range from minimally invasive procedures, such as arthroscopy, to major and complicated surgeries, such as joint replacements or spinal fusion. This book unravels the recent studies in the field of orthopedics. It will serve as a valuable source of reference for graduate and postgraduate students.

This book was developed from a mere concept to drafts to chapters and finally compiled together as a complete text to benefit the readers across all nations. To ensure the quality of the content we instilled two significant steps in our procedure. The first was to appoint an editorial team that would verify the data and statistics provided in the book and also select the most appropriate and valuable contributions from the plentiful contributions we received from authors worldwide. The next step was to appoint an expert of the topic as the Editor-in-Chief, who would head the project and finally make the necessary amendments and modifications to make the text reader-friendly. I was then commissioned to examine all the material to present the topics in the most comprehensible and productive format.

I would like to take this opportunity to thank all the contributing authors who were supportive enough to contribute their time and knowledge to this project. I also wish to convey my regards to my family who have been extremely supportive during the entire project.

Editor

1

Profunda Brachii Pseudoaneurysm following Supracondylar Fracture of Humerus Repair in an 8-Year-Old Boy: A Case Report and Review of Literature

Hamed Ghoddusi Johari,[1,2] **Mohammad-Ali Erfani**,[3] **Amirhossein Erfani**,[1,4] **Reza Shahriarirad**,[1,4] and **Mohammad-Mehdi Karami**[3]

[1]*Thoracic and Vascular Surgery Research Center, Shiraz University of Medical Sciences, Shiraz, Iran*
[2]*Trauma Research Center, General Surgery Department, Shiraz University of Medical Sciences, Shiraz, Iran*
[3]*Research Center for Bone and Joint Diseases, Department of Orthopedic Surgery, Chamran Hospital, Shiraz University of Medical Sciences, Shiraz, Iran*
[4]*Student Research Committee, Shiraz University of Medical Sciences, Shiraz, Iran*

Correspondence should be addressed to Amirhossein Erfani; ahnerfani@gmail.com

Academic Editor: Wan Ismail Faisham

Arterial pseudoaneurysm can manifest in almost all arteries, but peripheral ones such as brachial artery pseudoaneurysm are rare and typically happen after trauma or infections. We describe an 8-year-old boy who presented with a large nonpulsatile soft tissue mass-like lesion 20 days after supracondylar fracture of the humerus which was fixed using Kirschner wire. The neurovascular examination was normal; CT angiography revealed a large pseudoaneurysm arising from the left profunda brachii artery. The patient went under surgical repair and was discharged from the hospital with an uneventful postop course. A high index of suspicion is necessary in cases with humeral fractures for the early diagnosis of pseudoaneurysm where the delayed diagnosis may cause fatal outcomes.

1. Introduction

Arterial pseudoaneurysm can manifest in almost all arteries, but peripheral ones such as brachial artery aneurysms are rare and typically happen after trauma or infections [1, 2]. Supracondylar fracture of the humerus accounts for almost 17.9% of fractures in children aged under 16 and can lead to vascular injuries in 10-14% of cases [3, 4]. Brachial artery pseudoaneurysm can often present as a mass-like lesion with rapid expansion and pain or ischemic complications due to thrombosis or distal embolization [1]. There have been several reports of iatrogenic pseudoaneurysm of the brachial artery. However, to the best of our knowledge, this is the first report of profunda brachii pseudoaneurysm followed by pediatric supracondylar fracture of the humerus. Here, we present a case pseudoaneurysm of profunda Brachii caused by injury after treatment of the supracondylar fracture of the humerus using Kirschner wire fixation.

2. Case Presentation

An 8-year-old boy with no significant past medical history sustained a closed supracondylar fracture of the left humerus due to falling down. The initial X-ray demonstrated a type III fracture based on Gartland classification (Figure 1). He was admitted to the orthopedic ward in order to continue the treatment. Since closed reduction failed, the patient underwent surgery through posterior approach, patient being positioned in a lateral decubitus position and with the elbow held hyperflexed, in posterior aspect of elbow, a straight midline posterior incision was done, and medial and lateral skin flaps were created, elevated, and retracted.

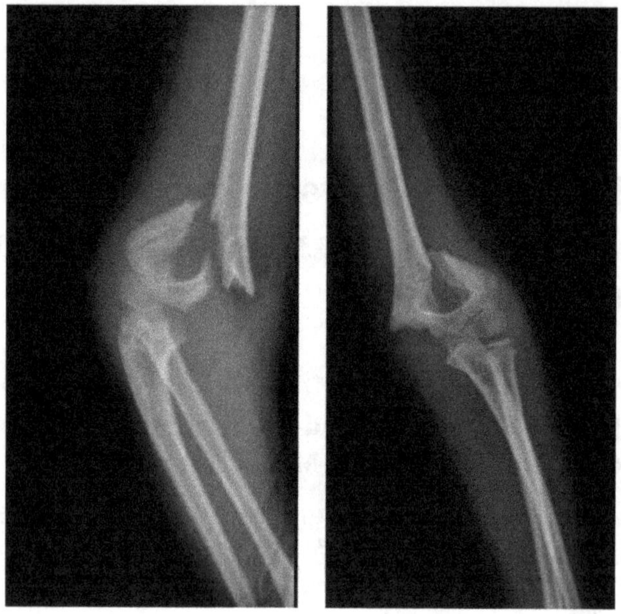

(a) (b)

Figure 1: Supracondylar fracture of humerus with posterior displacement on first admission. Lateral view (a) and anterior posterior view (b).

In medial aspect, ulnar nerve was isolated and protected, both medial and lateral paratricipital approach was done, and fracture site was exposed. Then, the fracture was reduced and with the first try, and 4 crossed Kirschner wires were inserted under direct visualization to achieve desired stability and rigidity. The patient was discharged the day after surgery (Figures 2 and 3). After 20 days, the patient was revisited due to pain and a large soft tissue mass-like lesion on the lateral aspect of the left elbow in site of surgery with no fever or other symptoms which was progressed gradually after being discharged. Physical examination revealed tense swollen sites of surgery with wound dehiscence and marginal necrosis with no evidence of infection or discharges. The patient was afebrile with a blood pressure of 110/70 mmHg, heart rate of 79, and a hemoglobin level of 8.3 g/dl. The neurovascular examination was normal with tenderness on a mass-like lesion without bruit. Based on preliminary assumption of hematoma formation versus pseudoaneurysm, soft tissue and duplex sonography were performed, which revealed normal arterial flow in all major arteries from the subclavian artery, brachial, and radial as well as ulnar arteries with a large collection in the posterior aspect of the elbow. However, based on the patient's history of recent trauma and physical examination, we were highly suspicious of pseudoaneurysm. Therefore, CT angiography was done, which revealed a huge pseudoaneurysm originating from the left profunda brachii artery with extravasation of contrast with the largest diameter of 54.96 mm (Figures 4 and 5).

Based on the necrotic overlying skin, the patient was emergently transferred to the operation room in which after heparinization and proximal control by a tourniquet, and the sac of pseudoaneurysm was opened and approached through a left lateral arm incision (Figure 6). The neck of pseudoaneurysm originated from the profunda brachial artery 2 cm above the line of fracture which was in close con-

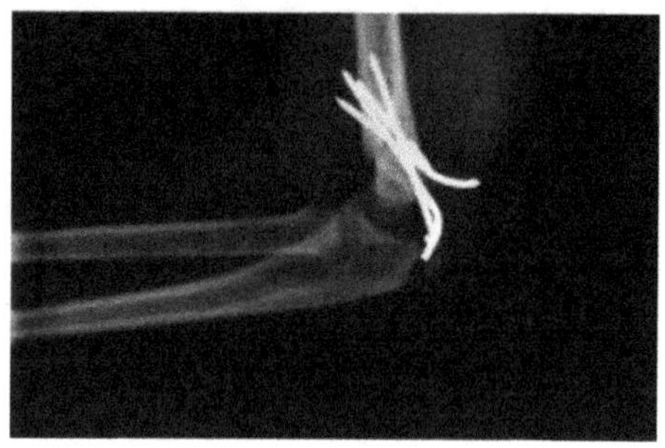

Figure 2: Lateral view of supracondylar fracture of humerus fixed with Kirschner wire (post-op).

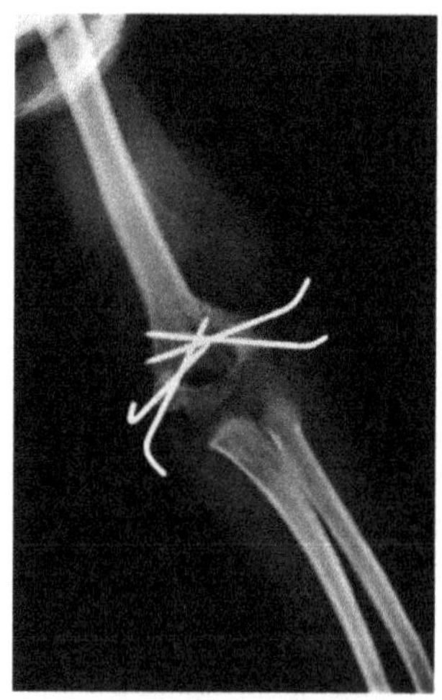

Figure 3: Anterior posterior view of supracondylar fracture of humerus fixed with Kirschner wire (post-op).

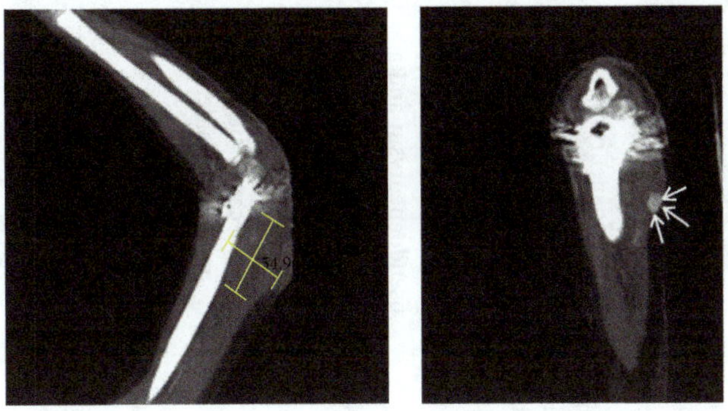

(a) (b)

FIGURE 4: (a) Coronal cut of CT angiography demonstrating maximum diameter of sac of pseudoaneurysm originating from left profunda brachii artery. (b) Extravasation of contrast in pseudoaneurysm of profunda brachii artery in CT angiography.

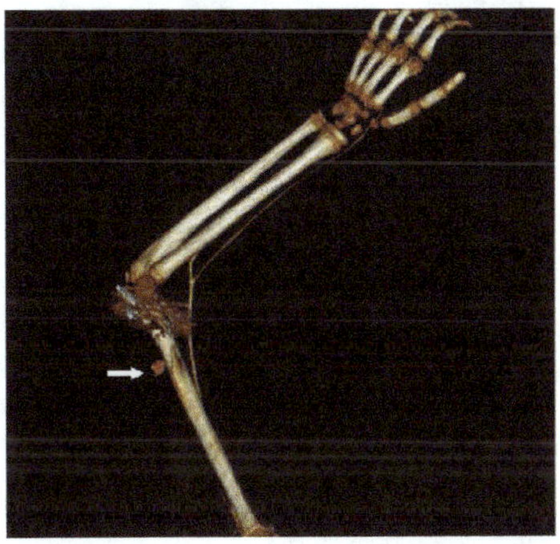

FIGURE 5: 3D reconstruction of CT angiography demonstrating a pseudoaneurysm of profunda brachii artery with extravasation of contrast (white arrow).

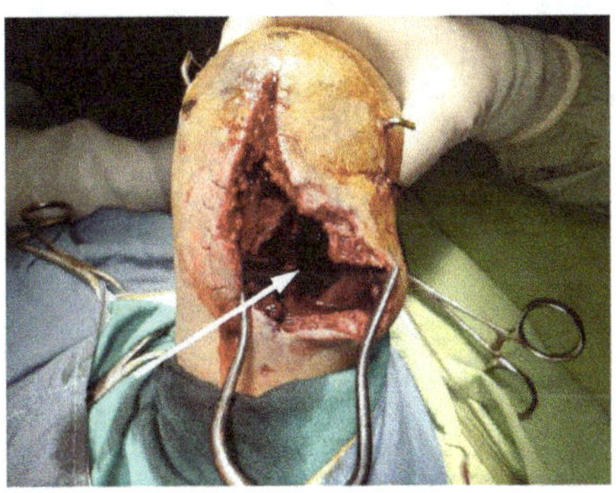

FIGURE 6: Open wound demonstrating the pseudoaneurysm sac through posterolateral approach. Neck of the pseudoaneurysm is visible in the depth of the wound (pointed by the arrow).

tact with the tip of Kirschner wire making an exit from the medical cortex of the bony structure. Furthermore, the punctured site of profunda brachial artery was repaired by prolene oversewing sutures, and the patient was discharged after 2 days of hospitalization with an uneventful postop course. In the patients' further follow ups, no neurovascular complications or signs of infection was reported, while also achieving full range of motion in examination.

3. Discussion

Although upper extremity peripheral pseudoaneurysm of the arteries is rare, they can happen iatrogenically and after trauma, especially in upper extremity fractures. Nowadays, the total rate of pseudoaneurysms has increased due to the widespread use of peripheral endovascular procedures from 0.04% before 2000 to 0.7% in 2019 [5, 6]. Arterial catheterization for blood gas, invasive monitoring, and diagnostic and therapeutic endovascular procedures are considered as the most common causes of iatrogenic injury to the brachial artery. Even though it is uncommon, the development of pseudoaneurysms is slow and can cause delayed diagnosis with further possible complications. Pseudoaneurysms, depending on the size, can be asymptomatic or present with symptoms ranging from pressure effect on the adjacent tissues such as pain, swelling, and nerve injury, or ischemic complications due to thrombosis or distal embolization with the management depending on the location, size, and causative pathogenesis of pseudoaneurysm [7, 8].

Table 1 demonstrates reported cases of pseudoaneurysm following supracondylar fracture of humerus after fixation. Most of the reported cases happened in close reduction and fixation with Kirschner wires, and in most cases in the first follow up of the patient, clinical suspicion to pseudoaneurysm formation was not made, and surgeons assumed that swelling and pain contribute to the postsurgery inflammation or postsurgery hematoma which further evaluation and follow ups revealed the diagnosis of pseudoaneurysm.

Asavamongkolkul and Ruangsetakit reported pseudoaneurysm of the brachial artery after supracondylar fracture in a 3-year-old boy. Similar to our case, the patient was treated using Kirschner wire fixation after an open reduction in the operating room. In this case, the patient presented with a slowly growing nonpulsatile soft tissue mass on the medial aspect of the left elbow with audible bruit. However, in contrast to our case, the interval of the initiation of symptoms was much longer, and it was found that the tip of the Kirschner wire was stuck in the pseudoaneurysm that could penetrate the brachial artery in some positions, which was not the case in our study. Also, the patient in their study developed malunion, while ours recovered after surgery without any complications in the follow-up visits [9].

Kemp et al. described an 82-year-old man who was referred to their clinic due to a painless pulsatile soft tissue mass with bruit following a comminuted fracture of the right humerus. He was treated with a hanging cast; however, since the incident, he developed loss of dexterity in his right hand and paresthesia. CT angiography confirmed the presence of a large brachial pseudoaneurysm. Therefore, he was transferred to the operating room for the surgical repair of the pseudoaneurysm. On close inspection during surgery, it was found that the sac contained a sharp fragment of the

Table 1: A review of reported cases of arterial pseudoaneurysm after supracondylar fracture of humerus fixation.

Firth author	Age (years)	Interval till initial presentation	Initial physical exam	Diagnosis	Type of fixation	Intraoperative findings agent
Asavamongkolkul and Ruangsetakit [9]	3	7 months	(i) 4 cm mass without erythema or warmth (ii) No pulsation, bruit on auscultation	Brachial angiography	OR via a posterior longitudinal incision and internal fixation with two-crossed K-wire.	Tips of the K-wire were stuck inside the aneurysm.
Chikande et al. [10]	6	11 days	(i) Painful tumefaction of the medial and distal part of the arm (ii) Fever (iii) Weak radial pulse (iv) Normal cutaneous hand perfusion	Duplex ultrasound and CT angiography	CRIF using 3 K-wire, 2 percutaneous from lateral condyle, and one by a mini-approach on medial epicondyle.	Brachial artery perforation without contacts with wires.
Hernandez et al. [11]	7	21 days	(i) Medial mass of the elbow, with no palpable thrill, or audible bruit (ii) Distal radial and ulnar pulses were present	Duplex ultrasound and CT angiography	CR and internal fixation with two lateral K-wires under fluoroscopic control.	Injury may be produced by punction humeral artery during the insertion of the wires.
Cunha et al. [12]	9	12 weeks	(i) Palpable, painless, and pulsatile mass (ii) Distal pulses were symmetric and palpable	Duplex ultrasound	Percutaneously using three K-wire placed divergently in a lateral-to-medial position.	Bone spicula perforating the artery during trauma or the maneuver reduction.
Got et al. [13]	6	5 weeks	(i) Diminished sensation and strength in the radial nerve distribution (ii) Diminished radial pulse (iii) Continued swelling in the antecubital fossa	Soft tissue sonography.	CR and percutaneous pin fixation of the supracondylar fracture with 3 lateral K-wire.	The pseudoaneurysm was a 1 cm segment of the posterolateral wall of the brachial artery.
Tepper et al. [4]	9	22 days	(i) Elbow mass, tender to palpation, and no pulsatile quality (ii) No overt palpable thrill (iii) Normal neurovascular examination	Intraoperative diagnosis was done during hematoma evacuation.	CR and percutaneous pin fixation with 2 K-wire inserted from the lateral condyle and divergent across the fracture site.	Ruptured left brachial artery pseudoaneurysm and a complex longitudinal arterial tear at the fracture site. The fixation pins were not near the pseudoaneurysm and were left in place because the fixation remained stable.
Bhandari et al. [14]	13 years old	2 weeks	(i) An expansile swelling of 5 cm diameter with thrill with normal radial pulse	—	CR and k-wire fixation (4 K-wire)	Brachial artery pseudoaneurysm

CR: closed reduction; CRIF: closed reduction and internal fixation; CT: computed tomography; OR: open reduction; K-wires: Kirschner wires.

humerus with a single puncture wound in the brachial artery which was the reason for pseudoaneurysm formation [8].

Moran et al. reported a 65-year-old female who presented with a large pulsatile soft tissue mass in the middle third of the left humerus 6 months after the humeral fracture which was fixed with an intramedullary nail. The patient presented with reduced sensation in the median nerve territory along with mild thenar muscle wasting. A pseudoaneurysm with the largest diameter of 5.8 cm was diagnosed with duplex sonography which was due to a break of proximal locking screw of the intramedullary nail. Although humeral fracture was fixed with an intramedullary nail, the patient developed brachial pseudoaneurysm [7].

It is worth mentioning that although orthopedic references put an emphasis on considering anterior approach for exploration and reconstruction. However, our patient developed iatrogenic pseudoaneurysm of the profunda brachii due to penetration of Kirschner wires used in open reduction and internal fixation through posterior approach. When utilizing posterior approach, persuasion should be taken to avoid neurovascular damage too while using Kirschner wires. Moreover, it should be mentioned that orthopedic surgeons must take the vascular complications in patients' follow-ups as well as other complications such as nerve damage, stiffness, and infection into consideration. This case emphasizes the importance of clinical suspicion to pseudoaneurysm even if the distal pulses were palpated and duplex sonography reveals normal arterial flow. Furthermore, close vascular observation must be done in the setting of well-perfused hand in cases of displaced supracondylar fractures before and after surgery.

4. Conclusion

Pseudoaneurysm is a complication that presents itself gradually and can be either asymptomatic or symptomatic, in which any external instrument or fragments of fracture with a sharp end can cause its formation. A high index of suspicion is necessary in cases with humeral fractures for the early diagnosis of pseudoaneurysm where the delayed diagnosis may cause further complications.

Abbreviations

CT: Computerized tomography.

Data Availability

Please contact the corresponding author for any further data.

Consent

Written informed consent was obtained from the patients' parents to write and publish the case as a report with accompanying radiological images.

Authors' Contributions

Mohammad-Ali Erfani was the orthopedist, and Hamed Ghoddusi Johari was the vascular surgeon in the described case. Amirhossein Erfani, Reza Shahriarirad, and Mohammad-Mehdi Karami collected the data. Amirhossein Erfani, Hamed Ghoddusi Johari, and Mohammad-Ali Erfani drafted the manuscript. Reza Shahriarirad revised and proofread the manuscript. All authors read and approved the final version of the manuscript.

Acknowledgments

The authors would like to thank Shiraz University of Medical Sciences, Shiraz, Iran, and also Center for Development of Clinical Research of Nemazee Hospital and Dr. Nasrin Shokrpour for editorial assistance.

References

[1] H. A. Hall, S. Minc, and T. Babrowski, "Peripheral artery aneurysm," *Surgical Clinics*, vol. 93, no. 4, pp. 911–923, 2013.

[2] T. Leite, M. Pires, L. Pires, C. Chagas, and A. C. Oliveira, "Giant iatrogenic pseudoaneurysm of the brachial artery: a case report," *International Journal of Surgery Case Reports*, vol. 37, pp. 193–195, 2017.

[3] S. Luria, A. Sucar, S. Eylon et al., "Vascular complications of supracondylar humeral fractures in children," *Journal of Pediatric Orthopaedics. Part B*, vol. 16, no. 2, pp. 133–143, 2007.

[4] S. C. Tepper, C. P. Gottlich, I. W. Nasr, and P. D. Sponseller, "Brachial artery pseudoaneurysm after supracondylar humerus fracture: a case report," *JBJS Case Connector*, vol. 10, no. 1, article e0218, 2020.

[5] Z. Tong, Y. Gu, L. Guo et al., "An analysis of complications of brachial and axillary artery punctures," *The American Surgeon*, vol. 82, no. 12, pp. 1250–1256, 2016.

[6] O. Borghese, A. Pisani, and M. D. Isabelle Di Centa, "Treatment of iatrogenic pseudoaneurysm of the brachial artery: case report and literature review," *Vascular Disease Management*, vol. 16, no. 7, pp. E87–E91, 2019.

[7] D. Moran, G. Roche-Nagle, R. Ryan, D. Brophy, W. Quinlan, and M. Barry, "Pseudoaneurysm of the brachial artery following humeral fracture," *Vascular and Endovascular Surgery*, vol. 42, no. 1, pp. 65–68, 2008.

[8] K. Kemp, R. Radwan, G. Shingler, and C. Davies, "Brachial artery pseudoaneurysm," *BMJ Case Reports*, vol. 2014, no. may23 1, article bcr2014203924, 2014.

[9] A. Asavamongkolkul and C. Ruangsetakit, "False aneurysm of the brachial artery in supracondylar fracture treated with Kirschner wire fixation: a case report," *Injury*, vol. 32, no. 3, pp. 256-257, 2001.

[10] J. Chikande, V. Rampal, N. Sadaghianloo, A. Voury-Pons, and F. Solla, "Pseudoaneurysm of the brachial artery after reduction and fixation of a displaced supracondylar elbow fracture in a child," *Annals of Vascular Surgery*, vol. 56, pp. 352.e9–352.e13, 2019.

[11] A. Hernandez-Fernandez, R. Vélez, F. Soldado, C. G. Fontecha, I. Barber, and M. Aguirre, "False aneurysm of the brachial artery secondary to K-wire fixation of a supracondylar fracture of the humerus," *European Journal of Pediatric Surgery*, vol. 23, no. 3, pp. 251–253, 2013.

[12] L. A. da Cunha, L. M. Ávila, J. R. Gonçalves, S. Pereira, C. M. Jamur, and B. M. de Souza, "Brachial artery pseudoaneurysm after fixation of supracondylar fracture in a 9-year-old child," *Journal of Pediatric Orthopaedics. Part B*, vol. 28, no. 6, pp. 559–563, 2019.

[13] C. Got, T. W. Tan, N. Thakur, E. J. Marcaccio Jr., C. Eberson, and I. Madom, "Delayed presentation of a brachial artery pseudoaneurysm after a supracondylar humerus fracture in a 6-year-old boy: a case report," *Journal of Pediatric Orthopedics*, vol. 30, no. 1, pp. 57–59, 2010.

[14] P. S. Bhandari, P. Bastola, and D. Gurung, "Case report on pseudoaneurysm of brachial artery: a rare complication of paediatric supracondylar humerus fracture pinning," *Journal of Institute of Medicine Nepal*, vol. 41, no. 3, pp. 95–97, 2019.

2

Free-Floating Scapular Spine: A Rare Shoulder Injury

John H. Cabot, Khang H. Dang, and Anil K. Dutta

Department of Orthopaedics, UT Health San Antonio, San Antonio, TX 78229, USA

Correspondence should be addressed to Khang H. Dang; dangk@uthscsa.edu

Academic Editor: Elke R. Ahlmann

A specific treatment protocol for managing scapular spine fractures does not currently exist. The purpose of our report is to describe this type of injury and detail our treatment management in order to better elucidate this rare pathology. We present a case of a 26-year-old female with an acute scapular spine and base fracture after a motor vehicle collision. Successful treatment of an acute free-floating scapular spine fracture was achieved with open reduction and internal fixation utilizing an elbow plate. Since scapular spine fractures are an unfortunate, rare injury, it may impose difficult challenges to the treating surgeon. With our case report, we hope to contribute to the overall knowledge of scapular spine fractures and offer our experience with a successful and appropriate treatment option in our patient.

1. Introduction

Acute scapula fractures are a rare injury accounting for 3-5% of fractures of the shoulder girdle and occurring at a rate of 0.7% for all fractures [1]. These injuries are generally a result of high-energy mechanisms, such as motor vehicle collisions, and are often associated with other upper extremity, thoracic, or pelvic ring injuries [2]. The most common scapula fractures involve the neck or the body, which represents two-thirds of all scapula fractures [3]. Conversely, scapular spine fractures are a rare subset accounting for only 6% of all scapula fractures and generally healed with conservative management [4, 5]. We present a case of a 26-year-old female with a fracture of the scapular body and spine with extension into the base of the acromion. Our case may shed light on what we believe is the first documented case report of free-floating scapular spine fracture, with consideration of a potential treatment option.

2. Case Report

A 26-year-old right-handed female with no pertinent medical history presented to our emergency department with left shoulder pain after a motor vehicle collision in early 2019. The patient was a restrained passenger in a high-speed motor vehicle rollover two days before her presentation, resulting in a fatality at the scene. She was initially seen at an outside facility who diagnosed her with a clavicle fracture and multiple rib fractures. Her physical exam showed no neurovascular deficits but significant pain and swelling over the scapula along with superficial abrasions. Radiographs showed a comminuted and displaced fracture of the scapular spine and body with an avulsion of the acromion base (Figure 1). Computed tomography 3-dimensional reconstruction revealed no glenoid involvement but a segmental fracture of the entire superior aspect of the scapula, including the acromion base and spine, which were free-floating fragments (Figure 2). Given the degree of displacement and increased risk of nonunion and poor functional outcome, the patient elected to proceed with open reduction and internal fixation one week following her injury.

Intraoperatively, the patient was positioned upright in the beach chair position. With an incision along the scapular spine, a posterior approach to the scapula was utilized. The trapezius muscle was elevated off the acromion and scapular spine while the posterior deltoid origin was maintained on the lateral aspect of the acromion. The supraspinatus and infraspinatus were elevated subperiosteally from their origin on the scapula towards their insertion thus allowing for full exposure of the entire superior body of the scapula. After adequate exposure, the posterior portion of the acromion was reduced to the scapular body with point of reduction clamps and stabilized with 2.7 mm lag screws (Figures 3 and 4).

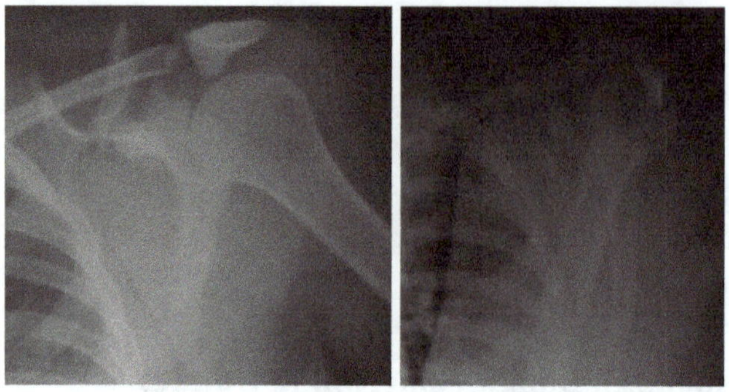

FIGURE 1: AP and lateral radiographic views of the scapula showing a comminuted and displaced fracture of the scapular spine and body with an avulsion of the acromion base.

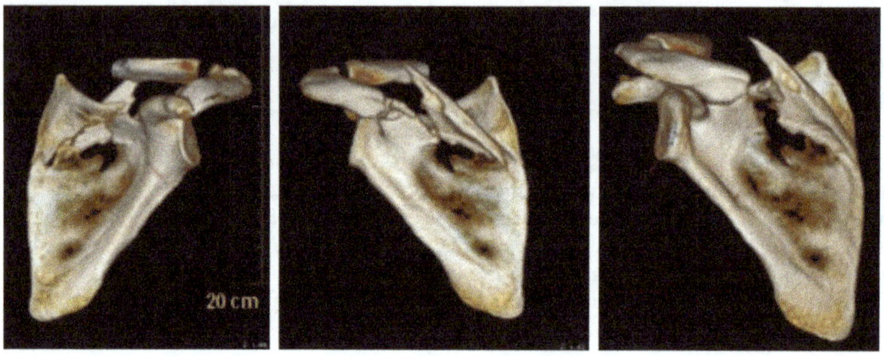

FIGURE 2: Computed tomography 3-dimensional reconstruction of the scapula showing a segmental fracture of the entire superior aspect including the acromion along with free-floating fragments of its base and spine.

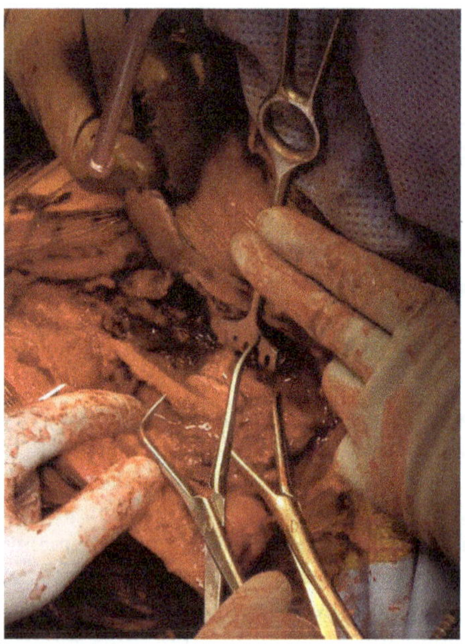

FIGURE 3: Intraoperative view of the temporary reduction of scapular spine fracture with forceps.

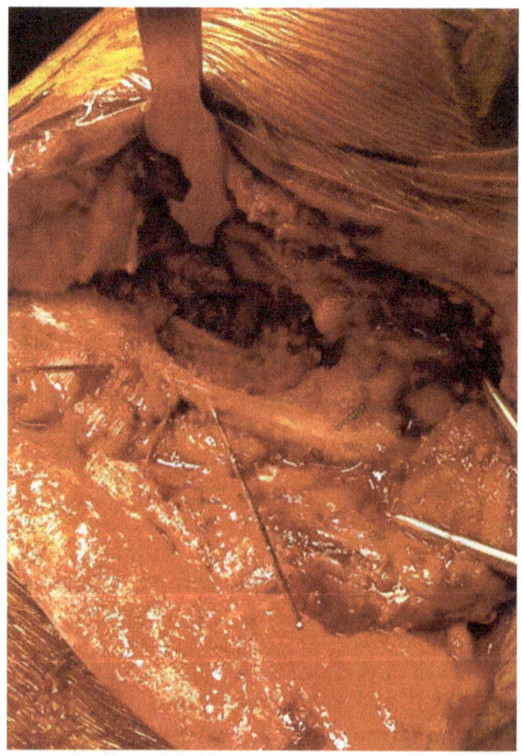

FIGURE 4: 2.7 mm lag screws and K-wires were used to provide temporary fixation and alignment of the scapular spine fracture.

Temporary reduction of the fractured scapular spine to the acromion was achieved with K-wires, and then, a Zimmer Biomet elbow plate was placed for definitive fixation

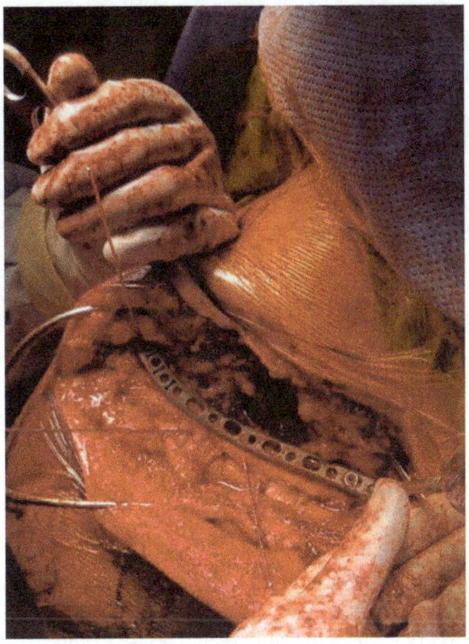

FIGURE 5: Intraoperative view of the placement of the Zimmer-Biomet elbow plate which matched the contour of the spine of the scapula.

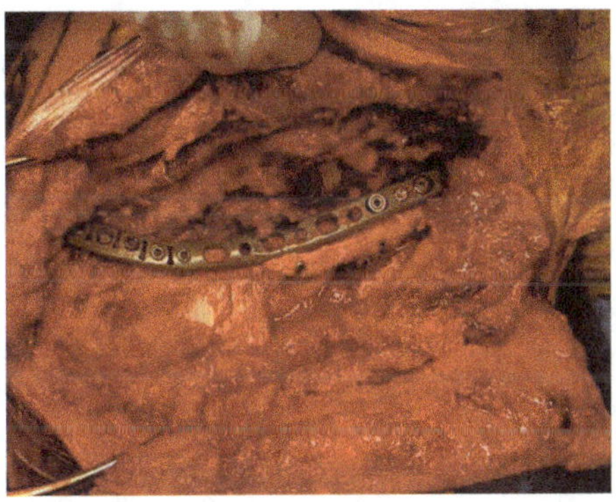

FIGURE 6: Intraoperative views showing our final plating construct which was supported with multiple cortical screws from superior and posterior to anterior and inferior.

(Figure 5). The curvature of the elbow plate matched the curvature of the acromion, and we were able to place multiple cortical screws from superior and posterior to anterior and inferior (Figure 6). Our plating construct had excellent bony purchase and maintained reduction of the acromion to the scapular body.

The patient had no perioperative complications and was discharged from her hospital stay without issues. She was briefly immobilized for two weeks and then started shoulder range of motion training followed by strengthening. Unfortunately, she did not follow up after seven months due to moving away from our location. At her last follow-up, she reported mild pain in her scapula with motion but otherwise had no complaints or neurovascular deficits. Regarding her function, she lacked terminal motion in all directions and has mild weakness compared to her contralateral side.

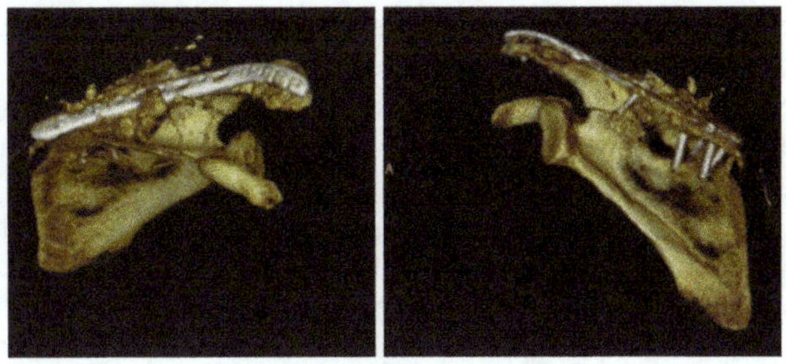

FIGURE 7: Postoperative computed tomography 3-dimensional reconstruction of the scapula showing our plate fixation of the scapular spine fracture.

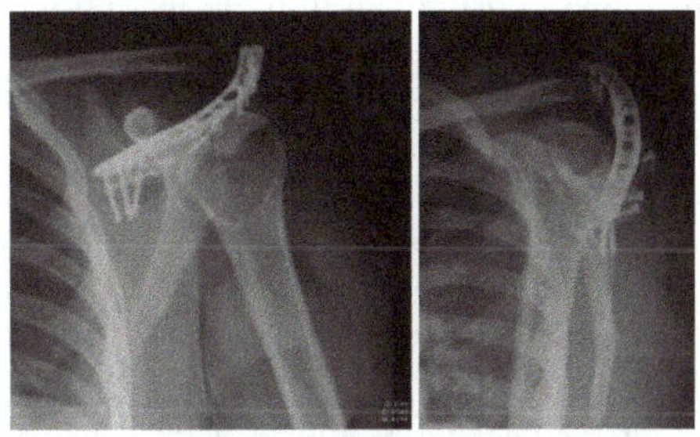

FIGURE 8: AP and lateral radiographic views of the scapula showing our fracture in appropriate alignment with evidence of implant failure or loosening.

However, she returned to all her daily activities without significant limitation to her sporting activities. Her last radiographic assessment showed maintained alignment of the acromion process without implant failure (Figures 7 and 8).

3. Discussion

Scapula fractures are an uncommon injury accounting for less than 1% of all fractures, with scapular spine accounting only 6% of these [4, 5]. The infrequency is due to the mobility of the scapula, allowing displacement of traumatic forces, as well as protection by the thoracic cavity anteriorly and the thick layer of soft tissue and muscles posteriorly [6]. Therefore, these fractures generally occur as a result of direct force from high-energy mechanisms such as motor vehicle collisions or autopedestrian accident. To the best of our knowledge, we present the first documented case of a free-floating scapular spine treated with our technique.

Scapular spines have a considerable amount of variability in their shape, thus adding to the difficulty of fixation. Wang et al. [7] developed a classification system of scapular spines, and according to this scheme, our patient's scapular spine fracture is classified as a Type IV or a "wooden club shape," the third most common morphology. Of note, patients with Type V or Type I classification have a more complex morphology that may result in more difficult fixation [7]. However, the literature on acute scapular spine fractures has been scarce.

Previous literature reported on the spontaneous occurrence of these fractures in the elderly or chronic scapular spine fractures. In elderly patients with poor bone quality, atraumatic scapular spine fractures have been reported as a result of chronic rotator cuff tear arthropathy or following reverse total shoulder arthroplasty. These fractures are usually nondisplaced and are treated conservatively [8–12]. Another etiology of atraumatic fractures of the scapular spine is avulsion fractures resulting from voluntary muscle contraction of the deltoid. These fractures are incredibly uncommon; current literature supports both conservative and operative management of these fractures [13, 14]. As-Sultany et al. [15] reported a case of a minimally displaced scapular spine fracture in a 39-year-old male that failed nonoperative management and developed a nonunion of the spine at the base of the acromion. He subsequently underwent plate fixation along with autograft placement from his iliac crest and eventually returned to full functional status post five months postoperatively. The excellent outcome achieved through their surgical treatment led the authors to have a low threshold for operative fixation of displaced scapular spine fractures, especially in healthy, younger patients [15]. Overall, there are no extensive studies on fractures of the scapular spine and their outcomes from various treatment options.

Our treatment consisted of open reduction and internal fixation of the scapular spine, and we achieved adequate fixation and good functional outcome. We stress the importance of proper exposure since we were able to assess the full extent of the fracture pattern for our fixation. While a modified Judet approach, as described by Cole and Dugarte [16], can be used for less extensive injuries to decrease soft tissue trauma, we opted to use the extensile Judet approach to raise the posterior musculature to evaluate this complex fracture pattern fully. Once we exposed the fracture site, 2.7 mm lag screws were used to reduce the posterior portion of the acromion to the scapular body and had excellent bony purchase. This temporary fixation was stabilized further with K-wires to allow for our definitive fixation. Scapular plating systems are not common for the scapular spine, and we found that an elbow plate matched the contour of the scapular spine. Additionally, this plating construct allowed us to place several cortical screws from superior and posterior to anterior and inferior, thus bolstering our fixation.

4. Conclusion

While scapular spine fracture is an unfortunate, rare injury that may impose difficult challenges to the treating surgeon, treatment guidelines for the management of these fractures currently do not exist. Here, we detailed the successful treatment of an acute free-floating scapular spine fracture after open reduction and internal fixation with an elbow plate. With our case report, we hope to contribute to the overall knowledge of scapular spine fractures and offer our experience with a successful and appropriate treatment option in our patient.

References

[1] P. A. Cole, G. Freeman, and J. R. Dubin, "Scapula fractures," *Current Reviews in Musculoskeletal Medicine*, vol. 6, no. 1, pp. 79–87, 2013.

[2] K. D. Baldwin, P. Ohman-Strickland, S. Mehta, and E. Hume, "Scapula fractures: a marker for concomitant injury? A retrospective review of data in the National Trauma Database," *The Journal of Trauma*, vol. 65, no. 2, pp. 430–435, 2008.

[3] T. P. Goss, "Fractures of the glenoid cavity," *The Journal of Bone and Joint Surgery. American Volume*, vol. 74, no. 2, pp. 299–305, 1992.

[4] C. P. Armstrong and J. Van der Spuy, "The fractured scapula: importance and management based on a series of 62 patients," *Injury*, vol. 15, no. 5, pp. 324–329, 1984.

[5] J. E. Kuhn, R. B. Blasier, and J. E. Carpenter, "Fractures of the acromion process: a proposed classification system," *Journal of Orthopaedic Trauma*, vol. 8, no. 1, pp. 6–13, 1994.

[6] M. A. Wirth, C. A. Rockwood, and S. B. Lippitt, *The Shoulder E-Book: Expert Consult-Online and Print*, Elsevier Health Sciences, Philadelphia, PA, USA, 2009.

[7] H.-J. Wang, H. Giambini, D.-B. Hou et al., "Classification and morphological parameters of the scapular spine: implications for surgery," *Medicine*, vol. 94, no. 45, p. e1986, 2015.

[8] D. C. Patterson, D. Chi, B. O. Parsons, and P. J. Cagle Jr., "Acromial spine fracture after reverse total shoulder arthroplasty: a systematic review," *Journal of Shoulder and Elbow Surgery*, vol. 28, no. 4, pp. 792–801, 2019.

[9] S. Mugikura, T. Hirayama, H. Tada, and Y. Takemitsu, "Avulsion fracture of the scapular spine: a case report," *Journal of Shoulder and Elbow Surgery*, vol. 2, no. 1, pp. 39–42, 1993.

[10] K. Karthik, J. Lau, J. Sinha, and A. Tavakkolizadeh, "Scapular spine stress fractures: to fix or not to fix, our experience in a patient with bilateral fractures and review of the literature," *International Journal of Shoulder Surgery*, vol. 8, no. 3, pp. 90–93, 2014.

[11] D. Groot, A. M. E. Giesberts, and J. B. A. van Mourik, "Spontaneous scapular spine fracture related to rotator cuff pathology: a report of two cases," *Strategies in Trauma and Limb Reconstruction*, vol. 7, no. 2, pp. 105–107, 2012.

[12] I. P. Mayne, S. N. Bell, W. Wright, and J. A. Coghlan, "Acromial and scapular spine fractures after reverse total shoulder arthroplasty," *Shoulder & Elbow*, vol. 8, no. 2, pp. 90–100, 2016.

[13] K. J. Burkholz, C. C. Roberts, and S. J. Hattrup, "Scapular spine stress fracture as a complication of reverse shoulder arthroplasty," *Radiology Case Reports*, vol. 2, no. 2, pp. 78–82, 2007.

[14] T. Morioka, T. Honma, and K. Ogawa, "Incomplete avulsion fractures of the scapular spine caused by violent muscle contraction," *The Keio Journal of Medicine*, vol. 63, no. 1, pp. 13–17, 2014.

[15] M. As-Sultany, A. Tambe, and D. I. Clark, "Nonunion of a scapular spine fracture: case report and management with open reduction, internal fixation, and bone graft," *International Journal of Shoulder Surgery*, vol. 2, no. 3, pp. 64–67, 2008.

[16] P. A. Cole and A. J. Dugarte, "Posterior scapula approaches: extensile and modified Judet," *Journal of Orthopaedic Trauma*, vol. 32, pp. S10–S11, 2018, Suppl 1.

3

Contiguous Multilevel Thoracic Ossification of Ligamentum Flavum in a Young Adult Spine

Tsuyoshi Yamada,[1,2] Ichiro Torigoe,[1] Kenichiro Sakai,[1] Atsushi Okawa,[2] and Yoshiyasu Arai[1]

[1]*Department of Orthopaedic Surgery, Saiseikai Kawaguchi General Hospital, Saitama 332-8558, Japan*
[2]*Department of Orthopaedic Surgery, Graduate School, Tokyo Medical and Dental University, 1-5-45 Yushima, Bunkyo-ku, Tokyo 113-8510, Japan*

Correspondence should be addressed to Tsuyoshi Yamada; yamada.orth@tmd.ac.jp

Academic Editor: Mark K. Lyons

The ossification of the ligamentum flavum (OLF) was characterized by the replacement of the ligamentum flavum by ectopic new bone formation. Although OLF is well known as one of the causes of thoracic myelopathy through the compression of the spinal cord from the posterolateral side, contiguous multilevel OLF is quite a rare cause of myelopathy. Severe ossifications were reported that only present in individuals aged over 25 years. External triggers of OLF might likely be increased as a consequence of biomechanical stress to the effect of posttraumatic ossification. The authors described one rare case of an enormous contiguous multilevel OLF in a 20-year-old female's thoracic spine after mild back trauma, to the extent that it was misdiagnosed as an old epidural hematoma initially. This female with obesity presented with a 6-month history of progressively worsening dorsal cord disorders. Resection or floating of the enormous OLF could be successfully achieved using O-arm-based navigation, and sensory loss, numbness, and gait disturbance were improved after operation.

1. Introduction

The ligamentum flavum may undergo various pathologic changes including hypertrophy, calcification, cyst formation, hematoma, and ossification [1, 2]. The ossification of the ligamentum flavum (OLF) was characterized by the replacement of the ligamentum flavum by ectopic new bone formation, and the most frequent OLF lesion is the thoracic spine. Although OLF is well known as one of the causes of thoracic myelopathy through the compression of the spinal cord from the posterolateral side [3], contiguous multilevel OLF is quite a rare cause of myelopathy, reported in a few cases [4–6].

Here, the authors described one case of an enormous contiguous multilevel OLF after mild back trauma, to the extent that it was misdiagnosed as an old epidural hematoma initially. Despite the high rate of perioperative complications in OLF resection, resection or floating of the enormous OLF could be successfully achieved using O-arm-based navigation in the present case.

2. Case Presentation

A 20-year-old female with obesity (body mass index: 33.3 kg/m^2) presented with a 6-month history of progressively worsening paresthesia of the lower limbs and gait disturbance. Moderate muscle weakness, severe spasticity in the lower limbs, a superficial hypoesthesia below the Th6 level, and severe dorsal cord disorders were noted on the first physical examination. There was a history of a contusion in the back following the drop from 2 meters height, treated with conservative therapy 2 years previously. She showed no feature of skeletal dysplasia. Laboratory data revealed no abnormality.

Magnetic resonance imaging (MRI) showed a dorsally located epidural lesion (Th6-Th9) which seemed a

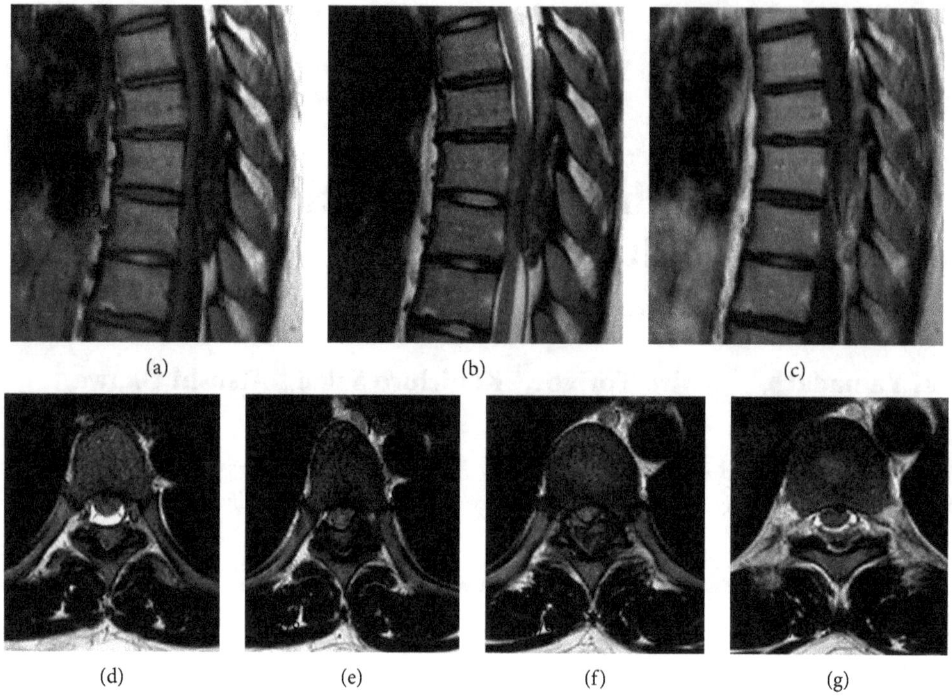

FIGURE 1: Preoperative thoracic MRI. Heterogeneous epidural posterior mass compressing the thoracic cord between Th6 and Th9 was revealed at the admission. Sagittal view of heterogeneous isointense mass of T1-weighted image (a), heterogeneous isointense mass of T2-weighted image (b), and nonenhancing mass of Gd-enhanced T1-weighted image (c). Axial view of epidural mass of T2-weighted image in Th6/7 (d), Th7/8 (e), Th8/9 (f), and Th9/10 (g) intervertebral levels. This epidural mass was considered as an old epidural hematoma initially.

heterogeneous mass hypointense on both T1- and T2-weighted images (Figure 1). These clinical courses and radiological findings suggested old epidural hematoma. Computerized tomography (CT) scans revealed that this dorsally located epidural lesion consisted of ossified components, which occupied about 50-80% of the spinal canal, and partially developed even to extraforaminal regions (bilateral Th7/8 foramen) or to the extent which integrated the lamina (Th7-Th8 laminas), leading to make the spinal cord compressed severely. These ossification lesions seemed to have the bone marrow inside (Figure 2).

Thoracic pedicle screw insertions in Th5, 6, 10, and 11 levels preceding thoracic cord decompression and the surgical excision of ossified lesion or floating of ossified lesion with the slight adhesion to dura matter were performed under O-arm-based navigation system (O-arm Surgical Imaging System and StealthStation; Medtronic, Inc., Minneapolis, MN, USA). When Th6-Th10 laminectomy was performed, the posterior epidural space was filled with an ossified mass. Between Th6-Th9 laminas and the ossified mass, there was a part of denatured flavum with abundant blood vessels. In particular, these ossified lesions developed in Th7-Th8 levels, where this mass adhered to bilateral pedicles of Th7 and Th8 (Figure 3). To float these lesions, pediculectomy of Th7 and Th8 was performed. We found bilateral OLF in Th9/10 level, separated from Th6-9 epidural ossified mass. This separated beak lesion was considered as the dynamic factor to mainly cause thoracic myelopathy through the compression of the spinal cord. The resection or floating of these extremely ossified components made compressive dura matter swollen (Figure 4). After the resection of ossified lesions, an autologous local bone graft harvested during decompressive laminectomy was placed between decorticated transverse processes or remained laminas as posterolateral spinal fusion from Th5 to Th11. The operation took 303 minutes. In spite of denatured enormous lesions, the intraoperative blood loss was no more than 420 mL, by repeating vigorous hemostasis by electrocoagulation, bone wax, and FLOSEAL hemostatic matrix (Baxter Healthcare Corp, Fremont, CA, USA).

Ossification of the ligament tissue was observed in the resected tumor. Contiguous multilevel OLF was diagnosed and confirmed by pathology (Figure 5). After operation, sensory loss, numbness, and gait disturbance were improved. Her Japanese Orthopaedic Association (JOA) score for thoracic myelopathy recovered from preoperative 5.0 points to 8.0 points out of 11 points. Following examinations indicated the absence of recurrence or neurological deterioration.

3. Discussion

The onset of OLF-related symptoms with consecutive surgical treatment ranges between 55 and 65 years, as the prevalence increases with age. The formation of OLF in the population is strongly considered due to degenerative wear-and-tear. There are reports on OLF manifestations in relation to diabetes mellitus, activity patterns (heavy manual labour in males), body weight (high-BMI values

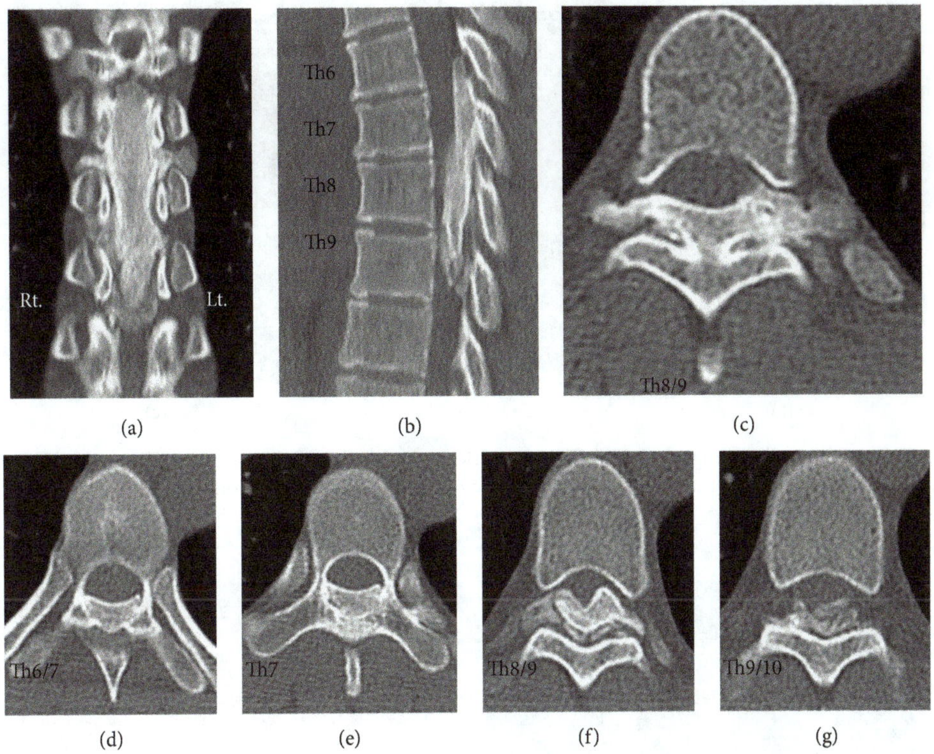

FIGURE 2: Preoperative thoracic CT. Ossified epidural posterior mass compressing the thoracic cord between Th6 and Th9 was revealed in coronal view (a) and sagittal view (b) of thoracic CT. Ossified lesion reached to extraforamen at Th7/8 intervertebral levels (c). Axial view of epidural ossified mass in Th6/7 (d), Th7 (e), Th8/9 (f), and Th9/10 (g) levels, which occupied about 50-80% of the spinal canal.

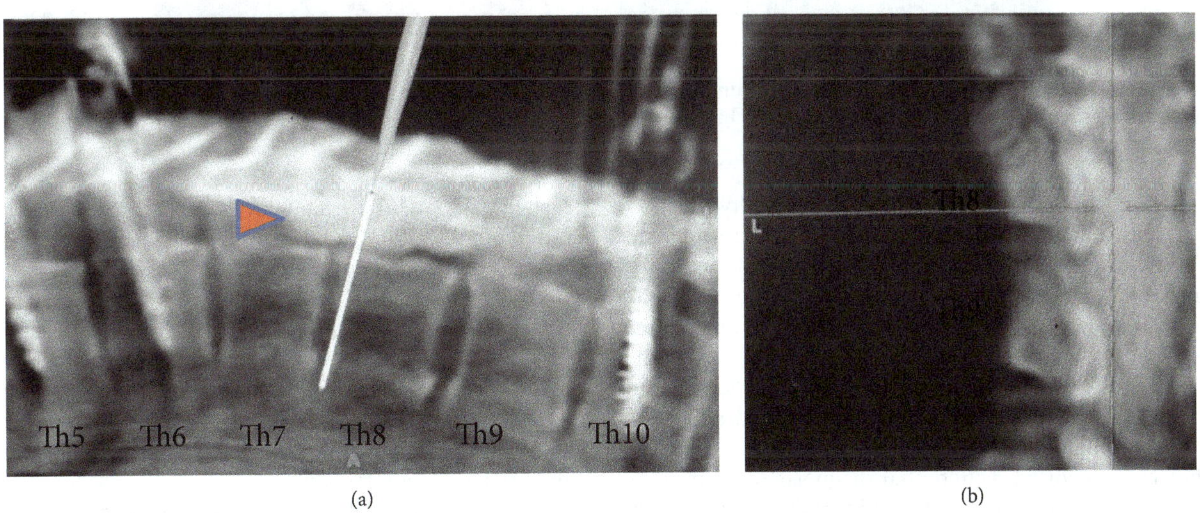

FIGURE 3: Surgical excision of ossified lesion under O-arm-based navigation system. After performing Th6-Th10 laminectomy, the posterior epidural space was filled with an ossified mass. To float the adhered ossified mass, pediculectomy of Th7 and Th8 and posterior spinal fusion from Th5 to Th11 were performed. Surgeons can resect or float an enormous contiguous ossified mass safely (arrowhead), confirming the thickness of ossification and the adhesion to circumferential tissues under O-arm-based 3D navigation (sagittal view (a), coronal view (b)).

in females), fluorosis, increased bone density, hyperparathyroidism, diffuse idiopathic skeletal hyperostosis (DISH), ankylosing spondylitis, acromegaly, and achondroplasia [7]. External triggers of OLF might likely to be increased as a consequence of biomechanical stress to the effect of posttraumatic ossification [8].

OLF can significantly contribute to a spatial reduction of the thoracic spinal canal, resulting in slowly progressive or acute paraplegia after trauma to the back. Given a 2-year-ago history of trauma and her young age, the formation of OLF in the present case could be attributed to the effect of posttraumatic ossification, in addition to the influence of

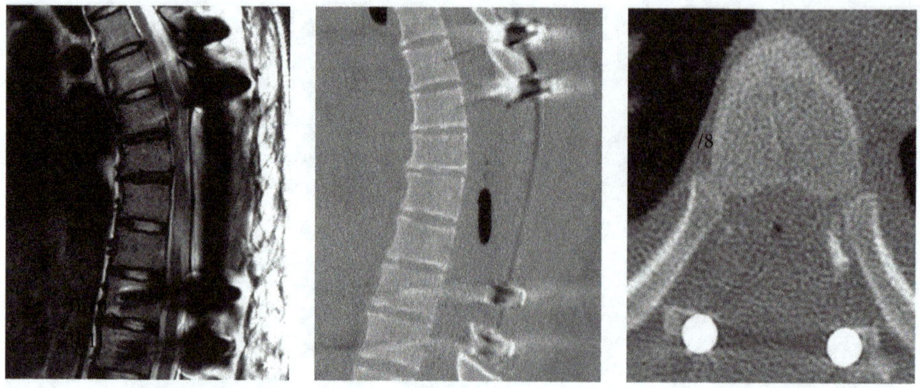

(a) (b) (c)

Figure 4: Thoracic spine radiological findings post Th5-Th11 posterior spinal fusion. Postoperative MRI showed the dura matter swollen (sagittal view (a)), while CT demonstrated the total resection of these extremely ossified components (sagittal view (b), axial view in Th7/8 level (c)).

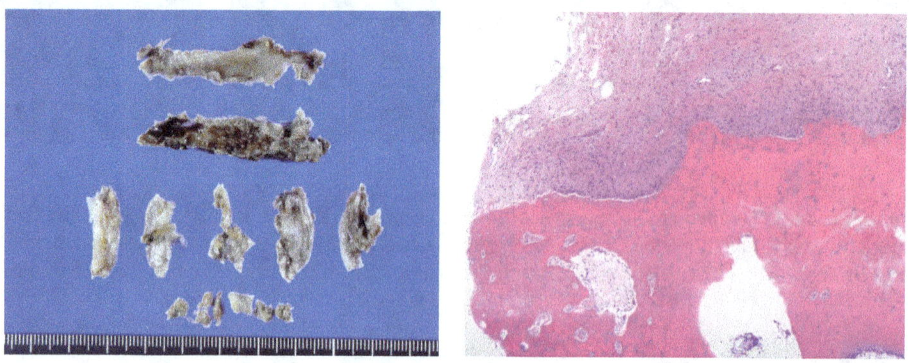

(a) (b)

Figure 5: Histopathological analysis of the resected tumors. Macroscopic findings of the resected epidural mass (a). Ossification of the ligament tissue was observed in the resected tumor. This mass was diagnosed as a contiguous multilevel OLF according to microscopic findings (hematoxylin and eosin stained) (b).

intrinsic high-BMI values. Because of the difficulty in clinically monitoring contusion in the back without fracture or neurological deterioration when we take the attributed risks of imaging radiation exposure and medical expenses into consideration, the exact incidence of epidural hematoma and much more epidural hematoma ossification is unknown. Although the posttraumatic or postoperative ossified epidural hematomas in cranial, especially in children, were discussed in a few reports [9–11], the thoracic spine lesion has not been reported. Differential diagnosis must include some epidural tumors and spinal epidural hematomas. All the cases of spinal epidural hematomas which needed emergent surgery in our institute (8 cases, from 2010 to 2016) showed hypointense mass on T1-weighted imaging while the intensity on T2-weighted images seemed variable. The epidural mass in this case was misdiagnosed as an old epidural hematoma initially, based on MRI findings. The diagnosis of this ossified mass had not been unconfirmed until we saw the result of pathology.

According to the previous classification on axial CT scan and T2-weighted sagittal MRI image [12], we could regard the present thoracic OLF in a young adulthood as bridged and round types. These bridged and round ossifications reached from Th6 to Th9 levels, shaping an enormous contiguous multilevel OLF with thickness over 4 mm. Grade 3 (≧4 mm) ossifications were reported that only present in individuals aged over 25 years, and a later progression of the condition that would almost exclusively have occurred in old age (≧46 years) [7]. To our knowledge, we present the first case of such an enormous contiguous multilevel OLF in a young adult thoracic spine, to the extent which myelopathy advanced to need posterior decompression and fusion largely.

Thoracic myelopathy secondary to OLF can be treated with laminectomy. Further, laminectomy with partially internal fixation is safe and effective in treatment of patients with symptomatic multilevel OLF [5]. The overall perioperative complication rate reached to 35%, with dural tears and cerebrospinal fluid leaks most frequently [13]. In the present case, we could successfully avoid such a complication because we could resect or float an enormous contiguous OLF safely, confirming the thickness of ossification and the adhesion to circumferential tissues under O-arm-based navigation. The use of intraoperative navigation in spine surgery, particularly the O-arm, has increased rapidly in the past several years, and many authors has addressed the utility of the O-arm

[14]. In the case of a contiguous multilevel OLF, O-arm-based 3D navigation is one of the safe and effective measures during surgery.

The authors described quite a rare case of an enormous contiguous multilevel OLF in young female thoracic spine after mild back trauma. Asymptomatic chronic epidural hematomas even in young adult spine might undergo large ossification, and enormous OLF could prevent natural absorption, leading to cause myelopathy. If there is a chronic spinal epidural mass with ossification, we recommend surgery before irreversible change has been completed. The use of O-arm-based intraoperative 3D scans for navigation can make drilling and resection of an enormous contiguous OLF reliable.

Consent

Written informed consent was signed by the patient for participating in this study and for publication of this case report and any accompanying images.

References

[1] Y. S. Lee, J. S. Yi, H. J. Kim, J. O. Kim, and E. S. Choi, "Epidural block-induced ligamentum flavum hematoma mimicking epidural hematoma in the lumbar spine: a case report," *The Spine Journal*, vol. 11, no. 2, pp. e23–e27, 2011.

[2] H. C. Chen, P. W. Hsu, C. Y. Lin, and W. C. Tzaan, "Symptomatic hematoma of cervical ligamentum flavum: case report," *Spine*, vol. 30, no. 16, pp. E489–E491, 2005.

[3] K. Miyasaka, K. Kaneda, S. Sato et al., "Myelopathy due to ossification or calcification of the ligamentum flavum: radiologic and histologic evaluations," *American Journal of Neuroradiology*, vol. 4, no. 3, pp. 629–632, 1983.

[4] K. Wang and X. Chen, "Thoracic cord compression caused by contiguous multilevel ossification of ligamentum flavum in Chinese patients," *Chinese Journal of Traumatology*, vol. 10, no. 4, pp. 213–217, 2007.

[5] R. Gao, W. Yuan, L. Yang, G. Shi, and L. Jia, "Clinical features and surgical outcomes of patients with thoracic myelopathy caused by multilevel ossification of the ligamentum flavum," *The Spine Journal*, vol. 13, no. 9, pp. 1032–1038, 2013.

[6] Z. H. Nie, F. J. Liu, Y. Shen, W. Y. Ding, and L. F. Wang, "Lamina osteotomy and replantation with miniplate fixation for thoracic myelopathy due to ossification of the ligamentum flavum," *Orthopedics*, vol. 36, no. 3, pp. e353–e359, 2013.

[7] J. Geber and N. Hammer, "Ossification of the ligamentum flavum in a nineteenth-century skeletal population sample from Ireland: using bioarchaeology to reveal a neglected spine pathology," *Scientific Reports*, vol. 8, no. 1, p. 9313, 2018.

[8] L. Ren, H. Hu, X. Sun, F. Li, J. J. Zhou, and Y. M. Wang, "The roles of inflammatory cytokines in the pathogenesis of ossification of ligamentum flavum," *American Journal of Translational Research*, vol. 5, no. 6, pp. 582–585, 2013.

[9] N. Yoshida, H. Iseki, K. Amano, and K. Kitamura, "A case with postoperative calcified epidural hematoma," *No Shinkei Geka*, vol. 13, no. 11, pp. 1199–1203, 1985.

[10] H. Seyithanoglu, F. K. Guzey, E. Emel, N. Ozkan, and A. Aycan, "Chronic ossified epidural hematoma after ventriculoperitoneal shunt insertion: a case report," *Turkish Neurosurgery*, vol. 20, no. 4, pp. 519–523, 2010.

[11] A. Akhaddar and O. Boulahroud, "Ossified chronic epidural hematoma of the posterior fossa," *Pan African Medical Journal*, vol. 20, p. 238, 2015.

[12] S. U. Kuh, Y. S. Kim, Y. E. Cho et al., "Contributing factors affecting the prognosis surgical outcome for thoracic OLF," *European Spine Journal*, vol. 15, no. 4, pp. 485–491, 2006.

[13] N. S. Osman, Z. B. Cheung, A. K. Hussain et al., "Outcomes and complications following laminectomy alone for thoracic myelopathy due to ossified ligamentum flavum: a systematic review and meta-analysis," *Spine*, vol. 43, no. 14, pp. E842–E848, 2018.

[14] N. E. Epstein, "Commentary: utility of the O-arm in spinal surgery," *Surgical Neurology International*, vol. 5, Supplement 15, pp. S517–S519, 2014.

4

Patella Osteomyelitis Mimicking Sinding-Larsen and Johansson Apophysitis: A Pitfall Not to Miss

Aurélien Traverso, Benjamin Tschopp, Tristan Mekdade, Barbara Kwiatkowski, and Nicolas Lutz

Department of Pediatric and Adolescent Surgery, Lausanne University Hospital (CHUV) and University of Lausanne (UNIL), Lausanne, Switzerland

Correspondence should be addressed to Aurélien Traverso; auremt@gmail.com

Academic Editor: Wan Ismail Faisham

Background. Diagnosis of bony infection remains difficult during childhood. Osteomyelitis of the patella (OMP) is rare and produces few symptoms and no fever. A high level of suspicion is needed to avoid missing this uncommon type of bone infection. *Methods/Results.* We report an acute osteomyelitis of the patella treated by joint and patella puncture aspiration followed by antibiotics in a 12-year-old healthy boy. Clinical and radiological findings, orthopedic follow-up, and clinical outcome are presented. *Conclusion.* Making a diagnosis of acute osteomyelitis of the patella can be challenging especially in the pediatric population, as it produces few specific symptoms with mostly nonspecific biologic anomalies. The paucity in specific signs and symptoms, accompanied by the rare occurrence, often leads to incorrect initial diagnosis, such as overuse injury or apophysitis. Clinical examination with high suspicion for patella infection is key. Radiological exams including MRI are the main components of the adequate imaging studies. Computed tomography may be an excellent addendum to better visualize any bony lesion within the patella. Bone aspiration or biopsy is essential to confirm the diagnosis and offers a first step in the treatment of this infection, which can then be successfully treated with a normal course of antibiotics.

1. Introduction

Osteomyelitis (OM) during growth has a prevalence of 2.9 per 100,000 children, with declining values in "developed" nations [1]. The first case of acute osteomyelitis of the patella (OMP) was described by Thirion in 1829 [2]. Reaching the diagnosis can be challenging, due to the paucity of its nonstandard clinical presentation [3]. Involvement of the patella in OM is very uncommon, when compared to the typical long bones localization [4, 5]. To establish with certitude, the diagnosis of a musculoskeletal infection remains an invasive process. Standard radiographs may be normal or reveal nonspecific cortical condensation, erosion, or periosteal reaction. When present, they are usually secondary to a significant delay between the beginning of the infection and the diagnosis. Magnetic resonance imaging (MRI) is the gold-standard imaging study for the diagnosis of osteomyelitis [6]. MRI can demonstrate bone edema or periosteal inflation, abscesses, and possible adjacent joint effusion. It can delineate any extraosseous spread of the disease. Aspiration is mandatory for the identification of the causative agent.

Early diagnosis of OM in children is the key to implement adequate antibiotic treatment and prevent severe sequelae such as bone or joint destruction, which can produce lifelong disabilities [3].

The authors report on a case of acute osteomyelitis of the patella (OMP) in a healthy 12-year-old boy treated successfully by local aspiration followed by a course of intravenous and oral antibiotics. Clinical presentation and radiological findings mimicking the Sinding-Larsen and Johansson apophysitis are described. The investigation process and treatment modalities are explained and discussed, comparing them to published case reports.

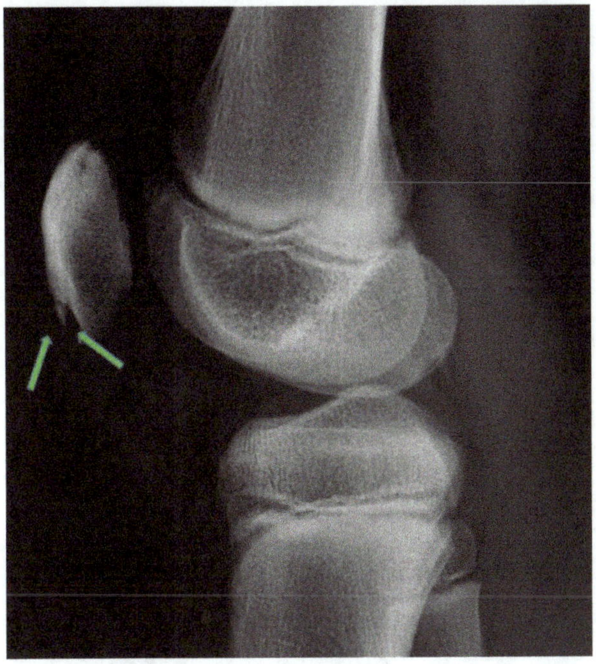

FIGURE 1: X-ray 1. Lateral view of the right knee. Green arrows shows the Sinding-Larsen and Johansson disease, initial radiological findings.

2. Statement of Informed Consent

The patient and his parents were informed that data concerning the case would be submitted for publication. The patient and parents agreed.

3. Case Report

A 12-year-old boy presented with a painful and swollen knee. He described anterior knee pain when walking and standing which had begun 48 hours prior to consultation. There was no history of acute fever, past trauma, or rheumatological history. Physical examination revealed antalgic gait and pain during compression of the inferior pole of the patella, mimicking a Sinding-Larsen and Johansson disease (SLJD), with limitation of the range of motion: active 140°-20°-0° (passive 140°-0°-0°). Full flexion of the knee was painful. The extensor apparatus was competent. Initial diagnosis was a SLJD due to localization of the symptoms and initial radiological findings on X-rays. Figures 1–3 (green arrows) show SLJD typical X-rays with calcifications plus irregular ossification of the lower pole of the patella and thickening and heterogeneity of the proximal patellar tendon. Blood tests showed a C-reactive protein (CRP) of 64 mg/l, sedimentation rate (SR) of 15 mm/h, and a normal leucocytes count (WBC) 72 hours after the beginning of the symptoms. The patient was treated with nonsteroidal antiinflammatory drugs (NSAIDs) and a brace for immobilization.

24 hours after initial diagnosis, the patient was reassessed as scheduled. There were no changes in the physical exam. CRP increased to 96 mg/l. The patient remained fever free.

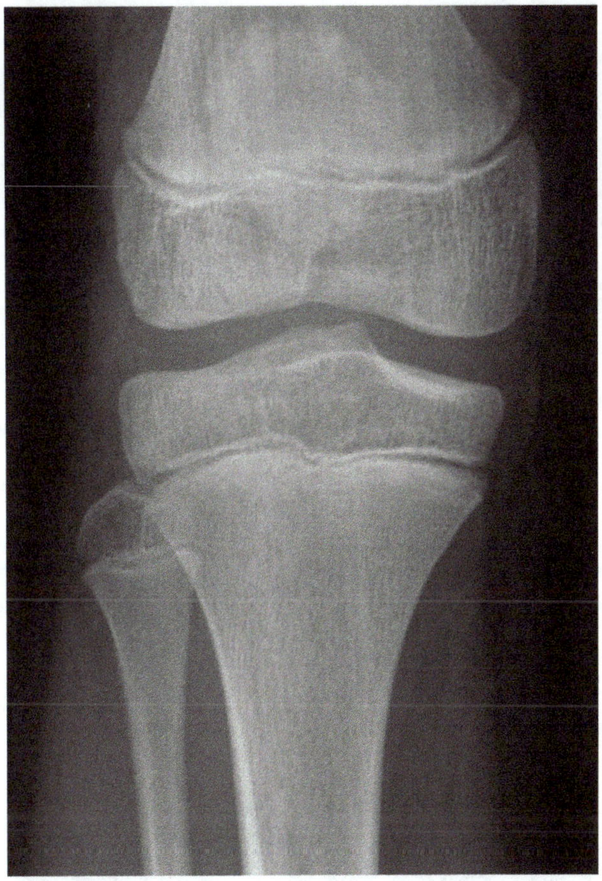

FIGURE 2: X-ray 2. AP view of the right knee, initial radiological findings.

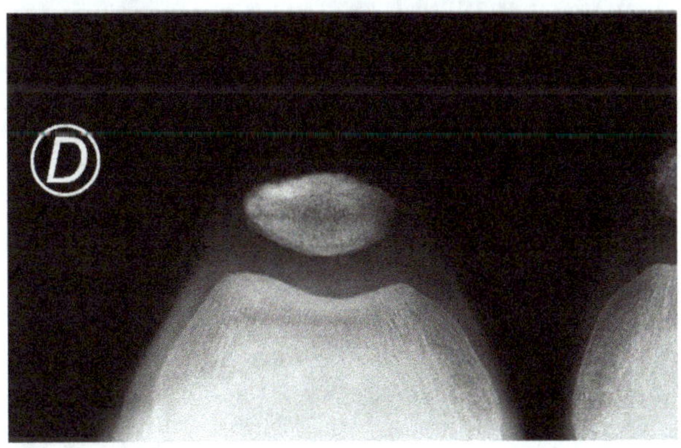

FIGURE 3: X-ray 3. Axial view of both knees (right knee on the left), initial radiological findings.

Because of the increased CRP, an infectious process and a magnetic resonance imaging (MRI) were performed, and the suspected diagnosis of OMP was established (Figures 4–6, blue arrows). An abscess of Hoffa's fat pad with circular fat pad infiltration was observed (Figures 4–6, red arrows). A puncture aspiration of the knee and the patella was performed in the operating theatre, under general anaesthesia, using a 17-gauge needle. First, a joint aspiration from a superolateral approach was performed, yielding a synovial fluid of physiological appearance, Then, a punction of Hoffa's

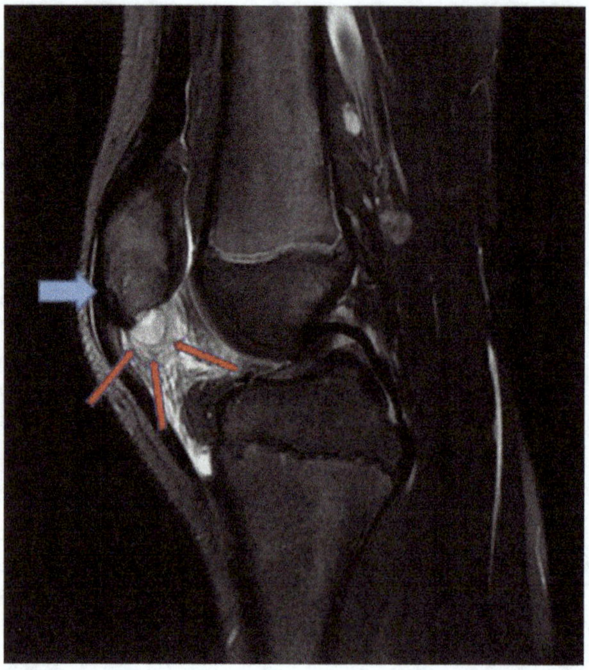

Figure 4: MRI 1. Sagittal T2 fat sat view. Osteomyelitis of the patella (blue arrow) and fat pad infiltration were observed (red arrows).

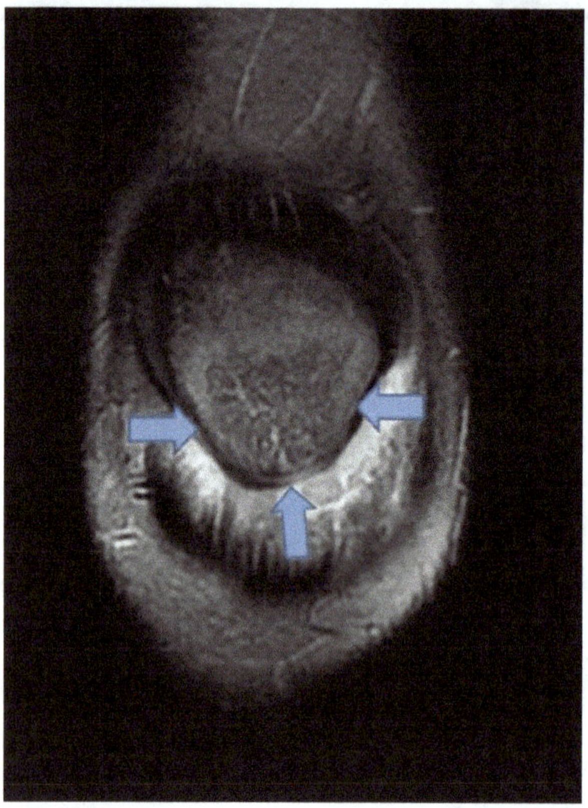

Figure 5: MRI 2. Coronal T2 fat sat view. Osteomyelitis of the patella (blue arrows).

fat pad and intraosseous lesion at the lower pole of the patella were performed, which yielded 1.5 ml of sanguine-purulent liquid. Directly after having collected the samples, empiric

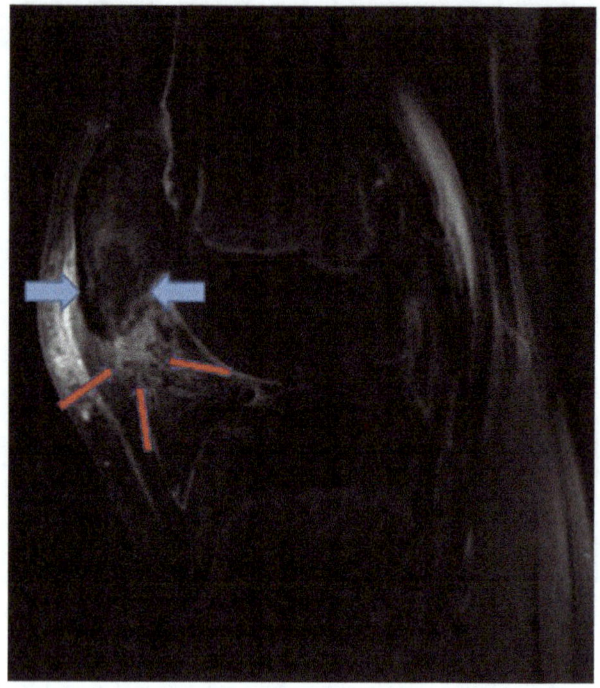

Figure 6: MRI 3. Sagittal T1 fat sat view. Osteomyelitis of the patella (blue arrows) and fat pad infiltration were observed (red arrows).

antibiotics were started intravenously (amoxicillin/clavulanate 50 mg/kg 3 times per day). The culture of the patella punction revealed a *Staphylococcus aureus* and so confirmed the presupposed diagnosis (>10 0000 germs/ml, methicillin sensible). Articular fluid analysis showed an inflammatory state with predominantly neutrophil polymorphonuclear cells. Two days after the puncture aspiration and the beginning of antibiotics, biological tests showed a significant decrease of the CRP at 58 mg/l and normal WBC count. Antibiotics were given intravenously for 5 days then changed for oral antibiotics (amoxicillin/clavulanate 30 mg/kg 3 times per day). At discharge, the patient was pain free with simple painkillers. The knee was immobilized in a full-extension brace for 15 days. Antibiotics were given for a total of four weeks according to Wagner et al. [7].

One week after the diagnosis, the follow-up examination was satisfactory, and the patient was pain free.

The six-week follow-up examination showed a full and symmetric range of motion of the knee (140°-0°-0°) without any pain neither during active mobilization. The patient reported return to daily life activities and was able to hop on the affected leg and run without pain. Knee Osteoarthritis Outcome Score (KOOS) (see Figure 7) and the Lower Extremity Functional Scale (LEFS) at 79/80 points were excellent. The radiograph of the knee showed a bone lysis area at the lower pole of the patella (Figures 8 and 9, orange arrows show the lysis area).

Clinical assessment at 6 months showed a normal knee function. KOOS and the LEFS score were both at the maximum.

There were no immediate or middle-term complications in this case.

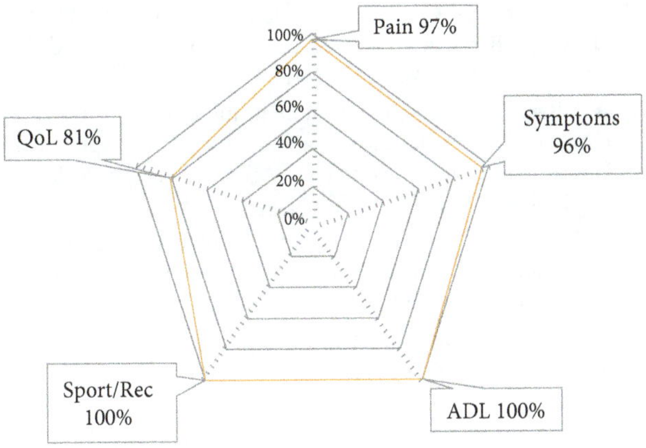

FIGURE 7: KOOS-child knee survey at 6 weeks postoperative.

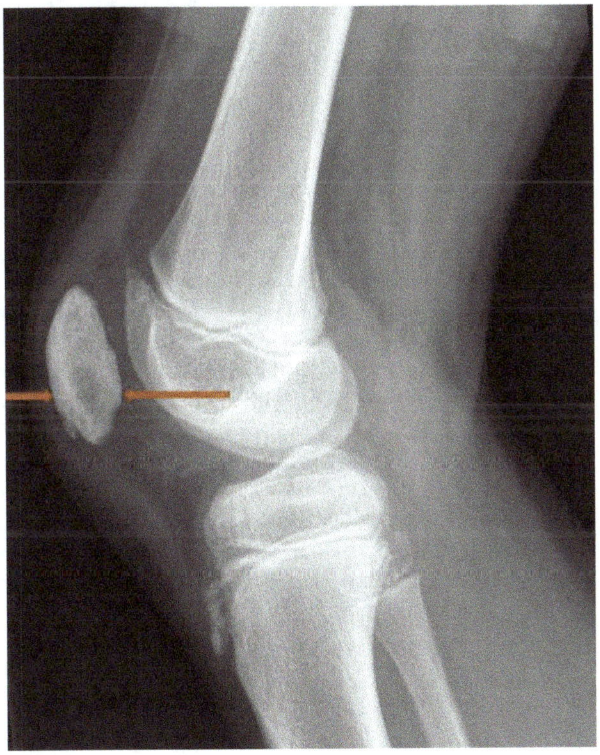

FIGURE 8: X-ray 4. Lateral view of the right knee, 6 weeks after diagnosis. Orange arrows show the lysis area at the lower pole of the patella.

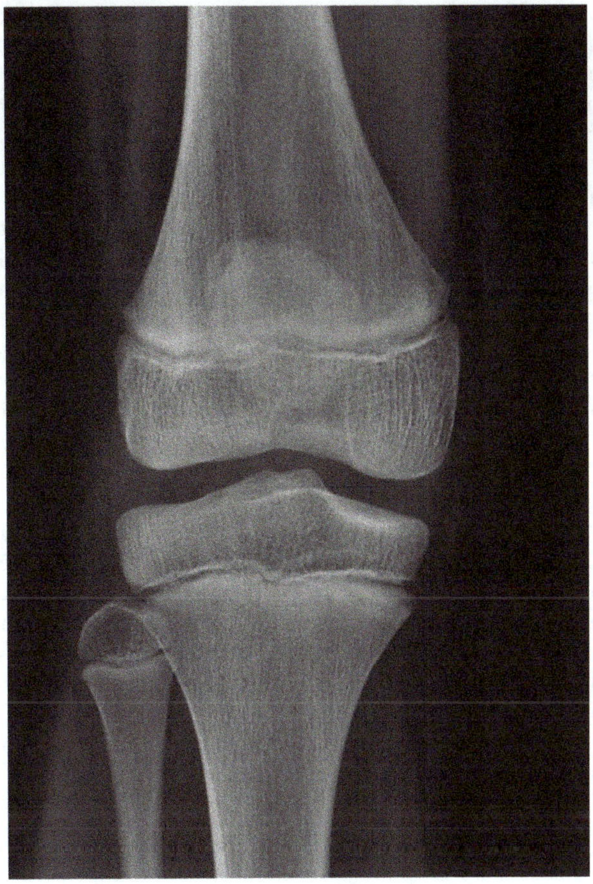

FIGURE 9: X-ray 5. AP view of the right knee, 6 weeks after diagnosis.

4. Discussion

Case series and review of the literature suggest a hematogenous origin for osteomyelitis of the patella, such as in this case. No local skin injury was recorded [8]. Its peak of prevalence seems to be between 5 and 15 years of age [4, 9–14]. Before the age of 5, the patella is primarily cartilaginous, which can explain the extremely low prevalence of OMP in the first years of life [11, 15]. The significant vascularisation, provided by an anastomotic extraosseous arterial network composed with the anterior tibial recurrent artery and the superior and inferior geniculate arteries, begins at the age of 4 to 5 [8]. The patella reaches its maximal blood supply by age 12. Radiological evidence of OMP may appear at a later stage of the disease because the patella is covered by a thin lamina with no real periosteum [12]. Therefore, the typical periosteal elevation found in other bone localizations may be absent in patellar infections [5].

Medical history should be reviewed accurately to detect congenital anomalies or past history of infection. The clinical exam, however, is the key when suspicion arises for OMP. Comparison of both sides is mandatory and can reveal asymmetries.

Septic arthritis of the knee is often suspected initially, which can delay the diagnosis of OMP. Synovitis, septic bursitis, and peripatellar cellulitis can also be confused whit OMP [9]. Differential diagnoses of patellar lesions, such as the Sinding-Larsen and Johansson disease, bipartite patella, and a variety of rare tumors (chondroblastomas, giant cell tumors, osteoid osteomas, and aneurysmal bone cysts) could mislead the surgeon [16].

Routine laboratory tests usually show normal WBC count even in the setting of acute osteomyelitis. SR and CRP are often elevated; however, they both lack specificity in the absence of other radiologic and microbiologic analysis. In cases of proven osteomyelitis, both tests (especially CRP) may be used to assess response to therapy or relapse [17].

Radiographs need to be performed as the first-line imaging. Computed tomography (CT) and magnetic resonance imaging (MRI) can be of great value in the diagnosis and evaluation of osteomyelitis. They show anatomic details, including cortical destruction and soft tissue extension of the infection which can be helpful to choose between a less (punction, biopsy) and a more invasive diagnostic and therapeutic act (open drainage and curettage) [17].

Staphylococcus aureus, like in this case, seems to be the most commonly found infecting organism [3, 5, 18].

No consensus exists concerning the optimal OMP treatment. In some simple cases, antibiotics may even be enough to treat OMP [3, 18]. The preferred routes of administration and the duration greatly vary between the different cases described in the litterature [3]. Debridement and curettage as surgical treatment represent the recommended therapy for OMP in case of absence of improvement despite antibiotic treatment [3, 4, 18]. There is clearly no evidence for arthrotomy in cases without joint involvment [3]. The punction aspiration as performed in this case is less invasive and offers a way to decompress eventual bone abscess and to withdraw sample for microbiologic analysis in order to get the exact diagnosis. It is also possible to make an articular punction of the knee in the same time when concomitant arthritis is suspected. It should be performed in the operating theatre under strict aseptic conditions, under general anaesthesia and fluoroscopy.

Diagnose and treatment of OMP provide challenges for the clinician as was shown in this case.

5. Conclusion

OMP continues to be a challenging diagnosis in children, especially with regard to unusual bacteria as well as unusual locations. In the emergency department, limping children without fever may still be affected by an uncommon OMP. A high grade of suspicion should arise for any painful knee with a slight effusion and mild ESR and CRP elevation. MRI remains the gold-standard imaging studies in such circumstances.

References

[1] M. J. G. Blyth, R. Kincaid, M. A. C. Craigen, and G. C. Bennet, "The changing epidemiology of acute and subacute haematogenous osteomyelitis in children," *Journal of Bone and Joint Surgery–Series B*, vol. 83-B, no. 1, pp. 99–102, 2001.

[2] M. Thirion, "Successful extirpation of the right patella for carieas," *Lancet*, vol. 2, p. 399, 1829.

[3] M. Sperl, M. Novak, D. Sperl, M. Svehlik, G. Singer, and T. Kraus, "Osteomyelitis of the patella in a 10-year-old girl: a case report and review of the literature," *Case Reports in Orthopedics*, vol. 2017, Article ID 6573271, 5 pages, 2017.

[4] H.-R. Choi, "Patellar osteomyelitis presenting as prepatellar bursitis," *The Knee*, vol. 14, no. 4, pp. 333–335, 2007.

[5] J. Gil-Albarova, V. E. Gomez-Palacio, and A. Herrera, "Hematogenous osteomyelitis of the patella," *Journal of Pediatric Orthopaedics Part B*, vol. 21, no. 5, pp. 411–414, 2012.

[6] Y. J. Lee, S. Sadigh, K. Mankad, N. Kapse, and G. Rajeswaran, "The imaging of osteomyelitis," *Quantitative Imaging in Medicine and Surgery*, vol. 6, no. 2, pp. 184–198, 2016.

[7] N. Wagner, D. Ceroni, A. Niederer, N. Ritz, and C. Relly, "Prise en charge des infections ostéoarticulaires aigües de l'enfant," *Paediatrica*, vol. 28, no. 1, 2017.

[8] A. J. Berg, M. C. Killen, A. Chauhan, and C. Bhatia, "Osteomyelitis of the patella: ensure a high index of suspicion and beware the negative aspirate," *BMJ Case Reports*, vol. 2014, no. 1, article bcr2014206630, 2014.

[9] D. R. Roy, W. B. Greene, and J. G. Gamble, "Osteomyelitis of the patella in children," *Journal of Pediatric Orthopaedics*, vol. 11, no. 3, pp. 364–366, 1991.

[10] B. R. Cahill, "Nontraumatic osteomyelitis of the patella," *Clinical Orthopaedics and Related Research*, no. 132, pp. 177–179, 1978.

[11] J. Vaninbroukx, M. Martens, M. Verhelst, and J. C. Mulier, "Haematogenous osteomyelitis of the patella: report of three cases," *Acta Orthopaedica Scandinavica*, vol. 47, no. 5, pp. 566–569, 1976.

[12] J. J. Angella, "Osteomyelitis of the patella," *American Journal of Diseases of Children*, vol. 113, no. 5, pp. 590–593, 1967.

[13] R. K. Kankate and T. P. Selvan, "Primary haematogenous osteomyelitis of the patella: a rare cause for anterior knee pain in an adult," *Postgraduate Medical Journal*, vol. 76, no. 901, pp. 707–709, 2000.

[14] D. R. Roy, "Osteomyelitis of the patella," *Clinical Orthopaedics and Related Research*, vol. 389, pp. 30–34, 2001.

[15] S.-S. Shim and G. Leung, "Blood supply of the knee joint. A microangiographic study in children and adults," *Clinical Orthopaedics and Related Research*, vol. 208, pp. 119–125, 1986.

[16] M. Song, Z. Zhang, Y. Wu, K. Ma, and M. Lu, "Primary tumors of the patella," *World Journal of Surgical Oncology*, vol. 13, no. 1, p. 163, 2015.

[17] J. M. Fritz and J. R. McDonald, "Osteomyelitis: approach to diagnosis and treatment," *The Physician and Sportsmedicine*, vol. 36, no. 1, article nihpa116823, 2008.

[18] J. Dartnell, M. Ramachandran, and M. Katchburian, "Haematogenous acute and subacute paediatric osteomyelitis," *Journal of Bone and Joint Surgery–Series B*, vol. 94, no. 5, pp. 584–595, 2012.

5

Acute Carpal Tunnel Syndrome Secondary to Amyloidosis

Ömer Serdar Hakyemez, Fatih Arslanoğlu, Murat Birinci, Mehmet Akif Çaçan, and Adnan Kara

Medipol Mega University Hospital, Istanbul, Turkey

Correspondence should be addressed to Ömer Serdar Hakyemez; hakyemezos@gmail.com

Academic Editor: Mark K. Lyons

Introduction. ACTS secondary to amyloidosis is a very rare situation in the literature, and here, we present a unique case of ACTS secondary to amyloidosis. *Case Report.* A 61-year-old male patient was admitted to our hospital with complaints of numbness in the lateral half of his 1, 2, 3, and 4 fingers of his right hand. These complaints started acutely, and the patient did not have a history of trauma. His clinical examination was suitable for acute carpal tunnel syndrome. *Discussion.* Carpal tunnel syndrome, as well as acute carpal tunnel syndrome, may occur based on different causes. ACTS is very rare, especially when it is not caused by a trauma. Here, we presented a unique case of ACTS based on amyloidosis. *Conclusion.* It should be kept in mind when ACTS may occur in patients with the diagnosis of amyloidosis.

1. Introduction

Amyloidosis is known to be associated with carpal tunnel syndrome (CTS) [1]. Amyloid deposition in the tendon and surrounding tissues further reduces the already low carpal tunnel volume, compressing the median nerve, and causes chronic CTS. However, this is not very expected to occur acutely. Here, we present a unique case of ACTS secondary to amyloidosis.

2. Case Report

A 61-year-old male patient was admitted to our hospital with complaints of numbness in the lateral half of the 1, 2, 3, and 4 fingers of the right hand and decreased range of motion which started 1 day earlier and increased in severity. With the in-depth analysis of the patient's, he did not have any similar complaints before. An immunohistochemical examination of the biopsy material obtained from the mass on the right shoulder 1 month before the patient's numbness in his fingers was consistent with secondary amyloidosis.

In the physical examination of the patient, active and passive flexions of the fingers were found to be limited and numbness was noticed in the 1st, 2nd, 3rd, and 4th lateral half of the fingers, which is the innervation area of the median nerve. Even though no atrophy was seen in the thenar muscles, it was observed that the palm of the effected hand was hypertrophic compared to the other palm, and the Tinel and Phalen tests were both positive.

Because the direct radiographs of the patient were interpreted as normal, MRI was requested for further examination. MRI revealed excessive fluid collection and intense synovitis in the intercarpal, radioulnar, and ulnocarpal joints and surrounding para-articular soft tissue planes at the wrist level. The findings were thought to be compatible with amyloidosis, but rheumatologic diseases could also be compatible with the same findings. Because of this, further investigation has been done with clinical examination and laboratory findings. No rheumatologic diseases has been diagnosed after the investigation.

In the patient's EMG, the following are found: (1) The compound muscle action potential of the right median nerve was found to be low amplitude, and the amplitude of the muscle action potential combined with wrist stimulation decreased by more than 50 compared to palm stimulation (partial conduction block). Motor transmission speed was low in the palm-wrist segment. Motor conduction studies of the other nerves of both upper and lower

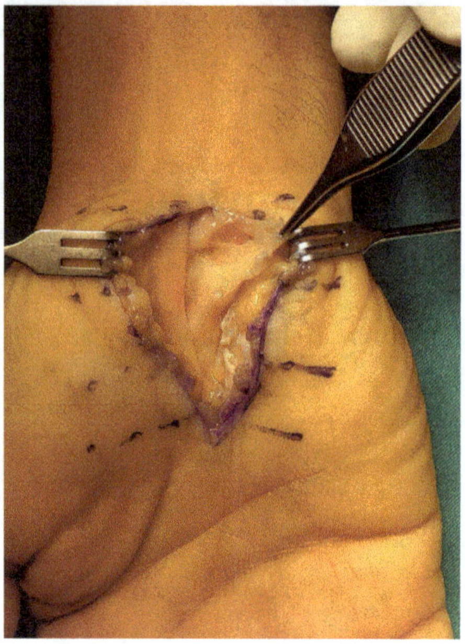

FIGURE 1: Hypertrophic synovial tissue.

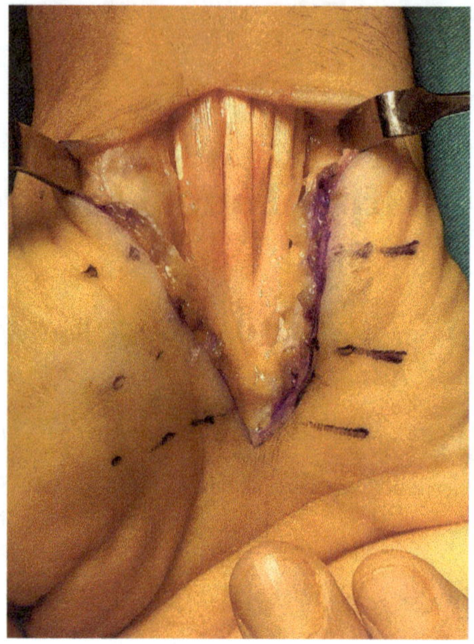

FIGURE 2: Loosened median nerve after synovectomy.

extremities were found to be normal. (2) Sensory action potential of the right median nerve could not be obtained. In conclusion, these findings were consistent with acute carpal tunnel syndrome causing axon and myelin damage on the right upper extremity.

The patient underwent surgery the day after he presented to our outpatient clinic. Incision has been done in the volar side of the right hand following the palmar crisis, and the transverse carpal ligament was loosened completely; afterwards, biopsy was taken for pathology. The median nerve appear to be swelled. It was assured that the nerve was completely decompressed distally and proximally. Neurolysis was performed after the median nerve was loosened. Diffuse synovial thickening has been observed around the flexor tendons which were hypertrophic (Figure 1). Synovectomy has been performed (Figure 2).

According to the results of the pathology samples sent during surgery, AA-type amyloidosis was detected in the samples taken from the median nerve sheath and from the synovial tissue on the flexor tendons (Figures 3 and 4).

The Tinel and Phalen tests were found to be negative, and numbness in the fingers disappeared and finger flexion movements were more comfortable after the operation.

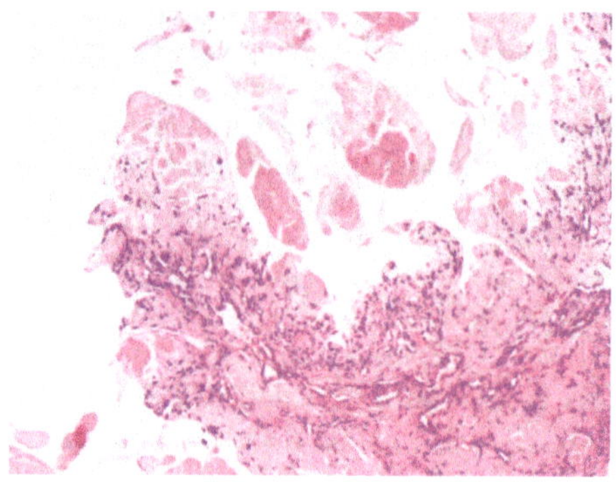

FIGURE 3: Amyloid deposits in the sample taken from the median nerve (HE stain ×100 magnification).

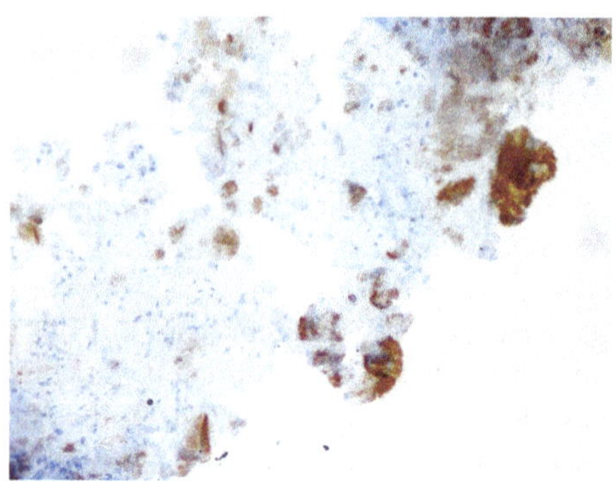

FIGURE 4: Amyloid deposits in the sample taken from the median nerve (IHC stain ×100 magnification).

3. Discussion

The carpal tunnel, which has a constant volume of 5 ml, is surrounded by carpal bones from 3 sides and surrounded by flexor retinaculum from the volar side. The problems occur in the structures passing through this small gap further narrowing the volume, leaving a minimal space for any expansion within the carpal tunnel [2].

Carpal tunnel syndrome develops due to the prolonged and intensive use of the wrist and some systemic diseases such as rheumatologic diseases, diabetes, and amyloidosis. CTS is the most common chronic compressive neuropathy [3]. There are many studies about chronic CTS as it is a common condition. But acute CTS is a much more rare condition. CTS symptoms progress in months to years, but in acute CTS, symptoms progress very quickly in hours to days.

This condition usually occurs after traumatic events [4]. Rarely, carpal tunnel syndrome may occur with atraumatic etiology such as infection, inflammation, and iatrogenic events that increase carpal tunnel pressure [4, 5].

ACTS is characterized by continuous pain and numbness along the median nerve track due to the sudden and rapid increase in pressure in the carpal tunnel. The patient complains numbness in the first 3 fingers on the affected side and in the lateral half of the 4th finger.

In the rapid process of ACTS, it is very important to make the diagnosis quickly and to plan the intervention early. The sooner the intervention is performed, the likelihood of undesirable conditions such as neural dysfunction, limitation of movement, disruption of microcirculation, and chronic pain is reduced [6].

Local amyloid deposits have been held responsible in CTS cases developing on the basis of amyloidosis, and this is not uncommon. According to Kyle et al., 1500 patients have been operated for carpal tunnel release and 124 of them had local amyloid deposits [7]. In another study, it has been shown that local amyloid deposition does not only occur in the tendons but may also occur in the transverse carpal ligament [8]. However, in these studies, no ACTS was developed on the basis of amyloidosis.

There are currently no guidelines for diagnosing ACTS or managing this process. But we know that early surgery and carpal tunnel loosening are the only ways to achieve good results. In one study, it was shown that patients who underwent surgery within 40 hours after the onset of ACTS symptoms have completely regained normal nerve function from day 4 postoperatively [9].

4. Conclusion

ACTS is less common than CTS. ACTS usually occurs due to trauma and begins to show serious symptoms within days to hours. Carpal tunnel decompression is always the first-line treatment in ACTS cases, whether trauma-induced or based on another etiology. As in our case, it should be remembered that acute CTS may develop while expecting chronic CTS in a previously diagnosed patient with amyloidosis.

References

[1] M. Nakagawa, Y. Sekijima, M. Yazaki et al., "Carpal tunnel syndrome: a common initial symptom of systemic wild-type ATTR (ATTRwt) amyloidosis," *Amyloid*, vol. 23, no. 1, pp. 58–63, 2016.

[2] J. D. Gillig, S. D. White, and J. N. Rachel, "Acute carpal tunnel syndrome: a review of current literature," *The Orthopedic Clinics of North America*, vol. 47, no. 3, pp. 599–607, 2016.

[3] R. M. Szabo and D. R. Steinberg, "Nerve entrapment syndromes in the wrist," *The Journal of the American Academy of Orthopaedic Surgeons*, vol. 2, no. 2, pp. 115–123, 1994.

[4] G. Kokosis, G. Blueschke, M. Blanton, H. Levinson, and D. Erdmann, "Acute carpal tunnel syndrome secondary to iatrogenic hemorrhage. A case report," *Hand*, vol. 6, no. 2, pp. 206–208, 2011.

[5] A. I. Mayne, A. Howard, M. Kent, and J. Banks, "Acute carpal tunnel syndrome in a patient with haemophilia," *BMJ Case Reports*, vol. 2012, p. bcr0320126152, 2012.

[6] G. A. Barbee, C. L. Haley, and C. S. Berry-Cabán, "A case of acute carpal tunnel syndrome," *Journal of the American Academy of Physician Assistants*, vol. 29, no. 1, pp. 31-32, 2016.

[7] R. A. Kyle, S. G. Eilers, R. L. Linscheid, and T. A. Gaffey, "Amyloid localized to tenosynovium at carpal tunnel release. Natural history of 124 cases," *American Journal of Clinical Pathology*, vol. 91, no. 4, pp. 393–397, 1989.

[8] R. Samões, R. Taipa, K. Valdrez, I. Gonçalves, and M. Melo Pires, "Amyloid detection in the transverse carpal ligament of patients with hereditary ATTR V30M amyloidosis and carpal tunnel syndrome," *Amyloid*, vol. 24, no. 2, pp. 73–77, 2017.

[9] D. J. Ford and M. S. Ali, "Acute carpal tunnel syndrome. Complications of delayed decompression," *Journal of Bone and Joint Surgery British Volume*, vol. 68-B, no. 5, pp. 758-759, 1986.

6

Traumatic Pelvic Ring Injury following Childbirth with Complete Pubic Symphysis Diastasis

Aaron Seidman[1] **Kelley Brossy,**[1] **Alfred Faulkner,**[1] **and Jeffrey Taylor**[2]

[1]*Department of Orthopedic Surgery, Beaumont Hospital, Farmington Hills, MI, USA*
[2]*Lake Erie College of Osteopathic Medicine, Erie, PA, USA*

Correspondence should be addressed to Aaron Seidman; ajerseid@gmail.com

Academic Editor: Eyal Itshayek

Case. Traumatic pelvic ring injury following childbirth is a rare but debilitating condition. We present a case of a 28-year-old female who sustained a traumatic pelvic ring injury following childbirth with a complete pubic symphysis separation of 5.6 cm treated successfully with nonoperative management. *Conclusion.* Operative and nonoperative treatments for traumatic pelvic ring injuries following childbirth have been described without universal adoption of a uniform treatment modality. We hope this case study adds to the collection of data to help guide medical decision-making in the future as surgeons encounter patients with similar orthopedic injuries.

1. Introduction

Traumatic pelvic ring injury with complete pubic symphysis diastasis following childbirth via vaginal delivery is a rare but debilitating condition. Widening of the cartilaginous joint during pregnancy prior to childbirth is physiologic and assists in widening the birth canal for successful delivery [1]. However, reports of nonphysiologic pubic diastasis exceeding that required for childbirth (typically greater than 1 cm) can leave mothers with debility and extreme pain. Incidence of complete separation of the pubic symphysis is reported to be within 1 in 300 to 1 : 30,000, with many instances likely undiagnosed [1, 2]. The orthopedic surgeon is presented with a difficult decision when managing these injuries as women are high-risk surgical candidates in the peripregnancy state, and prolonged debility can affect care for their newborn. We present the following case report of a 28-year-old female who sustained a traumatic pelvic ring injury with complete pubic diastasis of 5.6 cm that was successfully treated with nonoperative management, returning to full function one year out from injury. We present this case report in hopes to provide information to orthopedic surgeons presented with this challenging and debilitating diagnosis.

2. Statement of Informed Consent

Our patient was informed that data pertaining to her case and treatment would be submitted for publication and she agreed.

3. Case Report

Our patient is a 28-year-old G2PO female who presented to our institution in labor for the birth of her first child. At time of presentation, the position of the baby was cephalic. The patient denies antecedent pelvic pain or difficulty with ambulation prior to delivery. Active labor was initiated with Pitocin augmentation. She was provided an epidural spinal anesthesia. Following 3 hours of pushing, the patient delivered a baby boy of 6 lb 11.2 oz (3040 grams). The patient did sustain a grade 1 peroneal tear which was closed primarily with suture.

Two hours following delivery, the patient was evaluated by her obstetrics physician for persistent and worsening anterior pelvic pain and low back pain with inability to ambulate. She was then evaluated with an AP radiograph of the pelvis which revealed a complete pubic symphysis diastasis of 5.6 cm with widening of bilateral sacroiliac joints posteriorly

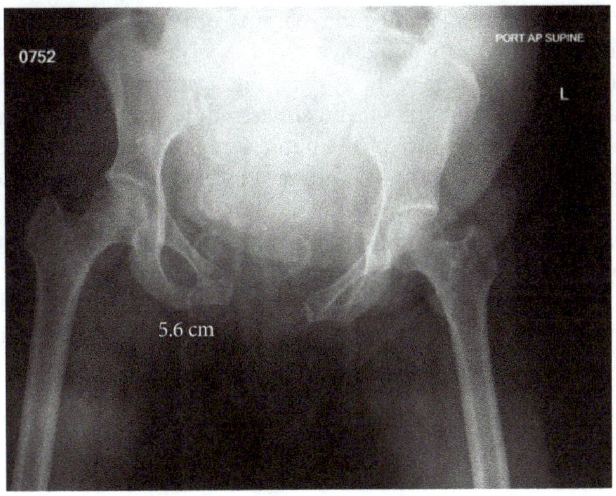

FIGURE 1: Diagnostic AP pelvis radiograph demonstrating a traumatic pubic ring separation of 5.6 cm.

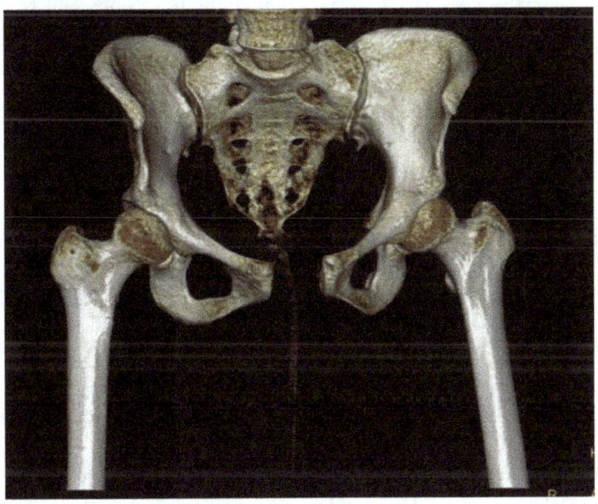

FIGURE 2: 3D CT reconstruction of the pelvis redemonstrating separation of the pubic symphysis.

(Figure 1) which is redemonstrated with 3D CT reconstruction (Figure 2). That evening, the orthopedic surgery team was asked to evaluate the patient. Following evaluation, a generic pelvic binder was placed on the patient and repeat imaging showed no significant improvement in her diastasis nor did the patient experience a reduction in her pain. The patient was left in a pelvic binder with constant skin assessments and was allowed to weight bear as tolerated. Considerations were given for both operative open reduction with anterior internal plate fixation and continued nonoperative management; however, the patient and family elected to continue nonoperative management with close observation.

The patient was transferred to the orthopedic surgery floor of our institution the following day where she worked with physical therapy twice daily for assistance with mobilization, beginning the following day post diagnosis. The patient had persistent pelvic pain and difficulty ambulating. On hospital day 8, as patient was only able to sit on the side of the bed and ambulate several feet with the assistance of a

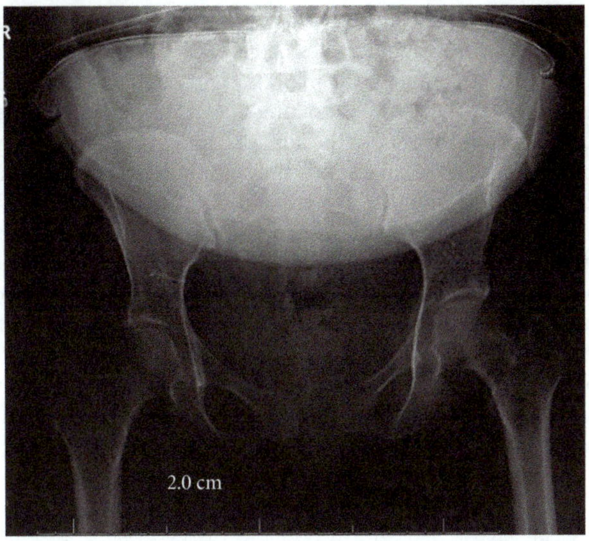

FIGURE 3: Follow-up AP pelvis radiograph at 6 weeks post injury demonstrating residual pubic symphysis widening of 2.0 cm.

walker device, she was transferred to inpatient rehabilitation where she spent 15 days before being discharged home able to walk with minimal pain with assistance of the walker device. The patient was seen back in office for her first clinic follow-up 6 weeks following her delivery. At that time, the patient's AP pelvic X-ray revealed 2.0 cm of residual pubic diastasis (Figure 3), and the patient was using an occasional walker when on uneven ground but able to do stairs and perform ADLs. She continued to work with outpatient physical therapy for a total of 6 months before returning to full-time work. At her 1-year follow-up, she is back to full-time work, ambulates both inside and outside the home without assistance, and is able to do stairs, perform ADLs, and care for her baby with only mild intermittent low back pain managed by over-the-counter anti-inflammatories.

4. Literature Review

There is currently much debate over the appropriate treatment modality for postpartum pubic symphysis diastasis. Kharrazi et al. described four patients with an average pubic symphysis diastasis of 6.4 cm all treated nonoperatively with a pelvic binder. These patients had a reduction of their diastasis to 1.7 cm; however, all four had persistent sacroiliac joint pain. They suggest considering operative treatment at a diastasis of >4 cm. Dunivan described the use of an external fixator successfully on a woman with a 6.2 cm diastasis with the ability to weight bear on her second post-op day and discharged on postpartum day four, able to ambulate with a walker.

Cases of open reduction internal fixation (ORIF) of pubic symphysis diastasis have also been described in the literature. Najibi et al. describe ten patients treated operatively with internal fixation [3]. Three patients had an excellent outcome, four had a good result, and three had a fair or poor result. Rommens described the successful internal fixation of three patients with diastasis ranging from 15 mm to

45 mm who failed conservative management. Yoo et al. identified that primigravid females had a higher risk for diastasis.

Physical therapy for the management of pubic symphysis diastasis has been well documented. Stretch and often complete rupture of both the superior and inferior pubic ligaments result in separation of the symphysis. Strengthening of the surrounding soft tissue, including the rectus abdominis, thoracolumbar musculature and fascia, and quadriceps and hamstrings, helps stabilize and reduce stress through the pubic symphysis [4]. A stable symphysis without recurrent stress through the joint allows a slow return towards anatomic position with scarring of the torn ligaments back towards their attachments. A combination of closed chain exercises targeting these muscle groups along with altered sleep positioning (pillow between legs during slumber) are recommended to expedite the healing process [5].

5. Discussion

Widening of the pubic symphysis during childbirth is physiologic and is an advantageous adaptation in widening of the birth canal for delivery. However, excessive widening of the pubic symphysis can be pathologic and lead to debilitating pain. A separation of more than 1 cm postpartum is historically noted to be pathologic and symptomatic [1]. Furthermore, literature suggests consideration of operative treatment for separations greater than 4 cm [6]. Relaxin, a hormone secreted by the placenta during pregnancy, peaks during the first trimester and again peripartum. A modulator of arterial compliance and cardiac output during pregnancy, relaxin also serves to relax the pelvic ligaments and contributes to softening of the cartilage of the pubic symphysis for preparation of the birth canal for delivery [7, 8]. Identified risk factors for postpartum pubic symphysis diastasis include primigravid women, multiple gestations, and prolonged active labor [2]. When considering operative management of postpartum symphysis diastasis, it is important to consider and respect the physiologic changes of pregnancy that could complicate surgery. Pregnancy and peripartum bed rest are associated with an increased risk of deep venous thrombosis [2]. In addition, pelvic anatomy can be distorted following birth and elevated relaxin levels have also been shown to be associated with increased uterine bleeding, which complicate surgical treatment [2, 9]. Treatments described for pelvis diastasis include nonoperative treatment with application of pelvic binder coupled with physical therapy and immediate weight bearing, non-weight bearing with bedrest, closed reduction with application of binder, application of anterior external fixator with or without sacroiliac screw fixation, and anterior internal fixation with plate and screws. While our patient initially presented with a diastasis of 5.63 cm, we pursued nonoperative management with application of a pelvic binder and immediate physical therapy with unrestricted weight bearing. At 6-week follow-up, repeat imaging showed improvement of diastasis to 2.0 cm with significant improvement in symptoms. At 1-year follow-up, our patient is ambulating without assistance and is back to performing all activities of daily living and caring for her child.

Prognosis is good for the majority of patients who experience postpartum pubic symphysis diastasis, and in most cases, full recovery without persistent pain is expected [1]. Follow-up radiographs in most case studies reviewed show near complete closure of the pubic symphysis and complete resolution of symptoms within 3 months. Some patients did require further physical therapy for up to 6 months including our patient presented above. No significant long-term sequelae have been identified. No definitive recommendations exist regarding alteration of care for future pregnancies, and this would be a good area for future study. We hope this case study provides insight for future treating physicians.

References

[1] J. J. Chawla, D. Arora, N. Sandhu, M. Jain, and A. Kumari, "Pubic symphysis diastasis: a case series and literature review," *Oman Medical Journal*, vol. 32, no. 6, pp. 510–514, 2017.

[2] J. J. Yoo, Y. C. Ha, Y. K. Lee, J. S. Hong, B. J. Kang, and K. H. Koo, "Incidence and risk factors of symptomatic peripartum diastasis of pubic symphysis," *Journal of Korean Medical Science*, vol. 29, no. 2, pp. 281–286, 2014.

[3] S. Najibi, M. Tannast, R. E. Klenck, and J. M. Matta, "Internal fixation of symphyseal disruption resulting from childbirth," *Journal of Orthopaedic Trauma*, vol. 24, no. 12, pp. 732–739, 2010.

[4] J. Borg-Stein and S. A. Dugan, "Musculoskeletal Disorders of Pregnancy, Delivery and Postpartum," *Physical Medicine and Rehabilitation Clinics of North America*, vol. 18, no. 3, pp. 459–476, 2007.

[5] E. R. Howell, "Pregnancy-related symphysis pubic dysfunction management and postpartum rehabilitation: two case reports," *The Journal of the Canadian Chiropractic Association*, vol. 56, no. 2, pp. 102–111, 2012.

[6] J. M. Miller, L. K. Low, R. Zielinski, A. R. Smith, J. O. L. DeLancey, and C. Brandon, "Evaluating maternal recovery from labor and delivery: bone and levator ani injuries," *American Journal of Obstetrics and Gynecology*, vol. 213, no. 2, pp. 188.e1–188.e11, 2015.

[7] E. R. Howell, "Pregnancy-related symphysis pubis dysfunction management and postpartum rehabilitation: two case reports," *The Journal of the Canadian Chiropractic Association*, vol. 56, no. 2, pp. 102–111, 2012.

[8] R. Hagen, "Pelvic girdle relaxation from an orthopaedic point of view," *Acta Orthopaedica Scandinavica*, vol. 45, no. 1-4, pp. 550–563, 1974.

[9] M. Shi, S. Shang, B. Xie et al., "MRI changes of pelvic floor and pubic bone observed in primiparous women after childbirth by normal vaginal delivery," *Archives of Gynecology and Obstetrics*, vol. 294, no. 2, pp. 285–289, 2016.

7

Retrograde Intramedullary Nail Fixation for Derotational Femoral Osteotomy for Recurrent Femoropatellar Instability

Maximiliano Barahona,[1] Alvaro Zamorano,[1] Cristian Barrientos,[1] Mauricio Guzmán,[2] Yoshiro Sato,[1] and Jaime Hinzpeter[1]

[1]*Orthopedic Department at Hospital Clinico Universidad de Chile, 999 Santos Dumont Street, Independencia, Santiago 8380456, Chile*
[2]*Radiology Department at Hospital Clinico Universidad de Chile, 999 Santos Dumont Street, Independencia, Santiago 8380456, Chile*

Correspondence should be addressed to Maximiliano Barahona; maxbarahonavasquez@gmail.com

Academic Editor: Dimitrios S. Karataglis

Axial alignment of the femur and tibia is often misdiagnosed in patients with patellofemoral stability problems. Femoral torsion is critical for patellofemoral biomechanics, so it must be evaluated in every patient before the plan of surgery is decided. This case describes a femoral derotational osteotomy due to excessive internal torsion of the femur fixed with a retrograde femoral nail. This type of fixation provides a biomechanical advantage compared to plates. At the two-year follow-up, the patient achieved excellent results, reaching a functional score of 91 points on the Lysholm scale. Derotational femoral osteotomy should be considered in patellofemoral pathology, and a retrograde femoral nail is a valid fixation method for this surgery.

1. Introduction

Patellofemoral instability is a multifactorial pathology, in which three main elements participate: lower limb malalignment, trochlear dysplasia, and the medial patellofemoral ligament (MPFL). Malalignment is a factor in a large percentage of patients who consult for this pathology, and the spectrum is broad. An increase in the distance between the intercondylar groove and the tibial tuberosity is just the tip of the iceberg; on the other end is the miserable malalignment syndrome, a rare condition that includes severe internal torsion of the femur [1, 2].

Femoral torsion is defined as the angle between the femoral neck axis and the condyle axis. The pathological cutoff value to perform a derotational osteotomy is a matter of current debate; one of the first values reported was those described by Cordier and Katthagen, who defined a normal range between 5° and 25° assuming a normal distribution of the data [3]. However, a range of two standard deviations from the mean sample does not imply a relation to a clinical problem like patella instability or pain.

Femoral torsion is a risk factor for patella instability [4]. A cadaveric study performed by Kaiser et al. [5] shows that a 10° increase of femoral torsion amplifies the lateral vector force to the patella, but a reconstruction of the MPFL alone can restore it; however, if the femoral torsion is now increased to 20°, the reconstruction of the MPFL alone is insufficient to decrease the lateral vector. This finding adds to the ever-growing evidence that supports the need to perform derotational osteotomies in patients with increased femoral torsion [6, 7].

Also, trochlea dysplasia may be a result of decreased contact between the femur and the patella due to an increased femoral torsion, emulating the proposed model in hip dysplasia [8]. So, when the trochlea angle is flat, femoral torsion must be evaluated and corrected if it is too high.

The knee surgeon must study the entire alignment in patella instability, including femoral and tibial torsion [9].

This case report is aimed at describing a femoral derotational osteotomy fixed by a retrograde femoral nail for recurrent patellar instability.

2. Case

The patient was a 17-year-old woman who complains of recurrent patellar instability in her left knee (5-7 episodes per year in the last three years) and in her right knee (two episodes). Physical examination revealed a full range of motion in both knees. The left knee had mild effusion and a positive apprehension test. On the right knee, no effusion or apprehension was noticed, but a pain in the medial retinaculum was found. The hip internal rotation was asymmetric, being greater in the left hip, so femoral malrotation was suspected. Tibial torsion, assessed by clinical thigh-foot angle, was normal. The preoperative patient-reported score was 19 on the Lysholm scale [10] and level 1 on the Tegner scale [11].

All patients with recurrent patellar instability are studied with full-length standing anteroposterior (AP) radiography, computed tomography (CT) of the lower extremities, and knee magnetic resonance imaging (MRI) in our institution. CT measurements are summarised in Table 1, and an increased femoral internal rotation was the main finding (Figure 1). Femoral torsion was measured according to the technique described by Jarrett et al. [12], with an expected value of 15°. Radiography shows mild symmetric valgus alignment in the coronal plane, a femoral-tibial mechanical angle of 1° of valgus, and a mechanical distal lateral femoral angle (mDLFA) of 86° on the left knee. Knee MRI shows a bilateral lesion of the MPFL and chondral type 2 damage in the lateral facet of the left patella. The trochlea was flat on both knees, which means that it corresponds to a type B according to Dejour's classification [13].

According to the classification of patellar instability by Frosch and Schmeling [14], the right extremity was a type 2: instability without malalignment as femoral torsion was below 25°. The authors use the upper limit to indicate a femoral derotational osteotomy according to the findings of Kaiser et al. [5]; therefore, a medial patellofemoral ligament (MPFL) reconstruction alone was planned. The left extremity was a type 3e (instability with femoral malrotation); therefore, a femoral derotational osteotomy was planned.

Our planning was estimating the perimeter of the femur at the level of the osteotomy. For the estimation of the perimeter, in an axial section of the CT scan at the level of the desired osteotomy, we measure the radius in the anteroposterior (2,98 cm) direction and in the midlateral direction (2,66 cm). With these two measurements, we obtained an average radius of 2,82 cm. Then, the perimeter calculation is based on the formula $2 * \pi *$ radius; therefore, the perimeter was 17,7 cm. The perimeter accounted for 360°, so for 17° of correction, a rotation of 0.8 cm should be made.

Both knees were operated on during the same surgery. The first step was to perform the femoral osteotomy; for this, a lateral approach in the thigh was performed. The lateral cortex of the distal third of the femoral shaft was exposed. Two clamps were positioned on both sides of the desired location for the osteotomy, and the bone was marked parallel to the long axis. A transverse bone cut, parallel to the shaft axis, was performed in between the clamps and in the middle of the horizontal line with fluoroscopy guidance. Then, a retrograde femoral nail (T2, Stryker®) was used to fix the osteotomy. To begin, a proximal blocking screw was placed in the dynamic hole, then the distal end of the osteotomy was externally rotated, as planned, using the clamps to apply the force to achieve a distance of 0.8 cm between the horizontal lines at both ends of the osteotomy cut. Immediately after the derotational maneuver, two distal locking screws were placed in the distal end of the nail (Figure 2).

Table 1: All CT measurements are shown. Femoral torsion was measured according to the method described by Jarrett et al. [12]. A femoral torsion of 32° was found in the left side, 17° higher than the expected value, so according to Kaiser et al. [5], a MPFL reconstruction alone is not enough to restore patellofemoral kinematics. The trochlea in both knees was type B according to the Dejour classification [13].

Measurement	Right	Left
Femoral torsion	**23.3°**	**32.2°**
Tibial torsion	**18°**	**21°**
Trochlea angle	**143°**	**147°**
TT-TG	**13 mm**	**14 mm**
Patellar height (Caton)	**0.98**	**0.87**

After the osteotomy was fixed, both the gracilis and the semitendinosus tendons of the left knee were harvested. The left MPFL was reconstructed with the gracilis autograft; it was fixed with two anchors in the patellar side and a biodegradable screw in the femur (BIORCI®, Smith & Nephew).

In the right knee, the MPFL was reconstructed with the semitendinosus of the contralateral knee using the same fixation method described for the left knee. In both knees, MPFL femoral attachments were selected using fluoroscopy as described by Schöttle et al. [15], and the grafts were fixed with 45° of knee flexion. In the left knee, while harvesting the hamstring tendon, an accidental partial lesion of the distal medial collateral ligament occurred and was repaired with an anchor.

After surgery, the patient did not present any complications. The rehabilitation protocol was weight bearing as tolerated, with two canes. Full knee extension was encouraged, and active flexion was limited to 60° for three weeks. After 10 weeks, she resumed walking without canes and gained full knee range of motion on the right knee and 100° in the left knee.

The eight-month postsurgery radiographs are shown in Figure 3 and are compared with the preoperative radiographs. It is remarkable how the patella looks medialised compared to the preoperative study (Figure 3), and as planned, the coronal alignment was not changed (Figure 4(a)) achieving a femoral-tibial mechanical angle after surgery of 0.51° of valgus. At the eight-month follow-up, the osteotomy was completely healed (Figures 4(b) and 4(c)). At the 18-month follow-up, a CT scan was performed, and femoral torsion was 6.4° (Figure 5). At the 24-month follow-up, the patient-reported outcome was 91 on the Lysholm scale

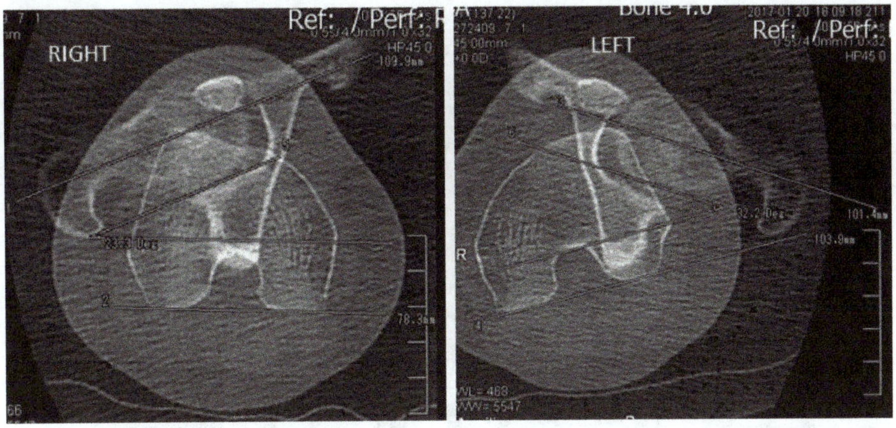

Figure 1: Preoperative CT scan femoral torsion measurements are shown. In the left leg, the femoral torsion is 32°; the right leg has a torsion of 23°. Measurements were made according to the technique described by Jarrett et al. [12].

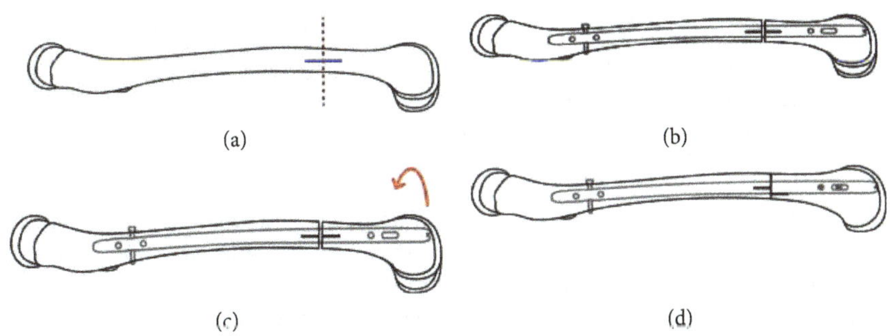

Figure 2: Illustrations that represent the surgery in the left femur. (a) The lateral cortex of the distal third of the femoral shaft was marked with a parallel line to the long axis to guide the correction (black line). A transverse bone cut (red line) parallel to the shaft axis was performed in the middle of the black line. (b) By a percutaneous approach to the knee, a retrograde femoral nail (T2, Stryker®) was placed. To begin with, a proximal blocking screw was placed in the dynamic hole. (c) The distal end of the osteotomy was externally rotated, as planned. (d) The parallel line to the axis of the diaphysis was the guide (black line), and the rotation was performed until both lines were separated by 0.8 cm. Immediately after the derotational maneuver, two distal locking screws were placed in the distal end of the nail.

[10] and level 4 on the Tegner scale [11]. The patient had no episodes of patella dislocation or instability complaints after the surgery.

3. Discussion

Axial alignment of the femur and tibia is often undervalued in patients with patellofemoral stability problems [9, 16]. Assessing femoral torsion is essential during the decision-making process for the surgical procedure to avoid poor surgical outcomes in patellofemoral pathologies [7]. Rotational alignment is crucial for knee biomechanics; knee arthroplasty is an excellent example of how patellar instability occurs when the femoral component is malrotated [17–20].

Recurrent patellofemoral instability is a multifactorial pathology; therefore, the evaluation should include the assessment of all factors that may be involved [21]. This must include MPFL, femoral torsion, tibial torsion, trochlea depth, patellar height, tibial tubercle to intercondylar groove distance (TT-TG), and coronal lower extremity alignment [2]. Femoral torsion plays an essential role in patellofemoral pathologies, so it must be evaluated in every patient before the surgery plan is defined for patellofemoral instability [2].

It is difficult to evaluate femoral torsion, both in the physical examination and in the radiological exams. In the former, an increase in passive internal hip rotation should raise a high suspicion for increased internal femoral torsion [22]. CT measurement is the gold standard to assess femoral torsion; however, MRI has been proposed, since it involves less radiation, despite having higher costs [23]. Also, some promissory findings have been reported with radiographs [24]. Another major problem lies in the lack of consensus on the anatomical landmarks chosen to perform the measurement. Kaiser et al. [25] showed that the six different methods of measurement proposed have a weak agreement. Our preference is to use the angle between the neck axis and the line that goes across both posterior condyles as proposed by Jarrett et al. [12].

The location in which to perform the derotational osteotomy in the femur is a matter of debate. According to findings of Seitlinger et al. [23], when patellar instability is due to excessive internal femoral torsion, the most critical factor is a lack of external rotation of the shaft of the femur which compensates for the normal or subtle excess of internal

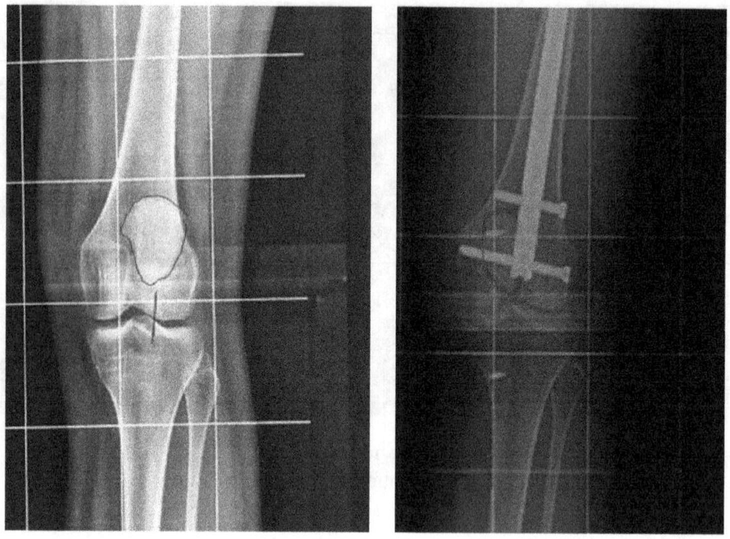

(a) (b)

FIGURE 3: The enlarged image of the left knee of the full-length standing AP radiography before surgery (a) and enlarged image 8 months after surgery (b) are shown. Both were taken with 15° of internal rotation of the foot. The perimeter of the patella is highlighted in red, and the medialization of the patella due to the derotational osteotomy is observed.

rotation of the femoral neck. Nevertheless, some studies have shown that the location of the derotational osteotomy in the femur may alter the coronal or sagittal alignment. Nelitz et al. [26] have proposed that if the coronal plane is in varus, the osteotomy must be performed in the distal metaphysis, and like in this case study, if the coronal alignment is neutral, a transverse osteotomy on the shaft of the femur must be done. However, Imhoff et al. demonstrated, in a cadaveric study, the importance of the orientation of the cut in the distal femur to avoid changes in the coronal orientation of the limb, when a distal femoral derotational osteotomy is performed [27]. More importantly, by a single cut in the distal femur, the coronal and the rotational problem of the patient can be addressed by choosing the patient-specific oblique cut [28]; these promising results must be validated in the operating room. In summary, the planning of the derotational osteotomy must consider the effects in the coronal and sagittal planes and the patient-specific segment of femur maltorsion. In this case, the distal shaft was chosen because the patient had normal coronal alignment, and according to Seitlinger et al., the problem must be the lack of external torsion of the shaft.

Few cases of femoral derotational osteotomy for patellofemoral instability are described in the literature; all of them are fixed with plates [29–33]. There are reports of successful cases of femoral derotational osteotomy, due to femoral fracture malunion, fixed with anterograde nails [34–36]. In this case report, a retrograde femoral nail was chosen for various reasons. First, biomechanically, the nail has a shorter lever arm than a lateral plate, making immediate weight bearing safer, and it can be allowed from day one after surgery. This was a significant factor, considering that both knees underwent surgery. Second, biomechanical studies have shown that nails have better torsion and axial stability compared to plates [37]. Bone healing after a femoral shaft fracture is 97% when fixed with a retrograde nail, and it is better when compared to plates and anterograde nails [38]. We believe that the same rate of bone healing can be expected in this type of osteotomy. Also, as the nail was first fixed in the proximal side and the distal end of the osteotomy was externally rotated, the presence of the nail inside the femur ensured that the fragment was rotated and not translated. In terms of cost, to use a plate or a nail is similar. The nail requires performing an arthrotomy; however, a minimum arthrotomy is also required for the MPFL reconstruction. Subtrochanteric fracture around the retrograde femoral nail is a well-known complication, and to leave the nail proximal to the lesser trochanter decreases the risk of this type of complication [39]. The nail's distal blocking screw placed 4 cm or lower from the knee articular line and blocking screws that radiographically extend to or beyond the medial cortex are more likely to cause pain and require removal, so it must be avoided [40]. In case of no union, it should be addressed in a similar way by using either a nail or a plate for fixation. Infection must be ruled out, and the need of bone grafting or additional mechanical stability should be evaluated [41]. Finally, if the patient requires a knee replacement in the future, since intramedullary guidance is needed to perform the cuts for the femoral component, both plate and nail must be removed. The nail can be removed by the same approach needed for the knee replacement; however, it requires an additional incision to remove the proximal blocking screw.

Femoral torsion correction was higher than planned; we aimed to correct at 17°, but instead, we corrected at 26°. According to our planning, instead of 0.8 cm, we made a rotation of 1.3 cm. Nevertheless, we still achieved a femoral torsion of 6.4° which is within our normal range of 5-25°, which is 10° lesser or higher [5] than the expected value of 15° according to the method described by Jarrett et al. [12].

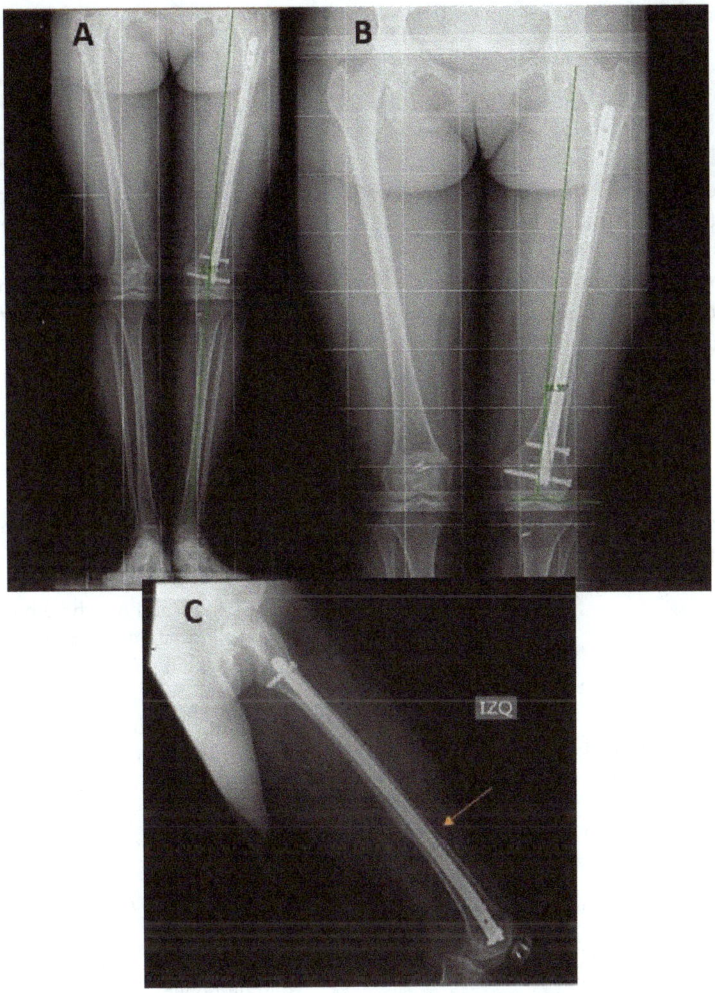

FIGURE 4: Radiographs at eight months after surgery are shown. (a) Full-length standing AP radiography of the lower extremity six months after surgery. Coronal alignment is symmetrical. (b) Femoral-tibial mechanical angle is 0.51° of valgus and mDLFA is 86°. (c) Lateral radiography of the femur. It shows complete healing of the osteotomy (red arrow). Also, the proximal locking of the nail and the entry point chosen in the distal femur for the LPFM can be observed.

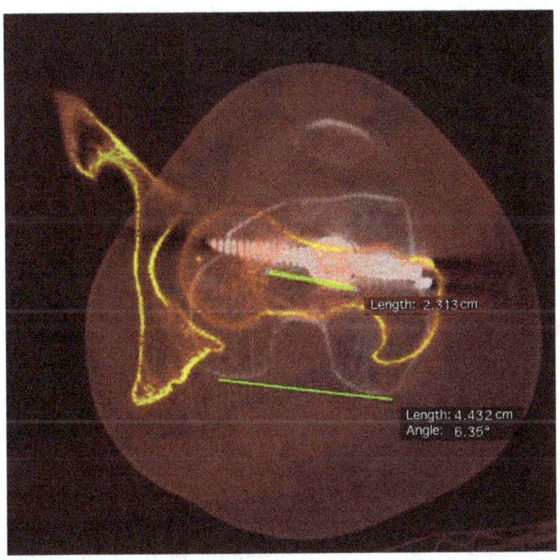

FIGURE 5: 13-month postsurgery CT scan. The final femoral torsion that was achieved is shown, measuring 6.4°. Femoral torsion according to the method described by Jarrett et al. was used [12].

To our knowledge, a precise method to achieve an excellent correlation between the correction planned and the correction obtained in derotational torsion has not been described. The accuracy of this method could be reported when we have more cases; however, we currently have not had a case outside 5°-25° of femoral torsion.

Derotational osteotomy can achieve a decrease in the load of the lateral patellofemoral compartment [8], as it was demonstrated in a cadaveric study by Liska et al. [42]. The decrease of the load in the compartment could at least avoid the progression of the chondral damage and even allow the cartilage to repair. This is also relevant to the case, in which the MRI showed ICRS chondral damage type 2 in the lateral facet of the left patella.

Postoperatory evolution was slower than expected; we think that the main reason was that both knees underwent surgery. After the 12-month follow-up, the patient showed excellent results and complete bone healing. Compared to the preoperative status, the patient now can ride a bike and has improved her performance in daily activities as Tegner and Lysholm scales show. Finally, the patient has not had any patellar dislocation or instability complain during the 24 months after surgery.

4. Conclusion

Femoral torsion has a crucial role in patellofemoral tracking; therefore, rotational alignment must always be assessed in recurrent patellofemoral instability. It may not be the most frequent finding, but if it is misdiagnosed, the treatment failure rate increases. Derotational femoral osteotomy is an excellent treatment option when internal femoral torsion is increased. The location on the femur where the osteotomy must be done ought to be chosen according to the segment of the femur that is more compromised and by the coronal and sagittal alignment of the femur. A retrograde femoral nail is a valid option for femoral derotational osteotomy fixation with biomechanical advantages compared to plates. The patient outcome after a two-year follow-up was excellent.

Acknowledgments

The first author acknowledges the support of Leonel Barahona in the elaboration of this paper. Also, the authors acknowledge the contribution of Paulina Barahona and Erin Dillinger for the English edition of this article.

References

[1] W. D. Bruce and P. M. Stevens, "Surgical correction of miserable malalignment syndrome," *Journal of Pediatric Orthopedics*, vol. 24, no. 4, pp. 392–396, 2004.

[2] R. A. Teitge, "Patellofemoral syndrome a paradigm for current surgical strategies," *The Orthopedic Clinics of North America*, vol. 39, no. 3, pp. 287–311, 2008.

[3] W. Cordier and B.-D. Katthagen, "Femoral torsional deformities," *Orthopade*, vol. 29, no. 9, pp. 795–801, 2000.

[4] P. Kaiser, W. Schmoelz, P. Schoettle, M. Zwierzina, C. Heinrichs, and R. Attal, "Increased internal femoral torsion can be regarded as a risk factor for patellar instability—a biomechanical study," *Clinical Biomechanics*, vol. 47, pp. 103–109, 2017.

[5] P. Kaiser, W. Schmoelz, P. B. Schöttle, C. Heinrichs, M. Zwierzina, and R. Attal, "Isolated medial patellofemoral ligament reconstruction for patella instability is insufficient for higher degrees of internal femoral torsion," *Knee Surgery, Sports Traumatology, Arthroscopy*, vol. 27, no. 3, pp. 758–765, 2019.

[6] F. B. Imhoff, M. Cotic, F. Liska et al., "Derotational osteotomy at the distal femur is effective to treat patients with patellar instability," *Knee Surgery, Sports Traumatology, Arthroscopy*, vol. 27, no. 2, pp. 652–658, 2019.

[7] P. M. Stevens, J. M. Gililland, L. A. Anderson, J. B. Mickelson, J. Nielson, and J. W. Klatt, "Success of torsional correction surgery after failed surgeries for patellofemoral pain and instability," *Strategies in Trauma and Limb Reconstruction*, vol. 9, no. 1, pp. 5–12, 2014.

[8] M. C. Liebensteiner, J. Ressler, G. Seitlinger, T. Djurdjevic, R. El Attal, and P. W. Ferlic, "High femoral anteversion is related to femoral trochlea dysplasia," *Arthroscopy*, vol. 32, no. 11, pp. 2295–2299, 2016.

[9] W. R. Post, R. Teitge, and A. Amis, "Patellofemoral malalignment: looking beyond the viewbox," *Clinics in Sports Medicine*, vol. 21, no. 3, pp. 521–546, 2002.

[10] J. Lysholm and J. Gillquist, "Evaluation of knee ligament surgery results with special emphasis on use of a scoring scale," *The American Journal of Sports Medicine*, vol. 10, no. 3, pp. 150–154, 1982.

[11] Y. Tegner and J. Lysholm, "Rating systems in the evaluation of knee ligament injuries," *Clinical Orthopaedics and Related Research*, vol. &NA;, no. 198, pp. 42–49, 1985.

[12] D. Y. Jarrett, A. M. Oliveira, K. H. Zou, B. D. Snyder, and P. K. Kleinman, "Axial oblique CT to assess femoral anteversion," *AJR. American Journal of Roentgenology*, vol. 194, no. 5, pp. 1230–1233, 2010.

[13] K. Tecklenburg, D. Dejour, C. Hoser, and C. Fink, "Bony and cartilaginous anatomy of the patellofemoral joint," *Knee Surgery, Sports Traumatology, Arthroscopy*, vol. 14, no. 3, pp. 235–240, 2006.

[14] K. H. Frosch and A. Schmeling, "A new classification system of patellar instability and patellar maltracking," *Archives of Orthopaedic and Trauma Surgery*, vol. 136, no. 4, pp. 485–497, 2016.

[15] P. Schöttle, S. Fucentese, and J. Romero, "Clinical and radiological outcome of medial patellofemoral ligament reconstruction with a semitendinosus autograft for patella instability," *Knee Surgery, Sports Traumatology, Arthroscopy*, vol. 13, no. 7, pp. 516–521, 2005.

[16] G. Pisani, "Some words about lower limb torsion and rotation problems," *Foot and Ankle Surgery*, vol. 15, no. 1, pp. 20-21, 2009.

[17] A. Keshmiri, G. Maderbacher, C. Baier et al., "The influence of component alignment on patellar kinematics in total knee arthroplasty," *Acta Orthopaedica*, vol. 86, no. 4, pp. 444–450, 2015.

[18] O. Kessler, S. Patil, C. W. Colwell Jr., and D. D. D'Lima, "The effect of femoral component malrotation on patellar biomechanics," *Journal of Biomechanics*, vol. 41, no. 16, pp. 3332–3339, 2008.

[19] J. H. Kim, B. W. Yoo, and C. W. Kim, "Influence of the rotational alignment of the femoral and patellar components on patellar tilt in total knee arthroplasty," *Knee Surgery & Related Research*, vol. 27, no. 3, pp. 163–167, 2015.

[20] J. Victor, "Rotational alignment of the distal femur: a literature review," *Orthopaedics & Traumatology, Surgery & Research*, vol. 95, no. 5, pp. 365–372, 2009.

[21] A. E. Weber, A. Nathani, J. S. Dines et al., "An algorithmic approach to the management of recurrent lateral patellar dislocation," *The Journal of Bone and Joint Surgery*, vol. 98, no. 5, pp. 417–427, 2016.

[22] V. Chadayammuri, T. Garabekyan, A. Bedi et al., "Passive hip range of motion predicts femoral torsion and acetabular version," *The Journal of Bone and Joint Surgery*, vol. 98, no. 2, pp. 127–134, 2016.

[23] G. Seitlinger, P. Moroder, G. Scheurecker, S. Hofmann, and R. P. Grelsamer, "The contribution of different femur segments to overall femoral torsion," *The American Journal of Sports Medicine*, vol. 44, no. 7, pp. 1796–1800, 2016.

[24] O. Meyrignac, R. Moreno, C. Baunin et al., "Low-dose biplanar radiography can be used in children and adolescents to

accurately assess femoral and tibial torsion and greatly reduce irradiation," *European Radiology*, vol. 25, no. 6, pp. 1752–1760, 2015.

[25] P. Kaiser, R. Attal, M. Kammerer et al., "Significant differences in femoral torsion values depending on the CT measurement technique," *Archives of Orthopaedic and Trauma Surgery*, vol. 136, no. 9, pp. 1259–1264, 2016.

[26] M. Nelitz, T. Wehner, M. Steiner, L. Dürselen, and S. Lippacher, "The effects of femoral external derotational osteotomy on frontal plane alignment," *Knee Surgery, Sports Traumatology, Arthroscopy*, vol. 22, no. 11, pp. 2740–2746, 2014.

[27] F. B. Imhoff, B. Scheiderer, P. Zakko et al., "How to avoid unintended valgus alignment in distal femoral derotational osteotomy for treatment of femoral torsional malalignment—a concept study," *BMC Musculoskeletal Disorders*, vol. 18, no. 1, p. 553, 2017.

[28] F. B. Imhoff, K. Beitzel, P. Zakko et al., "Derotational osteotomy of the distal femur for the treatment of patellofemoral instability simultaneously leads to the correction of frontal alignment: a laboratory cadaveric study," *Orthopaedic Journal of Sports Medicine*, vol. 6, no. 6, 2018.

[29] J. Dickschas, J. Harrer, B. Reuter, J. Schwitulla, and W. Strecker, "Torsional osteotomies of the femur," *Journal of Orthopaedic Research*, vol. 33, no. 3, pp. 318–324, 2015.

[30] J. Dickschas, A. Tassika, C. Lutter, J. Harrer, and W. Strecker, "Torsional osteotomies of the tibia in patellofemoral dysbalance," *Archives of Orthopaedic and Trauma Surgery*, vol. 137, no. 2, pp. 179–185, 2017.

[31] A. F. Kamath, R. Ganz, H. Zhang, G. Grappiolo, and M. Leunig, "Subtrochanteric osteotomy for femoral maltorsion through a surgical dislocation approach," *Journal of Hip Preservation Surgery*, vol. 2, no. 1, pp. 65–79, 2015.

[32] S. Hinterwimmer, P. Minzlaff, T. Saier, P. Niemeyer, A. B. Imhoff, and M. J. Feucht, "Biplanar supracondylar femoral derotation osteotomy for patellofemoral malalignment: the anterior closed-wedge technique," *Knee Surgery, Sports Traumatology, Arthroscopy*, vol. 22, no. 10, pp. 2518–2521, 2014.

[33] M. Nelitz, J. Dreyhaupt, S. R. M. Williams, and D. Dornacher, "Combined supracondylar femoral derotation osteotomy and patellofemoral ligament reconstruction for recurrent patellar dislocation and severe femoral anteversion syndrome: surgical technique and clinical outcome," *International Orthopaedics*, vol. 39, no. 12, pp. 2355–2362, 2015.

[34] N. Fiz, D. Delgado, X. Sánchez et al., "Application of 3D technology and printing for femoral derotation osteotomy: case and technical report," *Annals of Translational Medicine*, vol. 5, no. 20, p. 400, 2017.

[35] S. Jagernauth, A. J. Tindall, S. Kohli, and P. Allen, "New technique: a novel femoral derotation osteotomy for malrotation following intramedullary nailing," *Case Reports in Orthopedics*, vol. 2012, Article ID 837325, 2012.

[36] T. Mückley, C. Lerch, O. Gonschorek, I. Marintschev, V. Bühren, and G. O. Hofmann, "Compression nailing for posttraumatic rotational femoral deformities: open versus minimally invasive technique," *International Orthopaedics*, vol. 29, no. 3, pp. 168–173, 2005.

[37] I. Mehling, P. Hoehle, W. Sternstein, J. Blum, and P. M. Rommens, "Nailing versus plating for comminuted fractures of the distal femur: a comparative biomechanical in vitro study of three implants," *European Journal of Trauma and Emergency Surgery*, vol. 39, no. 2, pp. 139–146, 2013.

[38] R. E. Koso, C. Terhoeve, R. G. Steen, and R. Zura, "Healing, nonunion, and re-operation after internal fixation of diaphyseal and distal femoral fractures: a systematic review and meta-analysis," *International Orthopaedics*, vol. 42, no. 11, pp. 2675–2683, 2018.

[39] V. Mounasamy, S. Mallu, V. Khanna, and S. Sambandam, "Subtrochanteric fractures after retrograde femoral nailing," *World Journal of Orthopedics*, vol. 6, no. 9, pp. 738–743, 2015.

[40] M. Hamaker, N. N. O'Hara, W. A. Eglseder, M. F. Sciadini, J. W. Nascone, and R. V. O'Toole, "Radiographic predictors of symptomatic screw removal after retrograde femoral nail insertion," *Injury*, vol. 48, no. 3, pp. 758–762, 2017.

[41] J. R. Lynch, L. A. Taitsman, D. P. Barei, and S. E. Nork, "Femoral nonunion: risk factors and treatment options," *The Journal of the American Academy of Orthopaedic Surgeons*, vol. 16, no. 2, pp. 88–97, 2008.

[42] F. Liska, C. von Deimling, A. Otto et al., "Distal femoral torsional osteotomy increases the contact pressure of the medial patellofemoral joint in biomechanical analysis," *Knee Surgery, Sports Traumatology, Arthroscopy*, vol. 27, no. 7, pp. 2328–2333, 2019.

8

Median Nerve Entrapment after Supracondylar Humeral Fracture in a Young Child

C. Granier, E. Maury, B. Coulet, M. Delpont, J. Cottalorda, C. Sleth, R. Carré, and D. Louahem

Department of Pediatric Orthopedic Surgery, Lapeyronie Hospital, University of Montpellier, 371 Avenue Doyen Gaston Giraud, 34090 Montpellier, France

Correspondence should be addressed to C. Granier; clementgranier.mail@gmail.com

Academic Editor: Stamatios A. Papadakis

Median nerve entrapment after supracondylar humeral fracture in children is rare. We report a case of Gartland type III supracondylar humeral fracture complicated by an entrapment of the median nerve following closed reduction and percutaneous pinning in a 5-year-old child. The diagnosis of entrapment was made 14 months post injury following progressive motor and sensory palsy. Resection and end-to-end suture were performed, leading to complete sensory and motor recovery eight months later. This nerve complication is often unnoticed and should be suspected systematically before and after reduction of all displaced supracondylar humeral fracture in children. The indication of resection-suture or nerve graft depends on the entrapment and the delay of the palsy.

1. Introduction

Gartland type III supracondylar humeral fractures (SCHF) in children are known for their severe neurovascular complications. Extension-type fractures with posterolateral displacement are the most frequent and responsible for nerve or neurovascular injuries with a frequency of 9% to 17% [1–10]. The injury of the median nerve and particularly the anterior interosseous nerve (AIN) are the most frequently involved [1, 8, 10–13]. Its entrapment within the fracture site is rare and often left unnoticed especially in younger children. The diagnosis is delayed by 3 months to 2.5 years after the trauma and is characterized by progressive sensory-motor palsy [14]. Electromyogram (EMG), ultrasound, and MRI imaging are powerful tools to help in the confirmation of the nerve injury and its entrapment within the fracture site or the callus. The treatment is based on surgical exploration and neurolysis or end-to-end anastomosis or nerve graft. We report a case of a progressive sensory-motor palsy by entrapment of the median nerve within the fracture callus after type III SCHF in a 5-year-old child. The diagnosis and treatment of similar cases are discussed in light of the fairly scarce literature.

2. Case Report

The patient is a 5-year-old right-handed child, admitted to the pediatric emergency room for trauma of the left elbow after falling from a 1.5 meter height. Initial clinical examination found a deformity of the elbow with swelling, ecchymosis in the anterolateral side, and absence of the radial pulse but with a well perfused hand. Neurological examination was very difficult because of the child's young age and the painful trauma. Radiographic examination of the elbow revealed a Gartland type III SCHF with posterolateral displacement (Figure 1). Closed reduction of the fracture and its fixation by percutaneous lateral pinning were urgently performed (Figure 2). Postoperative X-ray control showed an imperfect reduction with moderate posterior translation but with no inter-fragment gap that could have suspected an entrapment of the median nerve. The return of the normal

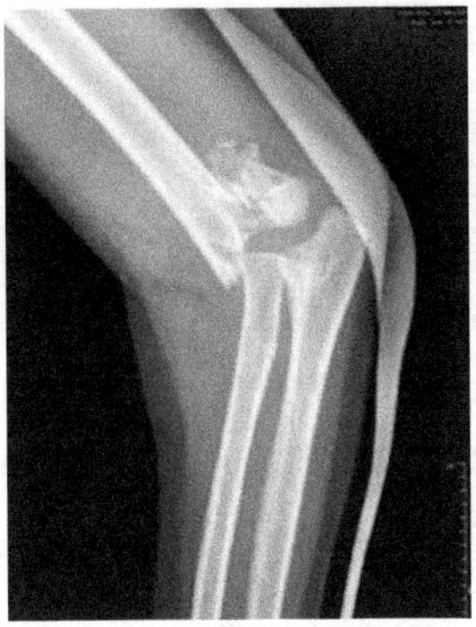

Figure 1: Gartland type III SCHF.

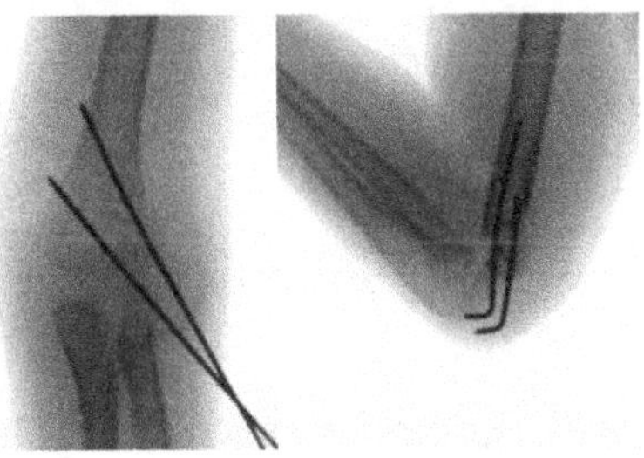

Figure 2: Lateral percutaneous pinning: front and side view.

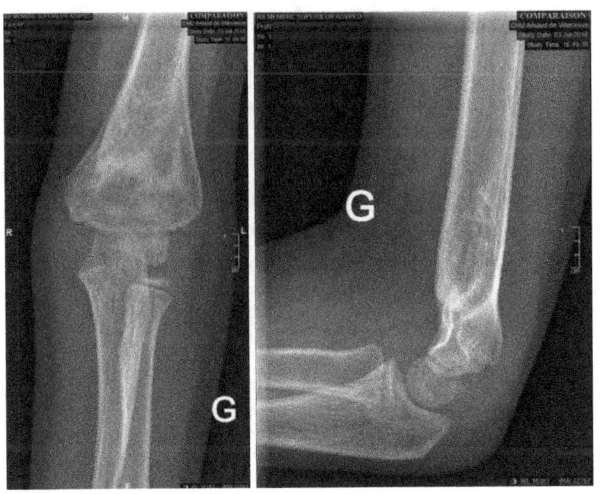

Figure 3: Complete remodeling of the distal end of the humerus: 6 months postoperatively—front and side view.

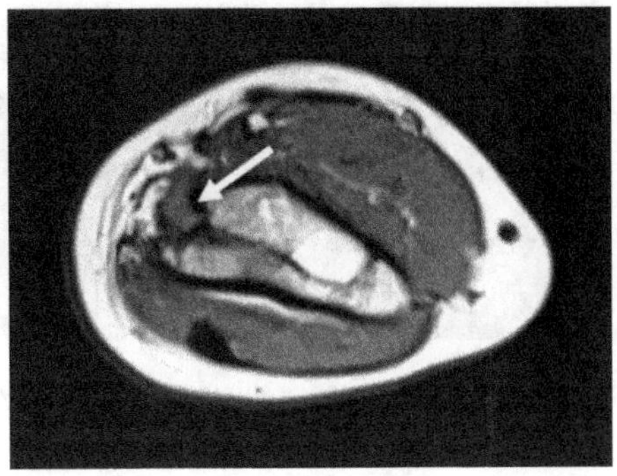

Figure 4: T1 MRI sequence showing median nerve entrapment upstream of the bone callus (white arrow).

radial pulse occurred two hours postoperatively. The healing fracture occurred one month later, followed by removal of the pins. Total remodeling of the distal humeral end was radiologically noticed six months later (Figure 3).

One year and two months later, the parents noted that their child had a functional discomfort when using the left hand and an amyotrophy of the thenar eminence and the forearm. Clinical examination found sensory-motor deficit in the median nerve with hypoesthesia and palsy of both the thumb opposition and AIN. Electroneuromyography confirmed severe truncal injury of the median nerve with an advanced denervation pattern of the abductor pollicis brevis muscle; the topography was in favor of a lesion nerve at the healed fracture site. Ultrasonography of the elbow revealed an entrapment of the nerve within the fracture callus. The median nerve was thickened (0.56 cm of diameter) entering the bone callus; invisible downstream along a 1.5 cm, it reappeared at the level of the elbow joint space with a normal diameter (0.18 cm). MRI confirmed the entrapment of the median nerve within the callus (Figures 4 and 5) with signs of nervous suffering as hypertrophy (0.5 cm of diameter against 0.2 cm at the same location on the contralateral side), hypersignal on DP fat sat sequences, and amyotrophy of the flexor, pronator quadratus, and pronator teres muscles.

Surgical exploration and dissection under a microscope following an anterior Henry approach revealed the presence of substantial fibrosis in the anteromedial side of the elbow facing the fracture callus. After careful dissecting and excision of the fibrosis, the proximal end of the median nerve was greatly thickened and entrapped within the bone callus. Its atrophic distal end was sheathed within a fibrosis facing the callus along a 1.5 cm section (Figure 6). The resected proximal end at the level of the callus and the regulation of the distal end by excision of all atrophic segment allowed for direct end-to-end suture, added to biological glue; the elbow was flexed at 60° to protect the suture from any tension (Figures 7 and 8). Postoperative immobilization was insured by a posterior splint for three weeks. Rehabilitation was performed by a physiotherapist specializing in the upper limb until complete recovery.

Follow-up at four months postoperatively showed normal mobility of the elbow and a travelling Tinel sign 3.5 cm below the elbow, demonstrating nerve regeneration. Partial motor recovery of the AIN was observed through the return of the distal interphalangeal joint flexion and the improvement of the thumb-index pinch. Eight months postoperatively, motor and sensory recovery was complete and amyotrophy of the thenar eminence and the forearm had disappeared. At the latest follow-up of twelve months, total return function was observed and the child could use normally again his left hand without discomfort or dysesthesia.

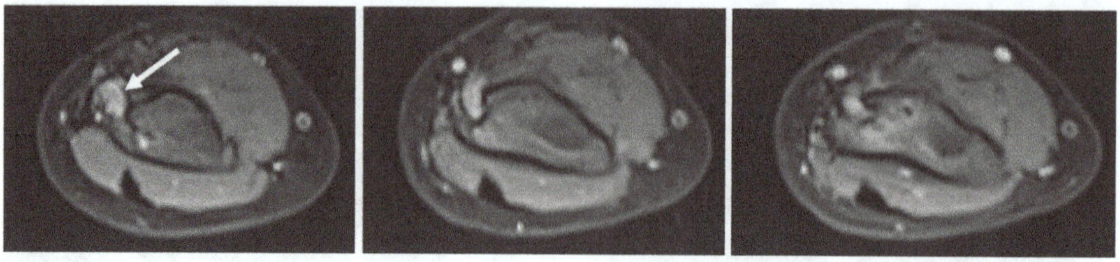

Figure 5: T2 DPFS MRI sequence showing hypertrophy (white arrow) and median nerve entrapment within the consolidated fracture.

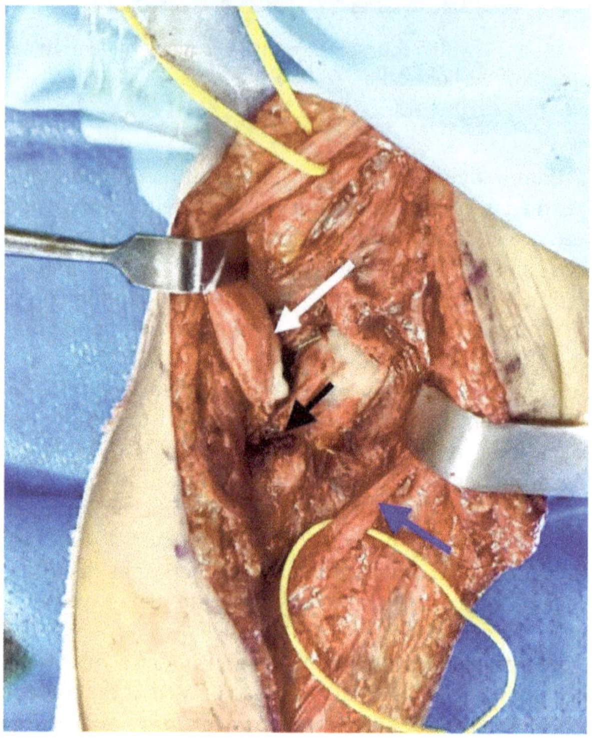

Figure 6: Entrapment of the hypertrophic proximal end of the median nerve (white arrow) within the consolidated fracture (black arrow) and fibrosis with atrophy of the distal end of the median nerve (blue arrow).

3. Discussion

Neurological complications in extension-type III SCHF in children represent 15% of cases [9], most of them involving damage of the median nerve and the AIN [1, 7, 10, 11]. Posterolateral displacement is generally incriminated [1]. These complications are often unnoticed, and their immediate postoperative diagnosis is difficult, particularly in young children [14]. It is most often neurapraxia, and spontaneous nerve recovery is ruled [1]. Entrapment of the median nerve within the fracture callus is exceptional in children. In 1974, Post and Haskell [15] published a case of median nerve entrapment after a displaced SCHF with an absence of radial pulse and complete motor palsy of the median nerve in a 5-year-old child. Three months after closed reduction and percutaneous pinning, persistence of the complete palsy was confirmed by electromyography. Surgical exploration revealed the entrapment of the median nerve within the callus. Nerve resection-reconstruction was followed by complete recovery. In 1986, Karlsson et al. [16] reported 4 cases of SCHF with entrapment of both brachial artery and median nerve within the fracture site. Nerve extrication and neurolysis allowed for complete recovery. In 1988, Thorleifsson et al. [17] described a case of entrapment of the median nerve after closed reduction of a displaced SCHF with acute injury of the median nerve. The absence of nerve recovery after ten weeks required surgical exploration confirming the nerve entrapment within the fracture callus. Dissection and neurolysis under a microscope allowed complete recovery of the nerve function. In 2006, Louahem et al. [1] reported 3 (11%) cases of entrapment of both brachial artery and median nerve within the fracture site among 28 cases of acute median nerve injuries, whether isolated or associated with brachial artery damage, in a series of 210 type III SCHF in children. In 2016, they compiled 3 (9%) other identical cases of neurovascular entrapment among 32 cases of median nerve lesions, associated with vascular injuries in a series of 404 type III SCHF in children [2]. In all these 6 cases, the entrapment diagnosis was established during the surgical exploration imposed by an imperfect closed reduction of the fracture and preoperative ischemia (white hand). Immediate extrication and neurolysis of the median nerve allowed for complete nerve recovery after a 3-month postoperative period. In 2014, Metineren et al. [18] reported a case of entrapment of the median nerve in the bone callus after a SCHF with acute palsy of the AIN in a 7-year-old child, initially treated by surgical reduction and pinning. The absence of recovery 6 months postoperatively needed surgical exploration, hence confirming entrapment of the nerve within the healed fracture site. After resection of

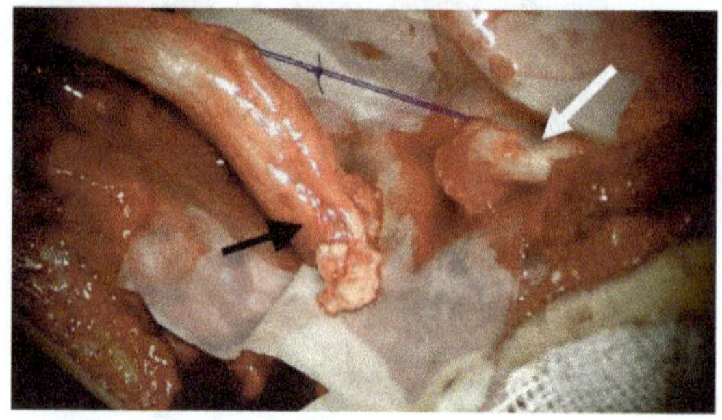

Figure 7: Post resection view flush of the bone callus of the proximal end (black arrow) and of the atrophic fibrosis part along a 1.5 cm section next to the distal end (white arrow) of the median nerve.

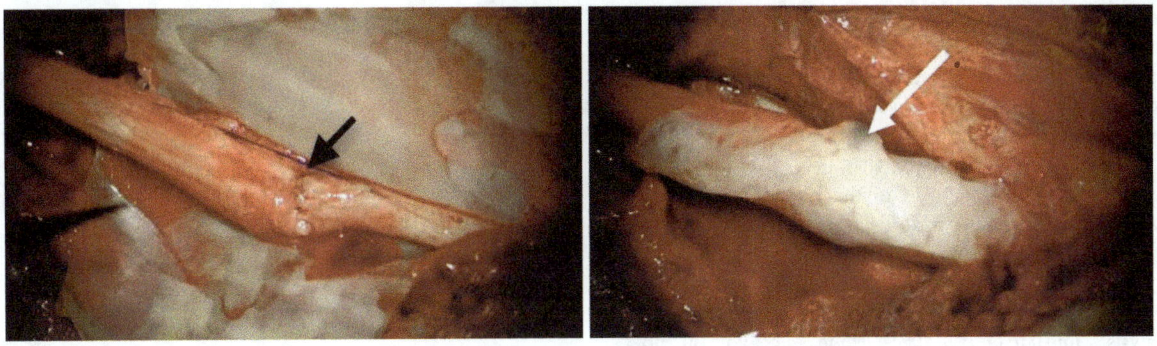

Figure 8: Terminoterminal direct type suture of the median nerve (black arrow) reinforced with biological sealant (white arrow).

the bone callus, the nerve was covered by fibrosis around the fracture site. Resection with the regulation of the nerve ends was followed by end-to-end anastomosis using Tisseel Fibrin Glue. Complete nerve and thumb opposition recovery was observed 12 months postoperatively.

The early diagnosis of the median nerve entrapment would reduce morbidity in such cases. The challenge of performing an urgent thorough examination of the neurological status, particularly in young children with type III SCHF, is responsible for the most part of diagnosis delay. Posterolateral displacement, vascular injury, imperfect reduction, and postreduction interfragment gap must encourage the search for median nerve entrapment [1, 2]. Repeated neurological examination postoperatively is crucial. The occurrence of dysesthesia, pain exacerbation, and motor or sensory deficit must require complementary investigations. Ultrasounds and especially MRI imaging reveal the course of the median nerve and signs of neuropathy and can also serve as an adjunct to electromyography in the evaluation of muscle denervation through the assessment of muscle atrophy. They allow to perform an early diagnosis of entrapment or lesion of the median nerve and thus for early, noninvasive treatment. In such cases, early extrication associated with neurolysis of the median nerve leads to complete and fast nerve recovery [1, 2, 16].

4. Conclusion

Median nerve entrapment after displaced SCHF in children remains rare but must not be underestimated, particularly in young children. Advances in noninvasive imagery, ultrasonography, and particularly MRI allow for an early and even preoperative diagnosis of entrapment within the fracture site and for rapid intervention by simple surgical exploration and neurolysis. At a later stage, resection-end-to-end suture of the nerve, when possible, may allow for complete recovery in a young child. Other surgical procedures reserved for old entrapment with extended nerve injuries such as nerve resection-graft do not always allow for a complete recovery, requiring further palliative surgery by tendinous transfer.

Supplementary Materials

The video is titled: "Preoperative video showing median nerve entrapment." Description of the video: This preoperative video shows, after dissection of the front side of elbow, the entrapment of the hypertrophic proximal end of the median nerve within the consolidated fracture and fibrosis with atrophy of the distal end of the median nerve. The flush resection of the bone callus of the proximal end and of the atrophic fibrosis part along a 1.5 cm section next to the distal end of the nerve allowed a terminoterminal type suture of the elbow flexed at 60°." *(Supplementary Materials)*

References

[1] D. M. Louahem, A. Nebunescu, F. Canavese, and A. Dimeglio, "Neurovascular complications and severe displacement in supracondylar humerus fractures in children: defensive or offensive strategy?," *Journal of Pediatric Orthopaedics B*, vol. 15, no. 1, pp. 51–57, 2006.

[2] D. Louahem and J. Cottalorda, "Acute ischemia and pink pulseless hand in 68 of 404 gartland type III supracondylar humeral fractures in children: urgent management and therapeutic consensus," *Injury*, vol. 47, no. 4, pp. 848–852, 2016.

[3] J. J. McGraw, B. A. Akbarnia, D. P. Hanel, L. Keppler, and R. E. Burdge, "Neurological complications resulting from supracondylar fractures of the humerus in children," *Journal of Pediatric Orthopaedics*, vol. 6, no. 6, pp. 647–650, 1986.

[4] K. E. Cramer, N. E. Green, and D. P. Devito, "Incidence of anterior interosseous nerve palsy in supracondylar humerus fractures in children," *Journal of Pediatric Orthopaedics*, vol. 13, no. 4, pp. 502–505, 1993.

[5] J. P. Dormans, R. Squillante, and H. Sharf, "Acute neurovascular complications with supracondylar humerus fractures in children," *The Journal of Hand Surgery*, vol. 20, no. 1, pp. 1–4, 1995.

[6] T. Gosens and K. J. Bongers, "Neurovascular complications and functional outcome in displaced supracondylar fractures of the humerus in children," *Injury*, vol. 34, no. 4, pp. 267–273, 2003.

[7] E. R. A. Joiner, D. L. Skaggs, A. Arkader et al., "Iatrogenic nerve injuries in the treatment of supracondylar humerus fractures: are we really just missing nerve injuries on preoperative examination?," *Journal of Pediatric Orthopaedics*, vol. 34, no. 4, pp. 388–392, 2014.

[8] I. H. Y. Kwok, Z. M. Silk, T. J. Quick, M. Sinisi, A. MacQuillan, and M. Fox, "Nerve injuries associated with supracondylar fractures of the humerus in children: our experience in a specialist peripheral nerve injury unit," *The Bone & Joint Journal*, vol. 98-B, no. 6, pp. 851–856, 2016.

[9] R. Tomaszewski, A. Wozowicz, and P. Wysocka-Wojakiewicz, "Analysis of early neurovascular complications of pediatric supracondylar humerus fractures: a long-term observation," *BioMed Research International*, vol. 2017, Article ID 2803790, 5 pages, 2017.

[10] E. T. Jones and D. S. Louis, "Median nerve injuries associated with supracondylar fractures of the humerus in children," *Clinical Orthopaedics and Related Research*, vol. 150, pp. 181–186, 1980.

[11] J. C. Babal, C. T. Mehlman, and G. Klein, "Nerve injuries associated with pediatric supracondylar humeral fractures: a meta-analysis," *Journal of Pediatric Orthopaedics*, vol. 30, no. 3, pp. 253–263, 2010.

[12] C. C. Campbell, P. M. Waters, J. B. Emans, J. R. Kasser, and M. B. Millis, "Neurovascular injury and displacement in type III supracondylar humerus fractures," *Journal of Pediatric Orthopaedics*, vol. 15, no. 1, pp. 47–52, 1995.

[13] B. J. Shore, B. T. Gillespie, P. E. Miller, D. S. Bae, and P. M. Waters, "Recovery of motor nerve injuries associated with displaced, extension-type pediatric supracondylar humerus fractures," *Journal of Pediatric Orthopaedics*, vol. 39, no. 9, pp. e652–e656, 2019.

[14] K. J. Noonan and W. F. Blair, "Chronic median-nerve entrapment after posterior fracture-dislocation of the elbow. A case report," *The Journal of Bone & Joint Surgery*, vol. 77, no. 10, pp. 1572–1575, 1995.

[15] M. Post and S. S. Haskell, "Reconstruction of the median nerve following entrapment in supracondylar fracture of the HUMERUS," *The Journal of Trauma: Injury, Infection, and Critical Care*, vol. 14, no. 3, pp. 252–264, 1974.

[16] J. Karlsson, T. Thorsteinsson, R. Thorleifsson, and H. Arnason, "Entrapment of the median nerve and brachial artery after supracondylar fractures of the humerus in children," *Archives of Orthopaedic and Traumatic Surgery*, vol. 104, no. 6, pp. 389–391, 1986.

[17] R. Thorleifsson, J. Karlsson, and T. Thorsteinsson, "Median nerve entrapment in bone after supracondylar fracture of the humerus," *Archives of orthopaedic and traumatic surgery*, vol. 107, no. 3, pp. 183–185, 1988.

[18] H. Metineren, "Median nerve entrapment at the fracture site following supracondylar humeral fracture: a case report," *European Journal of Medical Sciences*, vol. 1, no. 4, pp. 154–156, 2014.

9

Lesser Tuberosity Avulsion Fracture in an 11-Year-Old Baseball Player due to Batting

Ryan Cheng,[1] **Jay Moran**,[1] **Samantha Smith**,[1] **Don Li**,[1,2] **Christopher A. Schneble**,[1] **Shin Mei Chan**,[1] **and Elizabeth C. Gardner**[1]

[1]*Department of Orthopaedics and Rehabilitation, Yale University School of Medicine, New Haven, CT, USA*
[2]*Orthopedic Surgery, Hospital for Special Surgery-Weil-Cornell Medical School, New York, NY, USA*

Correspondence should be addressed to Ryan Cheng; ryan.cheng@yale.edu

Academic Editor: Georg Singer

Case. We report an 11-year-old male who sustained a lesser tuberosity avulsion fracture of the proximal humerus upon making contact with a baseball during an at-bat. This injury was neglected for 14 months and was eventually detected by an axillary radiograph and subsequent MRI. He successfully underwent an open surgical repair and regained full range of motion and level of activity at 1-year follow-up. *Conclusion.* In pediatric baseball players, lesser tuberosity avulsion fractures may occur upon striking a baseball with a bat. Even after being neglected for several months, these injuries can be treated successfully with an open surgical repair.

1. Introduction

Lesser tuberosity avulsion fractures in children and adolescents are relatively rare, with only a few cases reported in the literature [1–3]. Though most of these injuries tend to occur in 12 to 14-year-olds, incidents have been reported in patients as young as 8 years of age, with a predilection towards males [4–10]. These sports-related injuries have been reported in hockey, lacrosse, baseball, football, wrestling, and soccer and commonly occur from a contact mechanism of injury [10–12]. In Little League baseball, lesser tuberosity avulsion fractures have been reported in pitchers and are associated with poor pitching mechanics which place repetitive stress on the shoulder [10, 13].

In the pediatric population, lesser tuberosity avulsion fractures are often missed and can have unspecific findings on both physical examination and radiographic imaging [1–3, 8, 10, 14–16]. Despite these injuries being readily identified on magnetic resonance imaging (MRI), the varying clinical presentations associated with this injury can make it difficult to determine whether MRI or further workup is required [1, 2]. As a result, these injuries are commonly misdiagnosed as strains and are discovered weeks to months after the initial incident [2, 8, 17–20]. Understanding the various mechanisms of injury allows for a better understanding of patient presentations, prevents prolonged shoulder impairment, and enables a quicker return to activity.

This particular report describes the case of an 11-year-old patient who sustained a lesser tuberosity avulsion fracture from hitting a baseball during a Little League Baseball game.

2. Case Report

An 11-year-old male presented to the emergency department after injuring his shoulder in a baseball game. The patient expressed that he felt a "pop" in his right shoulder while swinging a baseball bat in a Little League game. He denied both a direct blow and any other trauma. On physical exam, he had full, pain-free passive range of motion of the right shoulder but experienced pain with active range of motion, particularly with internal rotation against resistance. Scapular Y and standard anteroposterior shoulder

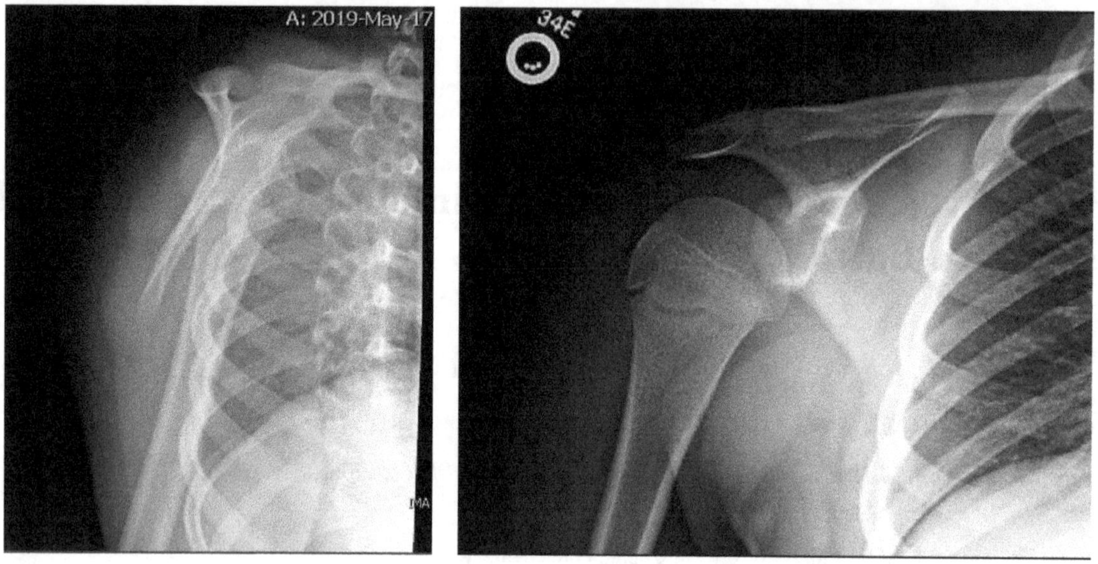

(a) (b)

Figure 1: (a) Scapular X-ray taken during patient's first visit to emergency department. (b) Anteroposterior X-ray taken during patient's first visit to emergency department.

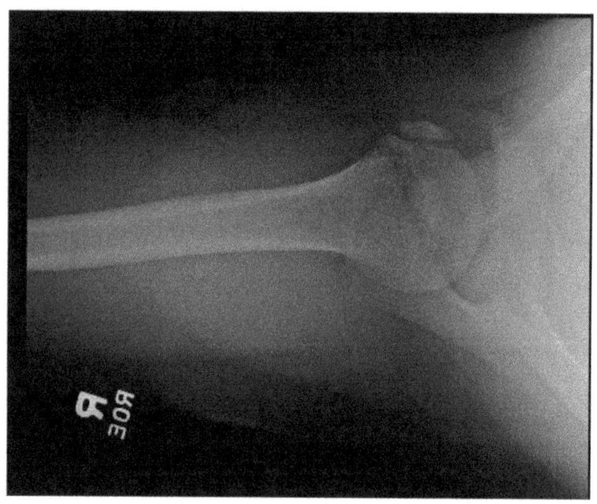

Figure 2: Axillary X-ray reveals age indeterminate fracture from the humeral head at the time of outpatient follow-up one year after injury.

radiographs were obtained and read as negative (Figures 1(a) and 1(b)). He was later discharged with a muscle strain.

Over the course of the following year, the patient had continued shoulder pain and tightness and was thus unable to throw the ball effectively. As a result, he switched positions from the 3rd base to the 1st base to limit the amount of stress placed on his injured shoulder. Despite this transition, he repeatedly experienced episodes of his right shoulder "popping," which were accompanied by pain.

Upon presenting to our institution 14 months postinjury, the patient was otherwise healthy and axillary X-rays demonstrated an age indeterminate fracture of the humeral head (Figure 2). Subsequent MRI showed heterogeneous signal and thickening of subscapularis fibers at the lesser tuberosity attachment as well as osseous fragmentation (Figure 3). These findings were suggestive of a prior avulsion fracture of the lesser tuberosity with interstitial tearing of the inferior subscapularis fibers. Surgery was recommended, and the patient and his family agreed to proceed accordingly. Repair of the subscapularis tendon was performed through the deltopectoral approach (Figures 4(a) and 4(b)). Four Mason-Allen sutures were used to anchor and stabilize the subscapularis tendon with excellent compression. The fracture fragment was tied down to the lateral aspect of the lesser tuberosity and attached to the periosteum with nonabsorbable Ethibond sutures. After the operation, the patient did not stay in the hospital. He was immobilized in a sling for 6 weeks and then rehabbed using a subscapularis tendon repair protocol. The patient had full range of motion at the 3-month follow-up appointment. At the 1-year follow-up, he was asymptomatic, had full range of motion, noted no feelings of locking, and was able to return to throwing and all baseball activities.

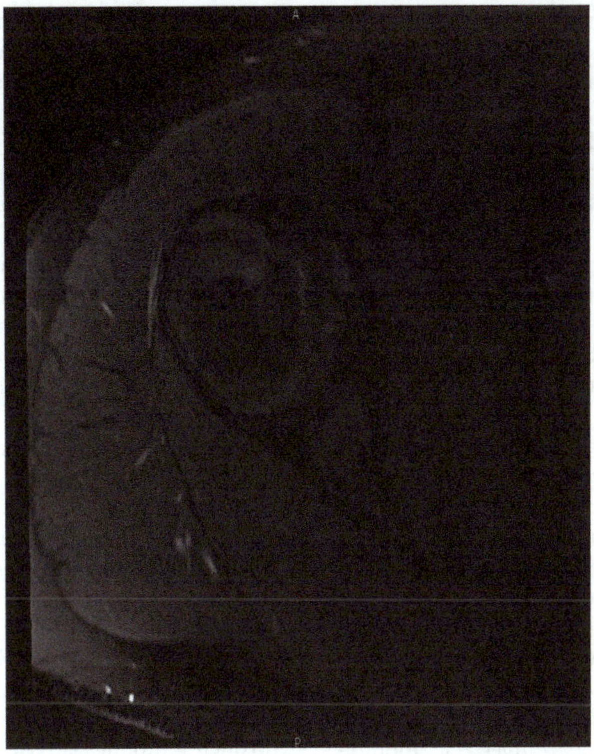

FIGURE 3: Axial proton density fat saturation image demonstrating the nonunited lesser tuberosity fragment without surrounding edema.

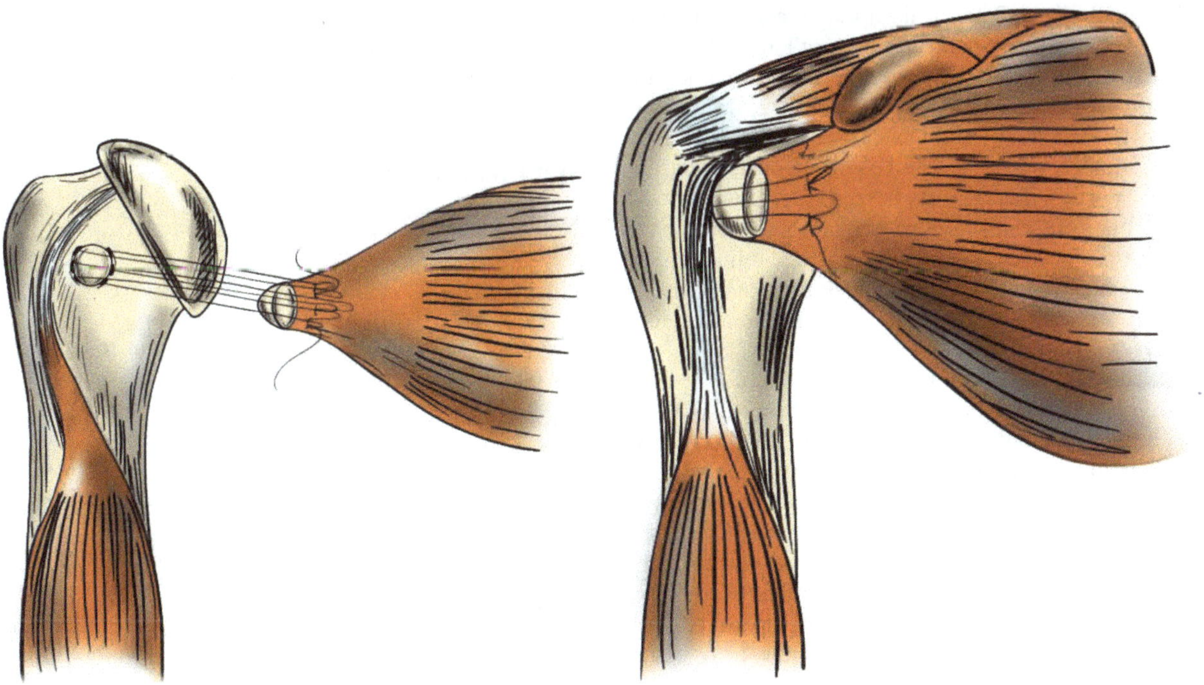

(a) (b)

FIGURE 4: (a) Anteroposterior view of suture placement for avulsion fracture repair; (b) finished repair.

3. Discussion

Lesser tuberosity avulsion fractures of the proximal humerus are rare injuries in children and adolescents [1–3]. These misdiagnosed injuries typically present as unspecific acute or chronic anterior shoulder pain, making them difficult to recognize on physical exam [3]. The mechanisms that lead to lesser tuberosity avulsion fractures can act a secondary sign for injury recognition and are important for clinical awareness. In this report, we describe a neglected lesser tuberosity fracture that occurred from a bat swinging mechanism in a Little League Baseball pediatric patient. To our knowledge, this mechanism of injury has not been reported in the literature.

Lesser tuberosity avulsion injuries have been previously identified in Little League pitchers [10]. Risk factors include poor pitching mechanics, increased number of curveballs thrown, and increased pitch counts as these variables may intensify the stress that throwing places on the shoulder and leave the lesser tuberosity at greater risk of avulsion [10, 21]. However, the presented case highlights an injury from a batting mechanism in a Little League baseball patient. We hypothesize that the mechanism of this injury may have resulted from external rotation of the humerus in an abducted position and eccentric contraction of the subscapularis upon striking a baseball with a bat. Similar to those who sustain avulsion injuries during contact sports, patients who are injured while batting could present with a sudden, rather than gradual, onset of pain [10]. We recommend further diagnostic workup if a pediatric patient describes a similar course of injury. In addition to Little League pitching, our reported bat swinging mechanism may be the first in developing more focused injury prevention efforts.

Lesser tuberosity avulsion fractures typically go, on average, 2 months (interquartile ranges: 1 month–7 months) before being diagnosed [22]. In our patient, the avulsion of the lesser tuberosity was diagnosed 14 months after the initial injury. Prompt diagnosis of lesser tuberosity avulsion fractures is advantageous, as very few patients are able to regain full range of motion and strength with nonoperative treatment alone [1, 2, 11, 13, 22, 23]. Moreover, timely diagnosis, through the use of MRI, may decrease shoulder impairment and enable continued participation in sports. While reports have showed that delayed treatment may not confer long term sequalae, some have suggested that delayed diagnoses of these injuries may predispose athletes to concomitant injuries, as there is diminished subscapularis strength and anterior shoulder instability [9, 11, 22, 24].

The detection of these injuries without the use of MRI has proven to be quite difficult because the majority of these injuries are not obvious on scapular Y and anteroposterior view radiographs. However, axillary radiographs have been shown to successfully identify many of these injuries [1, 2, 22, 25, 26]. Early MRI has been shown to have a higher sensitivity (0.95) compared to anteroposterior and axillary radiographs (0.16) in detecting lesser tuberosity avulsion fractures [1, 2, 22, 25, 26]. In our patient, axillary X-rays 14 months after the injury demonstrated the avulsion of the lesser tuberosity (Figure 2), whereas anteroposterior and scapular Y radiographs taken at patient's first emergency department visit failed to reveal the fracture (Figures 1(a) and 1(b)). His subsequent shoulder MRI, taken less than a week after the axillary X-rays identified the injury, ultimately revealed heterogeneous signal in the interior fibers of the subscapularis attachment on the lesser tuberosity with osseous fragmentation (Figure 3). If a lesser tuberosity avulsion fracture is suspected, an MRI should be considered for further workup, as demonstrated in our case.

Many pediatric patients who have elected to proceed with nonoperative care have reported the development of chronic shoulder pain, exostoses at the avulsion site, as well as inhibited internal rotation stemming from subscapularis muscle degeneration [1, 2]. Therefore, surgical intervention should be considered an effective method of treating lesser tuberosity avulsion fractures, including those that are only slightly displaced, as these fragments still pose a risk of anteromedial impingement, malunion, nonunion, and may limit shoulder strength and mobility [8]. Nevertheless, nonoperative treatment can be trialed for injuries with minimally displaced fragments or fragments that still retain adequate internal rotation [10]. When determining the appropriate course of treatment and the degree of compromise to subscapularis function, patient's athletic demands should also be taken into account. If persistent pain continues after 12 to 18 months of nonoperative care, this may serve as an additional sign to consider operative treatment [10]. In our case, surgical treatment with an open repair showed excellent results and return to full athletic function when conservative treatment failed.

In conclusion, lesser tuberosity avulsion fractures are difficult to diagnose due to the unspecific physical exam and imaging findings. The reported injury in this case occurred through a unique bat swinging mechanism in Little League baseball. The lesser tuberosity avulsion injury was eventually noticed on both MRI and axillary X-rays as opposed to anteroposterior and scapular X-rays [1, 2, 22, 25, 26]. Physicians should use this report to recognize this unique mechanism of injury and patient presentation to prevent delayed diagnoses in the future.

Data Availability

No data were used to support this study.

Consent

The patient's parent gave informed consent to use this case for publication.

References

[1] L. E. La Mont, D. W. Green, D. W. Altchek, R. F. Warren, and T. L. Wickiewicz, "Subscapularis tears and lesser tuberosity avulsion fractures in the pediatric patient," *Sports Health*, vol. 7, no. 2, pp. 110–114, 2015.

[2] K. Aagaard and K. Lunsjö, "Occult fracture of the lesser tuberosity in a 9-year-old female swimmer," *Journal of Surgical Case Reports*, vol. 2017, no. 1, 2017.

[3] M. A. Bendoya, C. A. Barrera, J. T. Bencardino, and V. Ho-Fung, "Humeral lesser tuberosity avulsion fractures – magnetic resonance imaging characteristics in the pediatric population," *Pediatric Radiology*, vol. 51, no. 8, pp. 1421–1430, 2021.

[4] J. D. Polousky and S. Harms, "Subscapularis tendon injuries in adolescents: a report of 2 cases," *Journal of Pediatric Orthopedics*, vol. 31, no. 5, pp. e57–e59, 2011.

[5] A. J. Provance and J. D. Polousky, "Isolated avulsion fracture

of the subscapularis tendon with medial dislocation and tear of biceps tendon in a skeletally immature athlete: a case report," *Current Opinion in Pediatrics*, vol. 22, no. 3, pp. 366–368, 2010.

[6] A. Bhalla, K. Higashigawa, and D. McAllister, "Subscapularis tendon rupture in an 8-year-old boy: a case report," *American Journal of Orthopedics*, vol. 40, no. 9, pp. 471–474, 2011.

[7] S. O. Paschal, K. S. Hutton, and P. T. Weatherall, "Isolated avulsion fracture of the lesser tuberosity of the humerus in adolescents. A report of two cases," *The Journal of Bone and Joint Surgery. American Volume*, vol. 77, no. 9, pp. 1427–1430, 1995.

[8] B. Levine, D. Pereira, and J. Rosen, "Avulsion fractures of the lesser tuberosity of the humerus in adolescents: review of the literature and case report," *Journal of Orthopaedic Trauma*, vol. 19, no. 5, pp. 349–352, 2005.

[9] R. Sikka, M. Neault, and C. Gaunche, "An avulsion of the subscapularis in a skeletally immature patient," *American Journal of Sports Medicine*, vol. 32, no. 1, pp. 246–249, 2004.

[10] M. Sugalski, J. Hyman, and C. Ahmad, "Avulsion fracture of the lesser tuberosity in an adolescent baseball pitcher: a case report," *American Journal of Sports Medicine*, vol. 32, no. 3, pp. 793–796, 2004.

[11] K. Ogawa and M. Takahashi, "Long-term outcome of isolated lesser tuberosity fractures of the humerus," *The Journal of Trauma*, vol. 42, no. 5, pp. 955–959, 1997.

[12] R. P. Teixeira, A. R. Johnson, B. T. Higgins, J. A. Carrino, and E. G. McFarland, "Fly fishing-related lesser tuberosity avulsion in an adolescent," *Orthopedics*, vol. 35, no. 5, pp. e748–e751, 2012.

[13] S. S. Kunkel and E. A. Monesmith, "Isolated avulsion fracture of the lesser tuberosity of the humerus: a case report," *Journal of Shoulder and Elbow Surgery*, vol. 2, no. 1, pp. 43–46, 1993.

[14] S. G. Park, B. J. Shim, and H. G. Seok, "Isolated avulsion fracture of the lesser tuberosity of the humerus in an adolescent amateur boxer," *JSES Int.*, vol. 4, no. 4, pp. 759–764, 2020.

[15] M. C. Koper and T. S. Jakma, "Case report of a proximal humeral fracture with an avulsion fracture of the lesser tuberosity in an adolescent girl," *Journal of Shoulder and Elbow Surgery*, vol. 24, no. 9, pp. e260–e263, 2015.

[16] B. E. Heyworth, C. C. Dodson, and D. W. Altchek, "Arthroscopic repair of isolated subscapularis avulsion injuries in adolescent athletes," *Clinical Journal of Sport Medicine*, vol. 18, no. 5, pp. 461–463, 2008.

[17] M. Caniggia, P. Maniscalco, and A. Picinotti, "Isolated avulsion fracture of the lesser tuberosity of the humerus. Report of two cases," *Panminerva Medica*, vol. 38, no. 1, pp. 56–60, 1996.

[18] J. C. Le Huec, T. Schaeverbeke, M. Moinard, M. Kind, D. Chauveaux, and A. Le Rebeller, "Isolated avulsion fracture of the lesser tubercle of the humerus in children," *Acta Orthopaedica Belgica*, vol. 60, no. 4, pp. 427–429, 1994.

[19] P. S. Vezeridis, D. S. Bae, M. S. Kocher, D. E. Kramer, Y. M. Yen, and P. M. Waters, "Surgical treatment for avulsion injuries of the humeral lesser tuberosity apophysis in adolescents," *The Journal of Bone and Joint Surgery. American Volume*, vol. 93, no. 20, pp. 1882–1888, 2011.

[20] N. N. Shah, A. Agarwal, R. Turner, and C. Hatrick, "Avulsion of the lesser tuberosity with a Salter-Harris type II injury of the proximal humerus: a case report," *Journal of Shoulder and Elbow Surgery*, vol. 15, no. 5, pp. e16–e18, 2006.

[21] S. Lyman, G. S. Fleisig, J. R. Andrews, and E. D. Osinski, "Effect of pitch type, pitch count, and pitching mechanics on risk of elbow and shoulder pain in youth baseball pitchers," *The American Journal of Sports Medicine*, vol. 30, no. 4, pp. 463–468, 2002.

[22] P. Vavken, D. S. Bae, P. M. Waters, B. Flutie, and D. E. Kramer, "Treating subscapularis and lesser tuberosity avulsion injuries in skeletally immature patients: a systematic review," *Arthroscopy*, vol. 32, no. 5, pp. 919–928, 2016.

[23] S. Goeminne and P. Debeer, "The natural evolution of neglected lesser tuberosity fractures in skeletally immature patients," *Journal of Shoulder and Elbow Surgery*, vol. 21, no. 8, pp. e6–e11, 2012.

[24] D. S. Neogi, N. Bejjanki, and P. M. Ahrens, "The consequences of delayed presentation of lesser tuberosity avulsion fractures in adolescents after repetitive injury," *Journal of Shoulder and Elbow Surgery*, vol. 22, no. 4, pp. e1–e5, 2013.

[25] B. Tosun and C. C. Kesemenli, "Isolated avulsion fracture of lesser tuberosity of the humerus: review of the literature and report of two cases," *International journal of shoulder surgery*, vol. 5, no. 2, pp. 50–53, 2011.

[26] G. J. Ross and M. B. Love, "Isolated avulsion fracture of the lesser tuberosity of the humerus: report of two cases," *Radiology*, vol. 172, no. 3, pp. 833-834, 1989.

10

Intrapelvic Femoral Head Dislocation without Associated Proximal Femur Fracture: A Case Report and Description of Closed Reduction Technique

S. Craig Morris,[1,2] Priyantha L. Wickramanayake,[2] Peter J. Wilton,[1,2] and Jonathan L. Allen[2]

[1]*Department of Orthopedic Surgery, Loma Linda University, Loma Linda, CA, USA*
[2]*Department of Orthopedic Surgery, Arrowhead Regional Medical Center, Colton, CA, USA*

Correspondence should be addressed to S. Craig Morris; stmorris@llu.edu

Academic Editor: Johannes Mayr

Traumatic hip dislocations are potentially devastating injuries, especially in young patients, and require emergent orthopedic treatment. Given the significant amount of energy required to cause these injuries, a high index of suspicion is necessary to identify related injuries. The associated injuries, direction of dislocation, and time between injury and reduction represent the known prognostic factors, based on limited available research. Intrapelvic hip dislocations represent an uncommon variant of the traumatic hip dislocation, with all previously reported cases involving ipsilateral proximal femur fractures. We present a case of intrapelvic femoral head dislocation without an associated proximal femur fracture, as well as the maneuvers used to treat the patient via a closed reduction.

1. Introduction

Traumatic hip dislocations are a serious orthopedic injury with increasing incidence, typically related to high energy trauma, most commonly motor vehicle accidents [1]. Due to the risk of osteonecrosis of the femoral head, many authors recommend that these injuries should be reduced emergently, especially in younger patients [1]. Other potential complications include sciatic nerve injuries and the development of posttraumatic osteoarthritis [2]. Hip dislocations are classified as simple if there is no associated fracture of the proximal femur or acetabulum, or complex if there is associated fractures. These injuries are also defined based on the direction of dislocation of the femoral head relative to the acetabulum, posterior, or anterior. Early reports also described a central dislocation, but these are thought to be more accurately defined as acetabulum fractures as opposed to traumatic hip dislocations. More detailed classification schemes for dislocations and fracture dislocations have been described previously by Thompson and Epstein [3], Stewart and Milford [4], and Brav [5]. Anterior dislocations are less common and are typically subdivided based on the position of the femoral head on an AP pelvic radiograph: obturator, pubic, and iliac [1–3]. Another subtype of anterior dislocation less frequently used is the perineal type, which describes a dislocation where the femoral head is more inferior than in the standard obturator dislocation [6]. A common complication of anterior hip dislocations is impaction of the femoral head on the anteroinferior rim of the acetabulum as it exits the acetabulum [2, 7]. Unique anterior hip dislocations through or into the scrotum have been reported in the literature [8, 9]. The anterior obturator class of dislocations has been reported in the literature to have a variety of presentations, including with associated femoral neck fractures [10, 11], with associated femoral head fracture [12], and with intrapelvic dislocation of the proximal femur through the obturator foramen [13–15]. Intrapelvic dislocations, while rare, have been reported previously, though always with associated proximal femur fracture [13–17], or fracture of both the proximal femur and the acetabulum or the pelvic ring

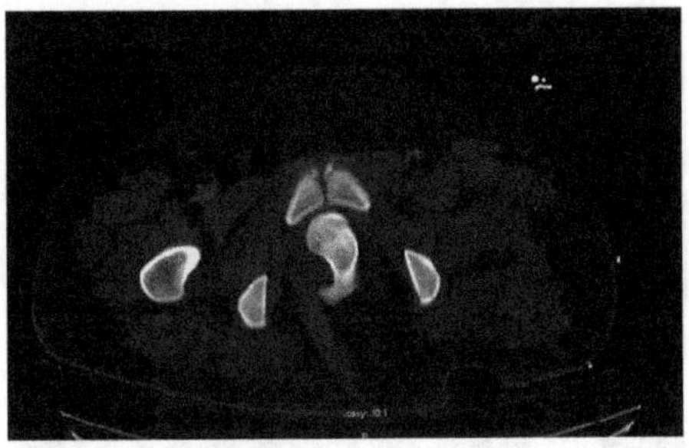

FIGURE 1: Axial slice of CT abdomen and pelvis with contrast demonstrating intrapelvic dislocation with the left femoral head just posterior to pubic symphysis.

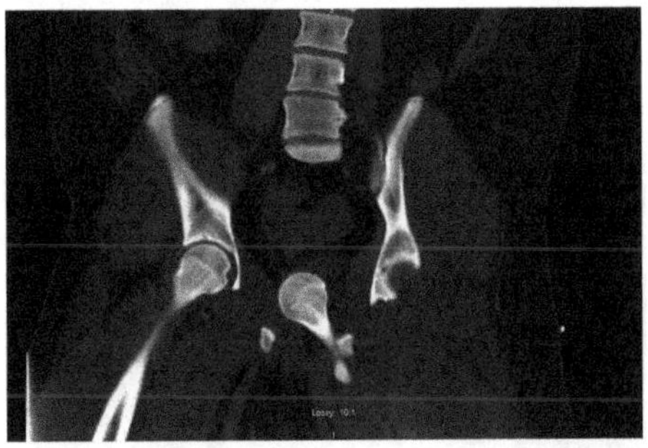

FIGURE 2: Coronal slice of CT abdomen and pelvis with contrast demonstrating medial displacement of femoral head into the true pelvis with empty acetabulum on the left.

[18–20]. There have been no reported cases in the literature of intrapelvic hip dislocation without associated proximal femur fracture. After discussion, the patient signed informed consent regarding the use of his medical information in this case report.

2. Case Presentation

An 18-year-old morbidly obese male with no reported past medical history presented to the emergency room after a high-speed motor vehicle collision (MVA). He had been positioned in the middle of the backseat and was ejected from the vehicle. The injury was reported to have occurred 1 hour prior to presentation at the hospital. Field responders had placed the patient on a backboard and placed a cervical collar. He was resuscitated with intravenous fluids during transport. No manipulation of the extremities was completed prior to arrival. Upon arrival to the emergency room, he was intubated and sedated for airway protection due to low Glasgow Coma Scale. He had sustained facial lacerations and closed head trauma. CT of the abdomen and pelvis was obtained showing a dislocated left hip, with the femoral head displaced into the intrapelvic space compressing the urethra (Figures 1 and 2). There was a small bony fragment noted, representing a minor acetabulum fracture, but no evidence of proximal femur fracture. He presented in critical condition due to subdural hemorrhage and was taken emergently to the operating room for a craniotomy performed by the neurosurgical team. Due to the acuity of his head injury, no other imaging of the orthopedic injuries was obtained prior to transfer to the operating room. He was already in the operating suite after completion of the craniotomy when the orthopedic team was able to evaluate the patient. Physical exam demonstrated gross deformity of bilateral lower extremities as both legs were externally rotated and shortened. On the right thigh, there was crepitus at the distal femur suggesting a distal femur fracture. Fluoroscopic imaging was obtained intraoperatively, confirming a right distal femur fracture and left hip dislocation. After receiving clearance from the trauma surgery and neurosurgery teams for further intervention on the patient at that time, the decision was made for emergent closed reduction of the left hip under general anesthesia given the intrapelvic dislocation of the femoral head in this young patient. Given the significant displacement of the femoral head, it was discussed that open reduction may be necessary, likely via a medial approach to the hip. Given the critical condition of the patient, closed reduction was preferred, if possible. The orthopedic surgery team began the closed reduction procedure approximately 3 hours and 30 minutes after presentation to the hospital and therefore approximately 4 hours and 30 minutes after injury.

Fluoroscopy was used to aid in the closed reduction. The primary surgeon began by applying gentle traction in line with the position of the left lower extremity. Due to his massive body habitus, more forceful traction was required, and a sheet was placed across his body at the level of iliac crests with an assistant pulling countertraction. Initial attempts at closed reduction using typical reduction techniques were ineffective given the position of the dislocated femoral head within the pelvis. After several minutes of traction, fluoroscopy revealed that the femoral head was still significantly displaced medially into the patient's intrapelvic region. At this time, additional countertraction, via another sheet, was placed around the left thigh and a laterally applied force was administered by another surgeon while the primary surgeon continued to apply longitudinal traction. Based off of the presumed injury pattern of hyperabduction in a frog leg position from being thrown forward into the front seats, hyperabduction and flexion combined with longitudinal traction were utilized to slowly mobilize the dislocation outside of the pelvis. Internal rotation was also used to manipulate the femoral head inferior to the ischium followed by external rotation to move the head out of the true pelvis. After significant time and effort, fluoroscopic images demonstrated that the hip was out of the pelvis and had effectively been converted to a more commonly encountered posterior dislocation. At this point, hyperabduction was no longer necessary. Instead, longitudinal traction, hip flexion, and external rotation were utilized until an audible clunk was appreciated, and a fluoroscopic image confirmed reduction of the left femoral head (Figure 3). Provisional treatment of the right distal femur fracture was then administered via skeletal traction to the right lower extremity through a tibial pin. The total operating time for the closed reduction as well as traction pin in the contralateral femur was approximately 1 hour and 15 minutes.

At this point, surgeons from other specialties took over care in the ongoing management of this polytraumatized patient and the urological surgery team was consulted to evaluate and manage any potential urethral injury from the dislocation. Placement of Foley in the trauma bay had been

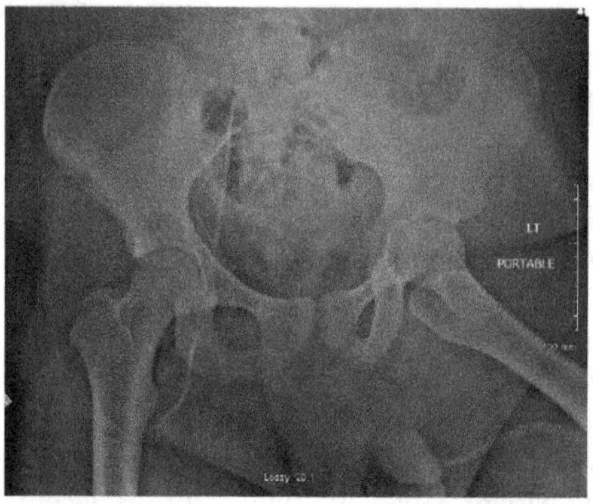

Figure 3: Intraoperative fluoroscopic AP pelvis demonstrating concentric reduction of the left femoral head.

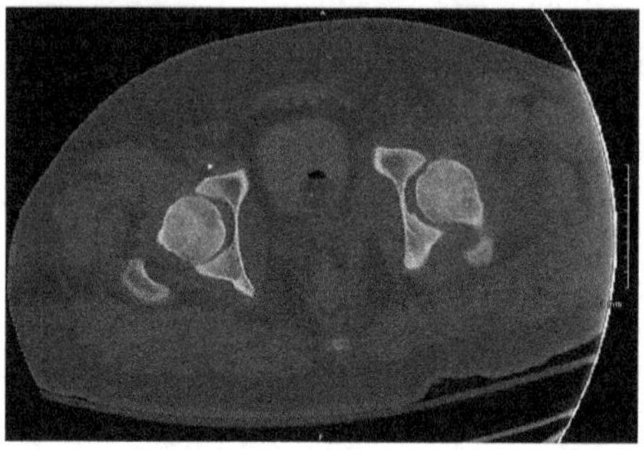

Figure 4: Postreduction axial slice of CT pelvis without contrast demonstrating concentric reduction of the left femoral head.

unsuccessful. After reduction of the hip, the urology team was able to place a Foley catheter without difficulty with return of normal-appearing urine without any evidence of hematuria. Given the ease of placement and benign appearance of the urine, no further imaging of the urinary tract was recommended by the urology service. The Foley catheter was removed later during hospitalization without complication.

The patient was admitted to the surgical intensive care unit after leaving the operating room. Postoperative radiographs and CT scan showed reduction of the left hip (Figures 4–5). An 8 mm bony fragment from the acetabulum was again noted, which was presumed to represent an avulsion fracture from the ligamentum teres, but the scan demonstrated concentric reduction of the femoral head and no evidence of femoral fracture. Three days after presentation, the patient was weaned from sedating medications and extubated. His right lower extremity remained in skeletal traction until definitive treatment could be completed in the form of retrograde intramedullary nailing of the femur on hospital day 4, which was completed without complication. His mental status continued to improve, and he began to work with physical and occupational therapists during his admission. He was made weight bearing as tolerated on the right lower extremity but kept nonweight bearing on the left lower extremity. The patient was discharged to an acute inpatient rehab facility on hospital day 21.

At a follow-up visit to the orthopedic surgery clinic 9 weeks after injury, the patient reported occasional pain to the left hip and lower back after extended sitting in the wheelchair. He had continued in physical therapy as an outpatient and had been ambulating with a walker. His mental status had improved as he was now not only alert and oriented but also conversant throughout the exam. Physical exam demonstrated left hip range of motion of 0-60 degrees flexion (0-90 degrees flexion contralateral side) and 4/5 strength with hip flexion (4/5 strength hip flexion contralateral side). Distally, he was able to actively dorsiflex and plantarflex the ankle as well as flex and extend the great toe with 5/5 motor strength throughout bilateral lower extremities. Sensation was intact to light touch in superficial peroneal, deep peroneal, sural, saphenous, and plantar nerve distributions. He had 2+ dorsalis pedis and posterior tibial artery pulses. His gait was antalgic with a walker with decreased stance phase on the left leg. Radiographs showed concentric left hip with some irregularity noted in the femoral head concerning for osteonecrosis without femoral head collapse, as well as heterotopic ossification in surrounding soft tissues (Figure 6). At this point, he was made weight bearing as tolerated on the left lower extremity and continued in outpatient physical therapy.

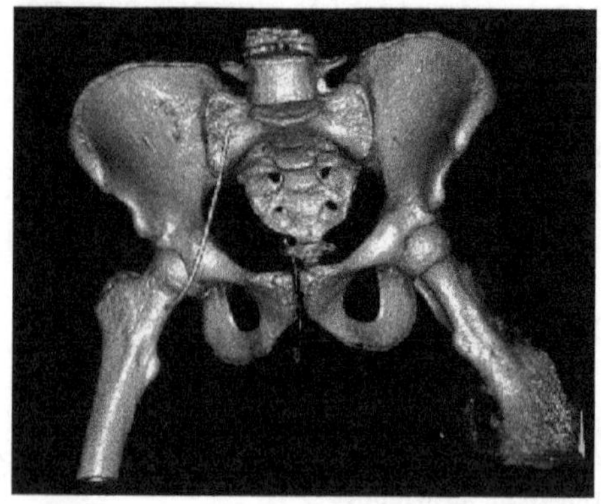

Figure 5: Postoperative 3D reconstruction from CT pelvis without contrast demonstrating reduced left femoral head without associated femoral fracture.

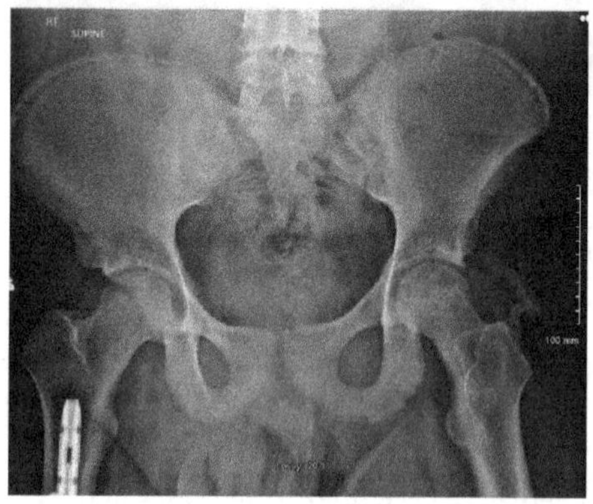

Figure 6: Follow-up AP pelvis radiograph at 9 weeks postinjury demonstrating concentric reduction of the left femoral head with heterotopic ossification without evidence of femoral head collapse.

The patient returned to follow-up in clinic 4.5 months after injury. At that time, he reported no left hip pain at rest. He had continued in physical therapy on an outpatient basis. Physical exam was notable for improved strength with hip

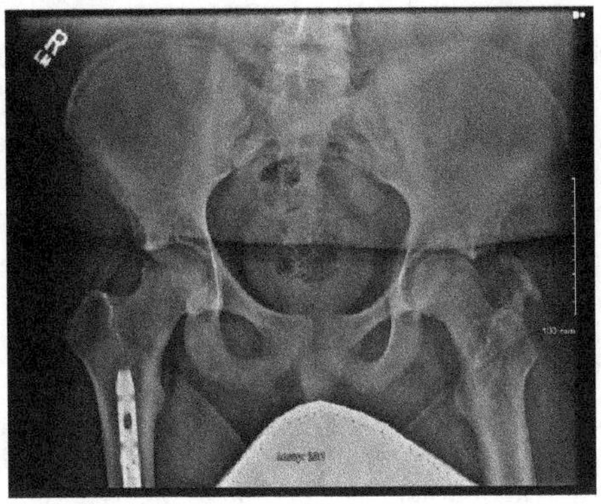

FIGURE 7: Follow-up AP pelvis radiograph at 4.5 months postinjury demonstrating further heterotopic ossification and some irregularity of the femoral head concerning for osteonecrosis.

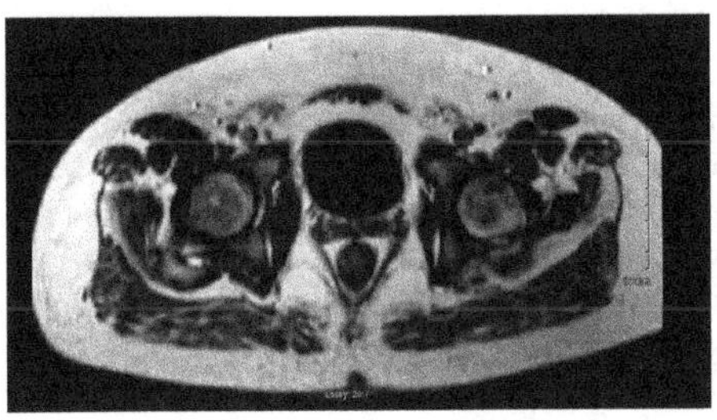

FIGURE 8: T1 axial image from MRI obtained 7 months postinjury demonstrating focal areas of hypointensity within the left femoral head consistent with osteonecrosis.

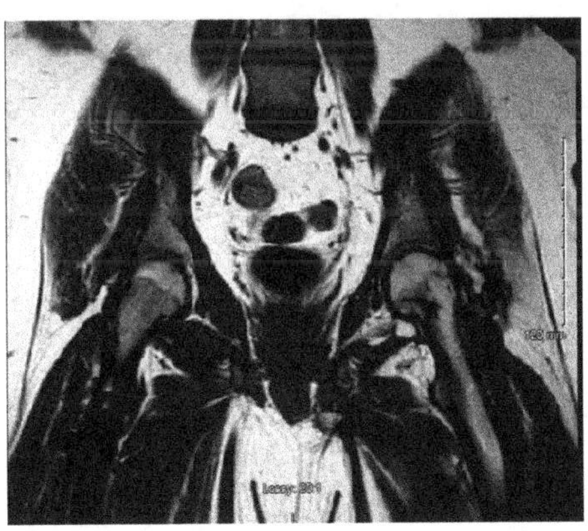

FIGURE 9: T1 coronal image from MRI obtained 7 months postinjury demonstrating focal areas of hypointensity within the left inferior femoral neck consistent with osteonecrosis.

flexion of 5/5 in bilateral lower extremities but otherwise was unchanged from prior exam. An AP pelvis X-ray was obtained which showed maturation of the heterotopic ossification adjacent to the left hip (Figure 7). Again noted was some irregularity in the femoral head but no evidence of femoral head collapse. An MRI of the pelvis was obtained 7 months postinjury, demonstrating focal areas of hypointensity on T1 images within the femoral head and inferior neck consistent with osteonecrosis, without evidence of femoral head collapse (Figures 8 and 9). Metal artifact from the right femur implant limited the ability of the MRI to evaluate the soft tissues in detail.

3. Discussion

Unfortunately, given the nature of the injury, the available literature on traumatic hip dislocations is largely limited to small, retrospective studies. In many of these cases, precise details regarding the time of injury to reduction and details of treatment are lacking given the retrospective nature. Moreover, results are conflicting as some have even reported good outcomes after reductions of chronic dislocations [21]. As such, conclusions regarding definitive treatment and prognosis are limited. Furthermore, given the unique displacement of the femoral head in our patient, it is unclear how the available literature will correspond to this patient's long-term prognosis. Based on available data, however, authors have reported that the most important factors in long-term prognosis for these injuries is the direction of the dislocation [22], time between injury and reduction [23], and the associated injuries [22, 23]. Associated injuries frequently occur with traumatic hip dislocations, involving up to 70.8% of patients [24], as was the case with our patient. Associated injuries can involve craniofacial and cervical spine fractures, closed head injuries, abdominal lacerations or organ injuries, lung contusions, and rib fractures, as well as fractures or dislocations of the upper and lower extremities [24, 25]. Due to the high energy required to produce a traumatic hip dislocation, a high suspicion for concomitant injuries must be maintained with thorough primary and secondary surveys completed according to advanced trauma life support protocols.

The presentation of our patient, with the femoral head located inside the pelvis without an associated proximal femur fracture likely resulted from a unique mechanism during the injury. It is suspected that the patient was thrown forward into the front seats prior to ejection from the vehicle. With a combination of hip flexion, hyperabduction, and internal fixation, the femoral head likely dislocated inferiorly from the acetabulum, then translated under the ischial tuberosity with subsequent external rotation bringing the femoral head superiorly up into the pelvis and ultimately resting behind the pubic symphysis. It is also likely that the patient's left leg became stuck momentarily during the ejection process resulting in the significant traction force required to clear the bony anatomy of the pelvis prior to dislocating medially. Given the strong sacrospinous and sacrotuberous ligaments, as well as lack of sacroiliac joint widening on imaging, it is less likely that the hip dislocated posteriorly and entered the pelvis from that direction. Significant energy and displacement, which resulted in the intrapelvic dislocation, likely caused significant injury to soft tissue structures, including but not limited to the ligamentum teres, hip capsule, short external rotators, and iliopsoas tendon. By visualizing the mechanism of injury and likely course of displacement into the pelvis, the operating surgeons were able to reduce the hip closed by reversing the suspected steps of dislocation. Reducing the hip with closed maneuvers was the ideal treatment for this polytraumatized patient who was still being resuscitated and treated for a traumatic brain injury. While the postoperative MRI demonstrates findings concerning for osteonecrosis, the patient has largely had a favorable outcome with no femoral head collapse, no hip pain at rest, and functional mobility.

Traumatic hip dislocations in young patients represent a true orthopedic emergency due to the potentially devastating complications including avascular necrosis and posttraumatic arthritis. Intrapelvic dislocations represent a very rare subset of these injuries and previously had only ever been reported with associated proximal femur fracture. This case demonstrates that not only can intrapelvic dislocations occur without femur fracture but that these injuries can be amenable to closed reduction despite their significant displacement into the true pelvis.

References

[1] D. M. Foulk and B. H. Mullis, "Hip dislocation: evaluation and management," *The Journal of the American Academy of Orthopaedic Surgeons*, vol. 18, no. 4, pp. 199–209, 2010.

[2] H. C. Epstein, "Traumatic dislocations of the hip," *Clinical Orthopaedics and Related Research*, vol. 92, pp. 116–142, 1973.

[3] V. P. Thompson and H. C. Epstein, "Traumatic dislocation of the HIP," *The Journal of Bone & Joint Surgery*, vol. 33, no. 3, pp. 746–792, 1951.

[4] M. J. Stewart and L. W. Milford, "Fracture-dislocation of the HIP," *The Journal of Bone & Joint Surgery*, vol. 36, no. 2, pp. 315–342, 1954.

[5] E. A. Brav, "Traumatic dislocation of the Hip," *The Journal of Bone and Joint Surgery. American Volume*, vol. 44, no. 6, pp. 1115–1134, 1962.

[6] J. C. DeLee, J. A. Evans, and J. Thomas, "Anterior dislocation of the hip and associated femoral-head fractures," *The Journal of Bone & Joint Surgery*, vol. 62, no. 6, pp. 960–964, 1980.

[7] R. E. Erb, J. R. Steele, E. P. Nance Jr., and J. R. Edwards, "Traumatic anterior dislocation of the hip: spectrum of plain film and CT findings," *American Journal of Roentgenology*, vol. 165, no. 5, pp. 1215–1219, 1995.

[8] A. Schicho and C. Riepl, "Images in clin medicine: femoral-head dislocation to the scrotum," *The New England Journal of Medicine*, vol. 372, no. 9, p. 863, 2015.

[9] T. Snoap, J. Habeck, and J. Roberts, "Open hip dislocation through the scrotum without osseous injury: a case report," *JBJS Case Connector*, vol. 7, no. 1, article e2, 2017.

[10] M. Allagui, B. Touati, I. Aloui, M. F. Hamdi, M. Koubaa, and A. Abid, "Obturator dislocation of the hip with ipsilateral femoral neck fracture: a case report," *Journal of Clinical Orthopaedics and Trauma*, vol. 4, no. 3, pp. 143–146, 2013.

[11] S. K. Jain, P. Aggarwal, and A. Yadav, "Obturator dislocation of hip with ipsilateral fracture neck femur-a case report," *Journal of Orthopaedic Case Reports*, vol. 7, pp. 16–19, 2017.

[12] B. S. Richards and D. J. Howe, "Anterior perineal dislocation of the hip with fracture of the femoral head," *Clinical Orthopaedics and Related Research*, vol. 228, pp. 194–201, 1988.

[13] A. S. Abdulfattah Abdullah, A. Abdelhady, and A. Alhammoud, "Bilateral asymmetrical hip dislocation with one side obturator intra-pelvic dislocation. Case report," *International Journal of Surgery Case Reports*, vol. 33, pp. 27–30, 2017.

[14] A. W. Farag and K. A. Shohayeb, "Intrapelvic dislocation of the head of femur through the obturator foramen associated with ipsilateral fracture femur," *The Journal of Bone and Joint Surgery. British volume*, vol. 85-B, no. 7, pp. 1056–1058, 2003.

[15] G. Prabhakar, N. Kusnezov, N. Rensing, and A. Abdelgawad, "Threading the needle: intrapelvic displacement of a femoral neck fracture through the obturator foramen," *Case Reports in Orthopedics*, vol. 2018, Article ID 2506187, 5 pages, 2018.

[16] C. Patrascanu and D. Cibu, "Anterior hip fracture dislocation with intrapelvic retention of the femoral head and ureter fistula," *Journal of Orthopaedic Case Reports*, vol. 4, no. 3, pp. 40–42, 2014.

[17] R. E. Polesky and F. A. Polesky, "Intrapelvic dislocation of the femoral head following anterior dislocation of the hip. A case report," *The Journal of Bone & Joint Surgery*, vol. 54, no. 5, pp. 1097-1098, 1972.

[18] T. Baba, K. Hitachi, and K. Kaneko, "Fracture-dislocation of the hip with ipsilateral femoral neck fracture," *European Journal of Orthopaedic Surgery and Traumatology*, vol. 12, no. 2, pp. 102–104, 2002.

[19] B. P. Meinhard, C. Misoul, D. Joy, and R. Ghillani, "Central acetabular fracture with ipsilateral femoral-neck fracture and intrapelvic dislocation of the femoral head without major pelvic-column disruption. A case report," *The Journal of Bone & Joint Surgery*, vol. 69, no. 4, pp. 612–615, 1987.

[20] V. Singaravadivelu, M. S. Mugundhan, and K. Sankaralingam, "Neglected intrapelvic dislocation of femoral head," *Indian Journal of Orthopaedics*, vol. 44, no. 2, pp. 224–226, 2010.

[21] P. Hoiness and O. Roise, "Successful open reduction of a 5-month-old hip dislocation associated with a femoral head fracture," *Journal of Orthopaedic Trauma*, vol. 17, no. 2, pp. 131–134, 2003.

[22] K. E. Dreinhofer, S. R. Schwarzkopf, N. P. Haas, and H. Tscherne, "Isolated traumatic dislocation of the hip. Long-term results in 50 patients," *The Journal of Bone and Joint Surgery. British volume*, vol. 76, no. 1, pp. 6–12, 1994.

[23] V. Sahin, E. S. Karakas, S. Aksu, D. Atlihan, C. Y. Turk, and M. Halici, "Traumatic dislocation and fracture-dislocation of the hip: a long-term follow-up study," *The Journal of Trauma*, vol. 54, no. 3, pp. 520–529, 2003.

[24] R. S. Yang, Y. H. Tsuang, Y. S. Hang, and T. K. Liu, "Traumatic dislocation of the hip," *Clinical Orthopaedics and Related Research*, vol. 265, pp. 218–227, 1991.

[25] C. A. Pietrafesa and J. R. Hoffman, "Traumatic dislocation of the hip," *JAMA*, vol. 249, no. 24, pp. 3342–3346, 1983.

11

Nonoperative Management of Proximal Tibiofibular Joint Synostosis after Tibial Intramedullary Nailing

David C. Ebbott, Alexander J. Johnson, and Christopher Haydel

Temple University, Department of Orthopaedics and Sports Medicine, 3401, N. Broad St. Zone B, 6th Floor, Philadelphia, PA 19140, USA

Correspondence should be addressed to David C. Ebbott; Dave.Ebbott@gmail.com

Academic Editor: Georg Singer

We report the case of a 28-year-old male semiprofessional basketball player who presented to an outside hospital with nonhealing stress fractures for which he underwent tibial intramedullary nailing (IMN). Two weeks after surgery, he developed pain proximal and lateral to the knee. As he returned to play, the pain worsened with jumping and lateral movement and improved with rest. He presented to our hospital one year after the operation with the same unresolved pain. Imaging one year after the surgery revealed proximal tibiofibular joint (TFJ) synostosis aligned with the drill path. Literature review showed that rare noncongenital cases of proximal TFJ synostosis cases were most often treated nonoperatively. However, two cases involved the removal of excessively protruding screws and two cases involved bone resection that resolved painful disruption of other joints, such as the ankle. The current patient had proper implant positioning and no other impacted joints, so he was managed without operative intervention. By the final 16-month postoperative follow-up, his symptoms had resolved completely. Although an unusual occurrence with limited data, we recommend nonoperative management for proximal TFJ synostosis caused by tibial nailing if implants are properly positioned and no other joints are affected.

1. Introduction

Proximal tibiofibular joint (TFJ) synostosis, as a complication of trauma or surgery, is an exceptionally rare occurrence with few reports available in the literature [1–7]. The literature more commonly reports synostosis occurring in the radioulnar joint [8], the distal TFJ [9, 10], or the tibiofibular diaphyseal area [11]. It also highlights congenital abnormalities and immature skeletal development as a common cause of synostosis [4]. In noncongenital cases, the interosseous bone growth is thought to occur from soft tissue damage, hemorrhage, or subperiosteal dissection [1]. Although rare, noncongenital proximal TFJ synostosis has been reported in two cases of excessive screw protrusion [1, 2] and nine nonsurgical cases [3–7]. Patients with proximal TFJ synostosis may be asymptomatic or they may present with knee pain or painful joint disruptions (e.g., ankle pain) with treatments ranging from nonoperative to screw removal or bone resections [1–7].

2. Case Report

A 28-year-old male semiprofessional basketball player presented to our orthopaedic practice with pain proximal and lateral to the left knee joint. He was treated for a tibial shaft stress fracture with tibial intramedullary nail (IMN) fixation 1 year prior at an outside hospital. He first noticed pain proximal and lateral to the left knee 2 weeks after surgery, and it persisted for the entire year. He had no complaints of pain in other joints and he denied any history of trauma since surgery. X-ray images taken during initial evaluation at our clinic showed no evidence of fractures, appropriate position of hardware, and presence of heterotopic bone at the proximal TFJ (Figure 1(a)). We ordered a CT scan to further evaluate the heterotopic bone and rule out implant problems including screw breakage, loosening, or prominent position. The CT scan demonstrated that the implant was properly positioned with no protruding or loosening screws (Figures 1(a)–1(d)). We posited that the implant likely had

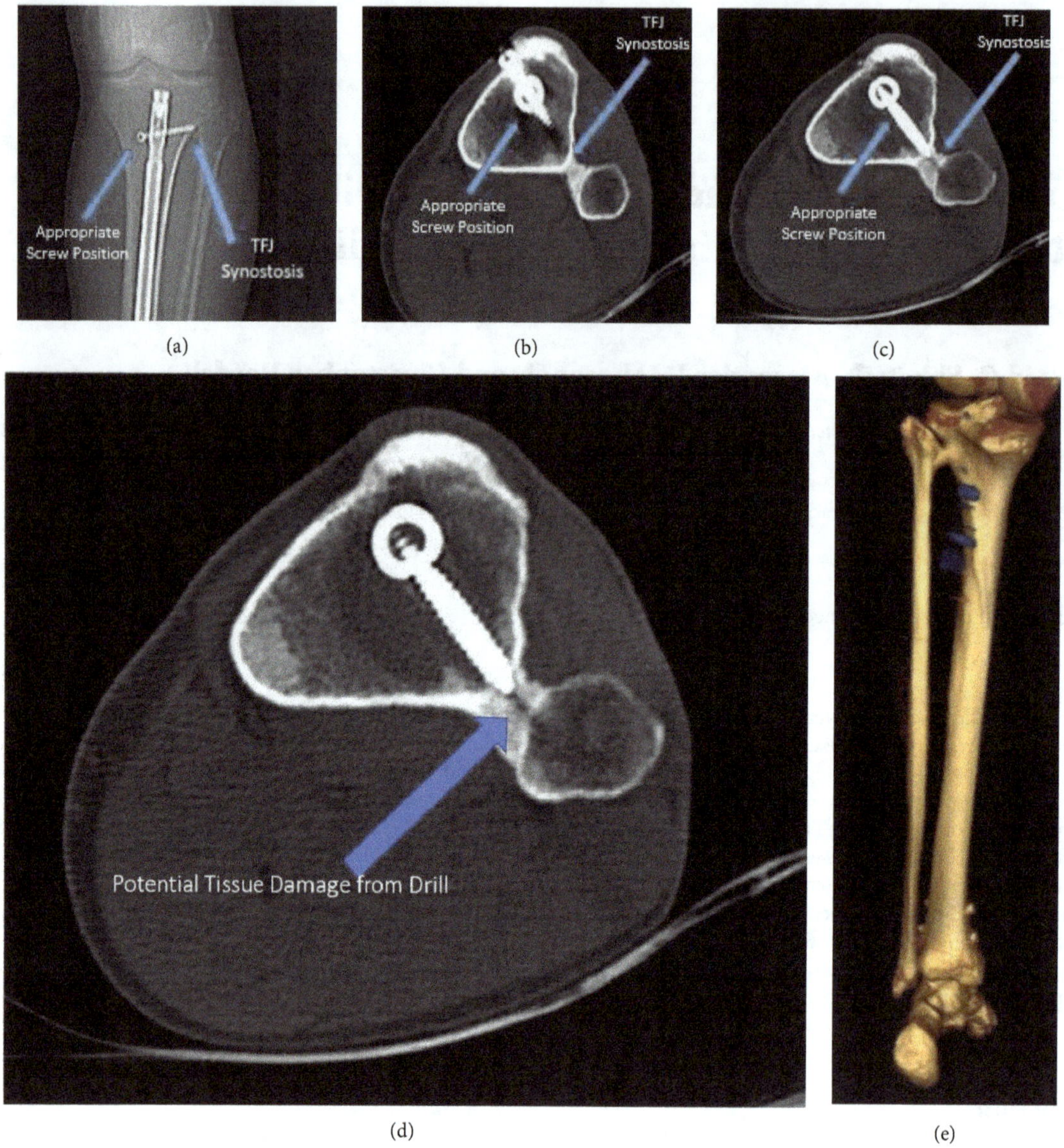

Figure 1: Proximal tibiofibular joint synostosis. (a) AP X-ray of the left proximal tibia show the tibial nail in an acceptable position with visible TFJ synostosis. (b) Axial CT scan showing appropriate position of the implant and TFJ synostosis. (c) Axial CT scan showing appropriate position of interlocking screw without excessive prominence. (d) CT scan demonstrating a potential soft tissue damage from drilling through the TFJ space into the fibula. (e) 3D reconstruction showing TFJ synostosis.

little to no impact on the patient's pain. The scan also displayed no acute fracture consistent with the patient's reported level of pain (Figures 1(a)–1(e)). However, it showed that the drill for the proximal locking screw may have penetrated through the tibia and into the fibula (Figure 1(d)). It also revealed proximal tibiofibular synostosis immediately distal to the proximal TFJ joint (Figures 1(a)–1(e)) aligned with the bone reaming along the drill path (Figure 1(d)). Following a literature review and a discussion with our patient, we decided to proceed with nonoperative management. The patient declined a steroid injection. The patient's knee pain resolved without intervention, and he was able to return to playing semiprofessional basketball. At 13 months postoperation, he reported intermittent, mild pain on the medial side of the knee while playing basketball, but this did not limit his participation. At the final follow-up 16 months postoperation, he reported no pain.

3. Discussion

Upon presenting with postoperative knee pain near the site of tibial proximal interlocking screws, there was a high suspicion of implant complications. IMN implant issues are very common and the source of many patients' postoperative pain [12, 13], especially with protrusion of interlocking screws beyond 5 mm [14]. While the consensus is not clear in the literature [15, 16], implant removal after tibial IMN may lead to symptomatic relief [12, 13]. The CT scan in the current case failed to show evidence of broken or loose implant that would clearly indicate surgical implant removal. Instead, the CT did show a synostosis aligned with the drill path.

No published case matched our patient's presentation, so we consulted several similar cases to aid in developing a treatment plan for the patient in this case. The most similar case involved a 14-year-old female who developed asymptomatic proximal TFJ synostosis secondary to tibial nailing; the new bone developed around the screw protruding well into the interosseous space. The patient had the screw removed at 48 weeks, and she remained asymptomatic at 5 years. Surgical excision was ruled out while the patient remained asymptomatic [1]. In a second similar case, a 62-year-old female developed asymptomatic proximal TFJ synostosis secondary to an osteotomy when a screw, later removed, penetrated well into the interosseous membrane [2]. While both cases bear similarities to the current case, the CT scan in the current case confirmed appropriate placement of the implant contributing to the decision to continue with nonoperative management.

Nine other noncongenital proximal TFJ synostosis cases were identified in the literature over the last 19 years, although none had a surgical etiology like the current case. Six of the nine identified related cases were asymptomatic and effectively managed nonoperatively [3, 4]. The asymptomatic trend casted doubt on the synostosis as the source of our patient's pain, suggesting that the synostosis acted as a red herring with the pain more likely resulting from the drilled tissue damage. However, in one case, proximal TFJ synostosis was associated with knee and ankle pain presumably by limiting the motion present at each of these joints [5], and in a second case, authors believed proximal TFJ synostosis was associated with referred low back pain (pseudoradicular syndrome) [6]. In both patients, surgical resection separating the tibia from the fibula led to complete symptom resolution [5, 6]. An additional case involved persistent ankle pain, but the patient refused the recommended resection [7]. Nevertheless, in the current case, no such adjacent joint disruption or radicular pain affected the patient, so surgical resection was not further considered.

Knee pain after tibial IMN is a well-known complication with poorly delineated etiology, and it is impossible to attribute the knee pain in the current case to any one factor [17, 18], so the prospect remains that the synostosis or the presence of the implant impacted the pain in the patient. Alternate low probability causes of pain in this case include metal allergies leading to nonspecific deep generalized pain and metal corrosion not seen on imaging [19].

After evaluating factors including imaging of the implant, drilled tissue damage, no painful disruption of adjacent joints, and the asymptomatic nature of the most similar synostosis cases, we surmised that patient's pain was most likely unaffected by the synostosis or the final position of the screw. These considerations along with a patient discussion guided us to the nonoperative approach that coincided with complete symptom resolution 16 months after the operation.

4. Conclusion

Proximal TFJ synostosis is an extremely rare finding post IMN fracture fixation. This is the first case where the penetration of the drill into the TFJ without screw prominence likely caused the synostosis and knee pain, the latter of which resolved without intervention. In post-tibial nailing proximal TFJ synostosis, we recommend nonoperative treatment if the screws are not excessively protruding and other joints are not affected pending additional data related to implant removal and this rare form of synostosis.

Consent

Signed informed consent from the patient was obtained for de-identified publication of the medical case.

References

[1] S. Mandal and N. Coleman, "Proximal tibiofibular synostosis following tibial nailing: a case report and review of literature," *Injury Extra*, vol. 36, no. 10, pp. 418–420, 2005.

[2] I. Esenkaya and K. Unay, "Proximal tibiofibular synostosis, an unexpected complication of a proximal tibial osteotomy," *International Journal of Case Reports in Medicine*, vol. 2013, article 113410, p. 6, 2013.

[3] L. Felli, M. Coviello, V. Seghezzo, M. Fiore, and L. Biglieni, "Proximal tibiofibular synostosis in a professional soccer player: a case report," *JBJSCase Connector*, vol. 2, no. 3, p. e46, 2012.

[4] N. K. Sferopoulos, "Synostosis of the proximal tibiofibular joint," *Case Reports in Medicine*, vol. 2010, Article ID 794594, 5 pages, 2010.

[5] M. Bozkurt, M. Dogan, and S. Turanli, "Osteochondroma leading to proximal tibiofibular synostosis as a cause of persistent ankle pain and lateral knee pain: a case report," *Knee Surgery, Sports Traumatology, Arthroscopy*, vol. 12, no. 2, pp. 152–154, 2004.

[6] B. van Ooij, A. van Ooij, J. W. Morrenhof, and C. N. van Dijk, "Proximal tibiofibular synostosis as a possible cause of a pseudoradicular syndrome: a case report," *Knee Surgery, Sports Traumatology, Arthroscopy*, vol. 19, no. 12, pp. 2115–2118, 2011.

[7] S. Takai, N. Yoshino, and Y. Hirasawa, "Unusual proximal tibiofibular synostosis," *International Orthopaedics*, vol. 23, no. 6, pp. 363–365, 1999.

[8] J. B. Jupiter and D. Ring, "Operative treatment of post-traumatic proximal radioulnar synostosis*," *The Journal of Bone and Joint Surgery (American Volume)*, vol. 80, no. 2, pp. 248–257, 1998.

[9] G. H. R. Albers, A. F. C. C. de Kort, P. R. J. M. Middendorf, and C. N. van Dijk, "Distal tibiofibular synostosis after ankle fracture," *The Journal of Bone and Joint Surgery British Volume*, vol. 78-B, no. 2, pp. 250–252, 1996.

[10] S. A. Kottmeier, G. A. Hanks, and A. Kalenak, "Fibular stress fracture associated with distal tibiofibular synostosis in an athlete: a case report and literature review," *Clinical Orthopaedics and Related Research*, vol. 281, pp. 195–198, 1992.

[11] B. Sonnery-Cottet, M. Alessio-Mazzola, B. F. Luz et al., "Diaphyseal tibiofibular synostosis in professional athletes:

report of 2 cases," *Orthopaedics & Traumatology: Surgery & Research*, vol. 102, no. 1, pp. 135–138, 2016.

[12] C. M. Court-Brown, T. Gustilo, and A. D. Shaw, "Knee pain after intramedullary tibial nailing: its incidence, etiology, and outcome," *Journal of Orthopaedic Trauma*, vol. 11, no. 2, pp. 103–105, 1997.

[13] J. F. Keating, R. Orfaly, and P. J. O'Brien, "Knee pain after tibial nailing," *Journal of Orthopaedic Trauma*, vol. 11, no. 1, pp. 10–13, 1997.

[14] P. C. Soraganvi, B. S. Anand-Kumar, R. Rajagopalakrishnan, and B. A. Praveen-Kumar, "Anterior knee pain after tibial intra-medullary nailing: is it predictable?," *Malaysian Orthopaedic Journal*, vol. 10, no. 2, pp. 16–20, 2016.

[15] T. O. Boerger, G. Patel, and J. P. Murphy, "Is routine removal of intramedullary nails justified?," *Injury*, vol. 30, no. 2, pp. 79–81, 1999.

[16] A. H. Karladani, P. Åke Ericsson, H. Granhed, L. Karlsson, and P. Nyberg, "Tibial intramedullary nails—should they be removed?: A Retrospective Study of 71 Patients," *Acta Orthopaedica*, vol. 78, no. 5, pp. 668–671, 2007.

[17] W. Obremskey, J. Agel, K. Archer, P. To, and P. Tornetta, "Character, incidence, and predictors of knee pain and activity after infrapatellar intramedullary nailing of an isolated tibia fracture," *Journal of Orthopaedic Trauma*, vol. 30, no. 5, article e185, 2016.

[18] P. Labronici, R. Santos Pires, J. Franco, H. Alvachian Fernandes, and F. dos Reis, "Recommendations for avoiding knee pain after intramedullary nailing of tibial shaft fractures," *Patient Safety in Surgery*, vol. 5, no. 1, p. 31, 2011.

[19] M. L. Busam, R. J. Esther, and W. T. Obremskey, "Hardware removal: indications and expectations," *Journal of the American Academy of Orthopaedic Surgeons*, vol. 14, no. 2, pp. 113–120, 2006.

12

Novel use of Joint Replacement in a Thumb Interphalangeal Joint

Desirae McKee and E. L. Domingo-Johnson

Department of Orthopaedic Surgery, Texas Tech University, 3601 4th Street, Mail Stop 9436, Lubbock, TX 79430-9436, USA

Correspondence should be addressed to Desirae McKee; desirae.mckee@ttuhsc.edu

Academic Editor: Paul E. Di Cesare

Arthrodesis of the interphalangeal (IP) joint of the thumb is widely acknowledged as the indicated treatment for trauma and osteoarthritis of this joint. Joint replacement was offered to a young patient as an alternative treatment after traumatic joint loss of the IP joint in her thumb. This allowed her to maintain motion of the joint as she did not wish to move forward with fusion. In the present case, a Humanitarian Use Device (HUD) was utilized in an off-label manner and placed into the interphalangeal joint of the patient's thumb. The patient did well postoperatively with reasonable pain-free range of motion of the interphalangeal joint with an arc of 40 degrees. We propose that joint replacement is a viable alternative to arthrodesis in select patients who do not wish to be fused. We believe this represents the first thumb IP joint replacement using a semiconstrained joint presented in the medical literature.

1. Introduction

The interphalangeal joint of the thumb provides the flexibility and range of motion necessary for activities that characterize modern living such as allowing for the use of a handheld cellular device as well as simple activities of daily living such as lacing up shoes. However, when the structural integrity of this joint is compromised, surgical immobilization of the joint is often required to prevent pain at the joint. Arthrodesis of the interphalangeal (IP) joint of the thumb is widely acknowledged as the indicated treatment for trauma and primary osteoarthritis of this joint [1]. Although standard treatment for interphalangeal joint trauma is IP arthrodesis, in the case of a 15-year-old female patient presenting with traumatic loss of the interphalangeal joint from a table saw, other treatment options were explored due to patient desire to avoid fusion. Small joint arthroplasty is a procedure typically reserved for use in the interphalangeal joints of the 2nd through 5th digits. In this procedure, the diseased or damage joint is removed and replaced with a metal/plastic or pyrocarbon implant that recreates the joint space. One other available option for small joint arthroplasty is a silicone joint implant. Given the patient's age, silicone implantation was ruled out due to the likelihood of implant breakage over time [2, 3]. Pyrocarbon implants have been used in proximal interphalangeal (PIP) arthroplasty with higher rates of survivorship shown at a long-term follow-up [4, 5]. The principle of using nonflexible material to increase longevity of a PIP joint implant was applied to the IP joint in the case we describe. In the present case, the patient's joint was traumatically damaged secondary to injury and subsequently replaced during treatment with a Humanitarian Use Device (HUD) consisting of high molecular weight polyethylene, cobalt chrome, and titanium. An HUD is a medical device which aids in the treatment or diagnosis of a disease or condition affecting less than 8,000 individuals in the United States per year [6]. Although placement of the prosthesis into the interphalangeal joint of the thumb is considered an off-label use of the HUD, we propose that our approach was the best method of treatment as it enabled this patient to retain some mobility of the joint rather than an arthrodesis which the patient did not desire. Current review of the published scientific literature did not reveal a similar case of joint replacement in the thumb although a newspaper article from the UK did comment on a silicone IP joint replacement in a thumb [7]. In that case, the patient specifically was able to regain function of the thumb for his professional requirements of being a magician.

2. Case Presentation

A 15-year-old Caucasian female presented with an intra-articular fracture and adjacent laceration at the distal portion of the proximal phalanx of the thumb resulting in near complete loss of the interphalangeal joint (Figures 1 and 2). The injury was incurred from a table saw accident. The patient had an initial pain level of 4/10 and was unable to flex her thumb. The patient and her family were offered a joint arthrodesis for joint stability, but they did not desire a fusion. The patient felt a fusion would limit activities important to her such as texting, playing video games, and applying cosmetics. Joint replacement was offered to the patient as an alternative treatment. In the present case, an HUD was utilized in an off-label manner and inserted into the interphalangeal joint of the patient's thumb. The patient and family were counseled that this was not a standard treatment option and that if fusion was needed in the future, it could be more complicated and require bone grafting compared to using fusion as the initial alternative.

The patient was followed for 22 months postoperatively and has remained happy with her choice of procedure. The patient's motion in the thumb IP joint is currently a 40 degree arc which is very reasonable given the repair of the flexor pollicis longus tendon and collateral ligament as well. There was excellent range of motion (ROM) in the metacarpophalangeal joint (MCP) which is comparable to the contralateral side. Radiographs demonstrated good seating of the joint implant with no evidence of loosening or periprosthetic fracture (Figures 3 and 4). The collateral ligaments were all stable at the IP joint, and the scar on the left volar thumb was well-healed. The patient reported pain of 0/10 at her most recent follow-up and recorded a DASH score of 6.82. No known complications have arisen as a result of the surgical reconstruction to this point in time.

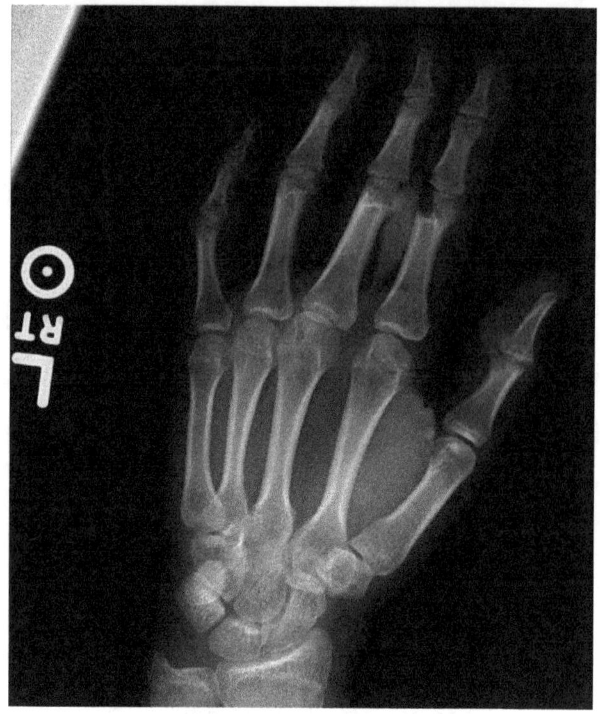

Figure 1: Preoperative AP view of the thumb.

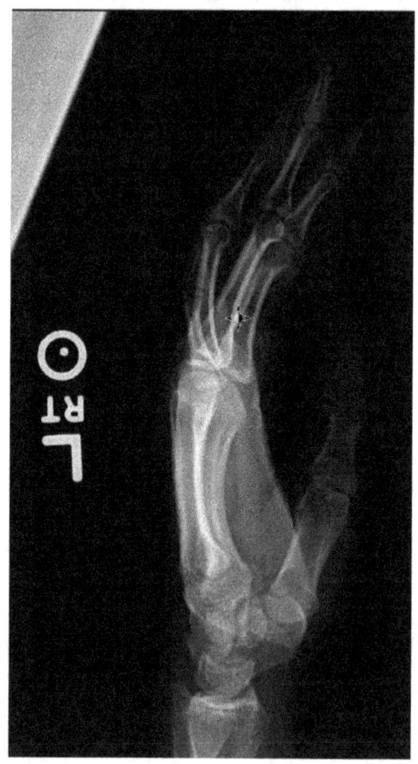

Figure 2: Preoperative lateral view of the thumb.

3. Discussion

A recent study demonstrated how the thumb's range of motion impacts certain activities of daily living [8]. It was shown that the position of the thumb influences both the efficiency of the task and the participants' evaluation of the task's ease. Specifically, power tasks were best completed at an angle of 0° for the nondominant hand and an angle between 0° and 30° for the dominant hand. Grip tasks were most efficient at 15° for the nondominant hand and between 0° and 15° for the dominant hand, and pinch tasks were best completed between 0° and 30° for the nondominant hand and between 15° and 30° for the dominant hand. These findings are in accordance with the more flexed posture typically utilized in gripping and strength tasks as these actions are likely to engage the extrinsic flexor pollicis longus (FPL) and increase total muscular involvement.

As previously discussed, arthrodesis of the interphalangeal (IP) joint of the thumb is widely acknowledged as the indicated treatment for trauma and osteoarthritis of this joint [1]. The current standard for interphalangeal joint arthrodesis is to place the thumb in 15-30 degrees of flexion. Given that the efficiency and ease of certain activities of daily living require a range of motion between 0° and 30° [8], it can be assumed that after undergoing arthrodesis, these movements will never be recovered.

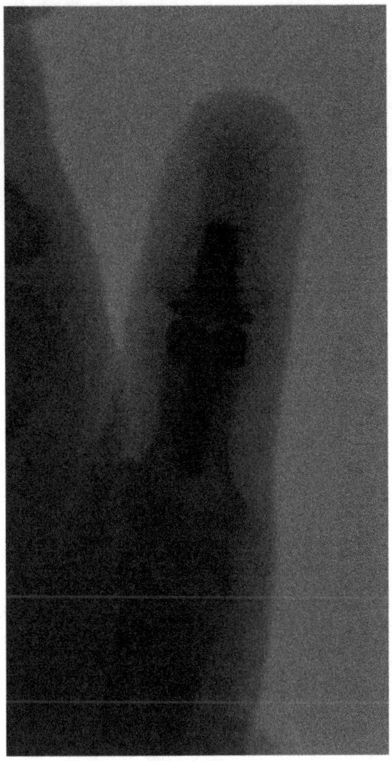

FIGURE 3: AP view of the thumb IP joint with the implant in place.

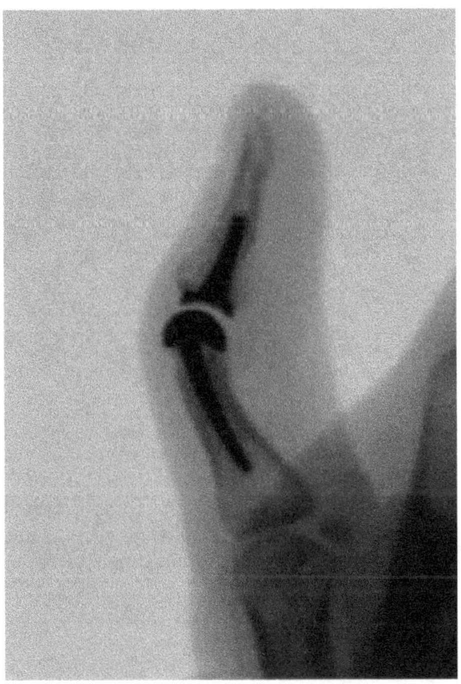

FIGURE 4: Lateral view of the thumb IP joint with the implant in place.

Arthrodesis is a standard acceptable method for treatment of damage to the interphalangeal joint of the thumb. It provides a stable, pain-free, motionless joint but can hinder some activities that are an essential part of an individual's activities of daily living. We hypothesized that our subject would benefit from retaining mobility at her thumb interphalangeal joint after joint replacement as she did not prefer fusion. The procedure initially has been a success and is allowing a patient, who is in a crucial developmental life stage, to lead a life closer to preinjury status. Long-term outcomes are unknown, and we will attempt to maintain a long-term follow-up with this patient.

This case is novel as there are no other reported thumb interphalangeal solid joint replacements found in the current literature. The educational value in this report is that it could demonstrate other possibilities and options for surgeons to offer patients who do not wish to move forward with fusion of that joint.

The authors recognize that this was an off-label use of the product in a minor individual. The patient and her parents were engaged in extensive discussions about moving forward with fusion vs. trying the implant. The patient and her mother were well educated about the risks associated with this procedure and understood that replacing the joint in the thumb IP region is not a traditional approach in this situation. Both the patient and her mother were made aware that a fusion may still be necessary in the future. Given the patient's desire to retain motion of her thumb, joint replacement was the only remaining course of treatment.

No adverse effects from the HUD have been noted to this point in time. We hypothesize that future outcomes will be analogous to using the implant in the other digit small joints. The major concern with arthroplasty in any joint is the possible need for revision surgery in the future. The implant that we used is composed of cobalt chrome, titanium, and polyethylene. A similar silicone implant is associated with an 18 percent revision rate in the proximal interphalangeal (PIP) joints [9]. There is low risk of a major adverse outcome associated with this procedure. Patient satisfaction and retained mobility of the joint have been established in this case. We understand that outcomes at 22 months of follow-up are considered short-term in the world of prosthetic joints, and this patient will continue to be closely monitored. A long-term follow-up and future case series will be critical in establishing efficacy and safety.

Acknowledgments

The authors would like to acknowledge Nancy Swinford, CCRC, Clinical Research Coordinator Texas Tech, and Cameron Cox, Research Assistant Texas Tech.

References

[1] M. Jakubek, M. Enzendorfer, R. Fiala, and K. Trieb, "Interphalangeal arthrodesis using an intramedullary nitinol implant: a prospective study," *Joint Diseases and Related Surgery*, vol. 28, no. 2, pp. 87–91, 2017.

[2] P. M. Murray, "Prosthetic replacement of the proximal interphalangeal joint," *Hand Clinics*, vol. 22, no. 2, pp. 201–206, 2006.

[3] F. Iselin and E. Conti, "Long-term results of proximal interphalangeal joint resection arthroplasties with a silicone implant,"

The Journal of Hand Surgery, vol. 20, no. 3, Part 2, pp. S95–S97, 1995.

[4] A. C. Watts, A. J. Hearnden, I. A. Trail, M. J. Hayton, D. Nuttall, and J. K. Stanley, "Pyrocarbon proximal interphalangeal joint arthroplasty: minimum two-year follow-up," *The Journal of Hand Surgery*, vol. 37, no. 5, pp. 882–888, 2012.

[5] D. R. Dickson, D. Nuttall, A. C. Watts, S. C. Talwalkar, M. Hayton, and I. A. Trail, "Pyrocarbon proximal interphalangeal joint arthroplasty: minimum five-year follow-up," *The Journal of Hand Surgery*, vol. 40, no. 11, pp. 2142–2148.e4, 2015.

[6] *Designating Humanitarian Use Device (HUD)*, U.S. Food & Drug AdministrationOctober 2018, https://www.fda.gov/ForIndustry/DevelopingProductsforRareDiseasesConditions/DesignatingHumanitarianUseDevicesHUDS/ucm232388.htm. Published October 24, 2017.

[7] A. Grebot, "A new thumb joint? That''ll do the trick! Magician''s op saves his slide of hand. Daily Mail Online," 2013, October 2018, http://www.dailymail.co.uk/health/article-2308523/A-new-thumb-joint-Thatl-trick.html. Published April 13, 2013.

[8] S. McGowan, M. Deisher, and K. S. Matullo, "Functional fusion angle for thumb interphalangeal joint arthrodesis," *Hand*, vol. 11, no. 1, pp. 59–64, 2016.

[9] L. Squitieri and K. C. Chung, "A systematic review of outcomes and complications of vascularized toe joint transfer, silicone arthroplasty, and PyroCarbon arthroplasty for posttraumatic joint reconstruction of the finger," *Plastic and Reconstructive Surgery*, vol. 121, no. 5, pp. 1697–1707, 2008.

13

A Rare T2-T3 Synovial Facet Cyst Causing Progressive Myelopathy

Mohamed F. Albana,[1] **Sean Z. Griffiths**,[1] **and Kris E. Radcliff**[2]

[1]*Department of Orthopedic Surgery, Inspira Heath, 1505 W Sherman Ave, Vineland, NJ 08360, USA*
[2]*Department of Orthopedic Surgery, The Rothman Institute, 2500 English Creek Ave. Egg Harbor Township, NJ 08234, USA*

Correspondence should be addressed to Mohamed F. Albana; albanam@ihn.org

Academic Editor: Eyal Itshayek

Intraspinal extradural synovial cysts are a rare occurrence at the spinal cord level and thus a rare cause of myelopathy. Synovial cysts usually present in the more mobile lumbar and cervical parts of the spine; however, they may also arise in the thoracic spine. We present a case of a 59-year-old male with a left upper thoracic synovial cyst at T2-3 causing disabling, progressive myelopathy, and an incomplete spinal cord injury syndrome with inability to ambulate. An urgent decompressive laminectomy with bilateral facetectomies, cyst excision, and posterior fusion was performed. Subsequently, the patient recovered full function. Synovial cysts should be considered in the differential diagnosis of progressive thoracic myelopathy. This is only the sixth reported case of a synovial cyst of this kind occurring between the levels of T1 and T7. Urgent surgical decompression is the recommended treatment.

1. Introduction

Intraspinal extradural synovial cysts are a rare cause of myelopathy, and when they occur, they most commonly present in the lumbar and cervical spine. Such cysts can also appear in the thoracic spine, although such cases are rare. We present a case of a 59-year-old male with a left-sided intraspinal, extradural synovial cyst at the T2-T3 levels on the left resulting in an inability to ambulate and paresthesia in bilateral lower extremities. A laminectomy and excision of the cyst with fusion from T2-T4 was performed resulting in complete resolution of symptoms. There are only 5 reported cases of synovial cysts in the upper thoracic spine. Laminectomy, with cyst excision, is the treatment of choice, although steroid injections and percutaneous drainage have been described in the literature.

2. Case Report

2.1. History. Patient is a 59-year-old male who sustained a minor impact to his back one month prior to presentation. He was evaluated by a pain management specialist for chief complaint of back pain and ambulatory dysfunction. An MRI of the lumbar spine was performed which demonstrated mild, multilevel spondylosis. He was referred for physical therapy of the lumbar spine and was prescribed NSAIDs and muscle relaxers. He was reevaluated and reported worsening gait and an improvement in pain. He was referred for a lumbar epidural injection. He was reevaluated again two weeks after the epidural (approximately six weeks following the initial injury). At that time, he was completely wheelchair bound. He endorsed difficulty with bladder control for two days. He was referred to the emergency department for an immediate evaluation. At that time, he reported mild (3/10) pain in the lumbar spine. He denied neck pain, thoracic pain, arm pain, or leg pain. He denied numbness or paresthesia in any distribution including the chest wall.

2.2. Examination. The patient's physical examination revealed 2/5 strength in the left iliopsoas, quadriceps, tibialis anterior, EHL, and gastrocnemius. His right lower extremity strength was 4/5 in the left iliopsoas, quadriceps, tibialis anterior, EHL, and gastrocnemius. He had decreased sensation below the nipple line bilaterally. He had normal digital rectal tone. He had no sensory loss in the perineal region. He had

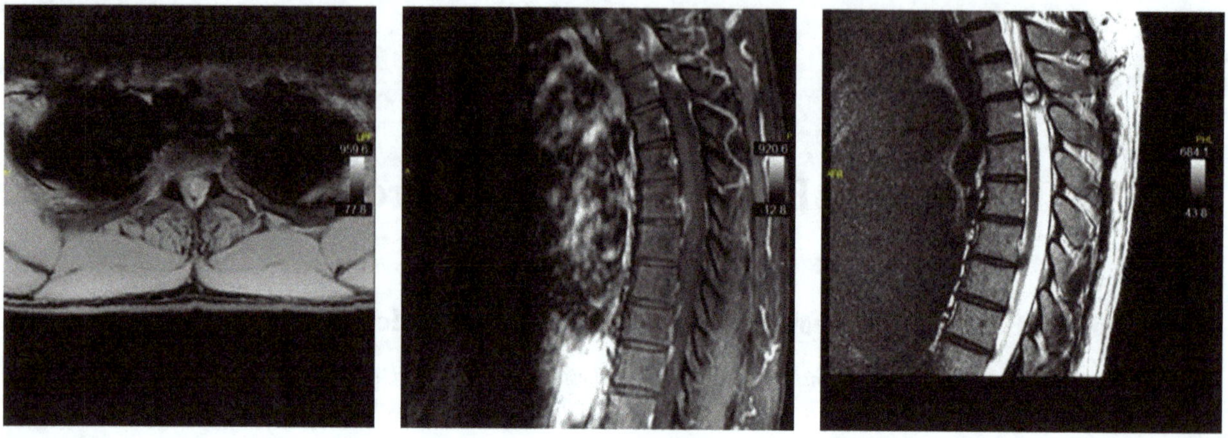

(a) (b) (c)

Figure 1: (a) Axial T1-weighted MRI, (b) sagittal T1-weighted MRI, and (c) sagittal T2-weighted and short tau inverted recover MRI images demonstrating a large left T2-T3 synovial facet cyst within the spinal canal.

no clonus or Babinski sign. He had 1+ reflexes in all distributions.

2.3. Imaging. A CT scan of the thoracic spine was ordered and found to be negative for any acute pathologic process. An MRI of the thoracic spine demonstrated a large high T2 intensity, low T1 intensity, heterogenous, and extradural round mass at the level of T2-T3 on the left side. There was no contrast enhancement. There was severe cord compression. There was acute cord signal change at the T2 level (Figure 1).

The patient was admitted to the intensive care unit, and intravenous steroids were administered with no significant improvement prompting surgical management.

2.4. Surgical Intervention. The patient was taken to the operating room for surgical intervention. Due to the location of cyst, as noted on preoperative imaging, a full laminectomy of T3 was performed first to define a normal region of dura. During the approach, the T3-4 interspinous ligament was resected. A midline laminectomy and decompression of T1, T2, and T3 was performed followed by complete excision of a large 3 cm × 1.5 cm synovial cyst (Figure 2). The cyst was noticed to be originating from the left T2-T3 facet and demonstrated adhesions to the dura but was clearly extradural. Medial facetectomies and foraminotomies from T2 to T4 were performed bilateral to help prevent cyst recurrence and ensure a wide decompression followed by instrumented spinal fusion from T2 to T4 with autograft and allograft. The fourth thoracic vertebra was included in the fusion to minimize risk of iatrogenic instability as the T3-4 interspinous ligament was resected during the approach. There were no intraoperative complications or adverse recorded signal changes on intraoperative monitoring from baseline.

2.5. Postoperative Course. Immediately after surgery, the patient was at his preoperative baseline level. He had an uneventful postoperative course. He was discharged to an inpatient rehabilitation facility and eventually home. Final pathology report resulted in a diagnosis of a benign synovial cyst. The patient was evaluated at 2, 6, and 10 weeks postoperatively. At his two-week follow-up, his strength had substantially improved to at least four out of five in all distributions. By the sixth week postoperatively, patient's strength was fully restored to five out of five strength bilaterally in all distributions with no remaining paresthesia. At the patients tenth week postoperatively, his strength had remained full with no recurrence of symptoms and complete resolution of symptoms. A follow-up MRI was obtained three months postoperatively and revealed persistently adequate decompression of the spinal cord with no cyst recurrence as compared to preoperatively (Figure 3).

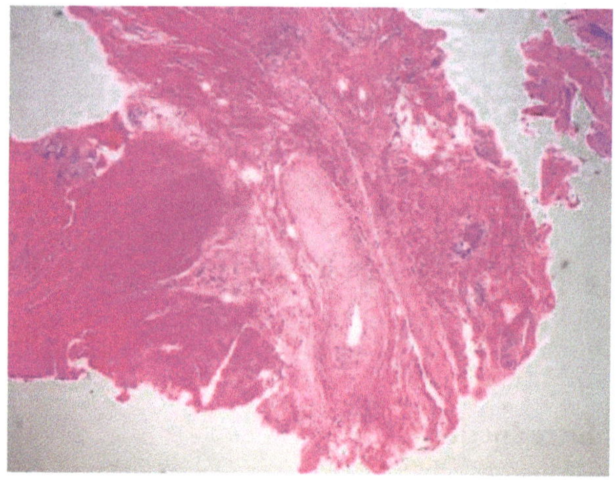

Figure 2: Microscopic image showing denuded cyst lining with focal synovium present. Gross specimen size 4.0 × 1.3 × 0.5 cm.

3. Discussion

We present a case of a relatively young male in the setting of a thoracic synovial cyst. Synovial cysts in themselves are rare in the spine; however, when they are identified, they typically arise in the lumbar spine [1–4]. When they do present in

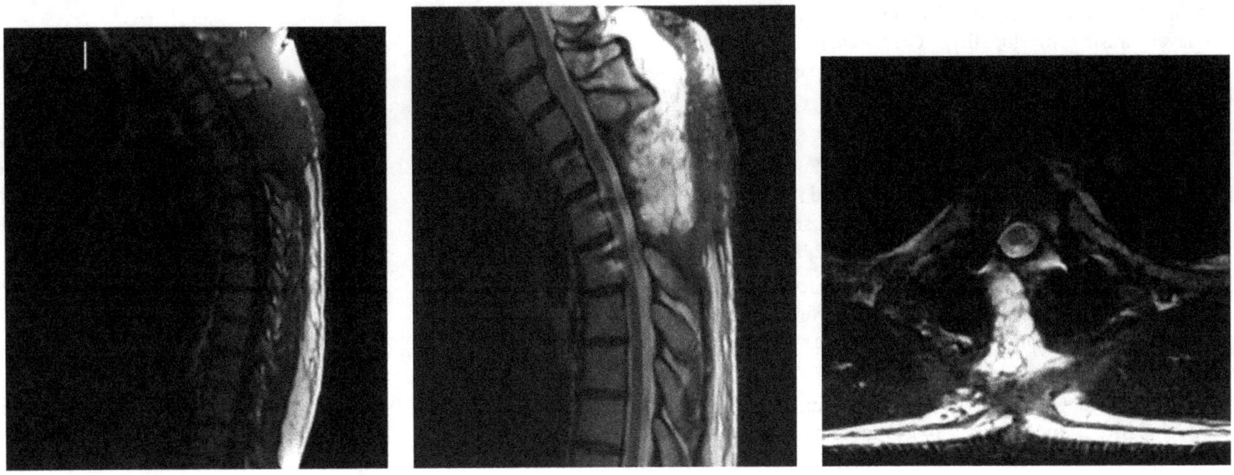

(a) (b) (c)

Figure 3: Sagittal, precontrast (a) and postcontrast (b), and axial postcontrast (c) MRI sequences 3 months postoperatively demonstrating maintained surgical decompression and no recurrent cyst formation.

the cervical or thoracic spine, they often arise in locations of increased motion such as the cervicothoracic junction or lower thoracic vertebra [5, 6]. There have been 6 reported cases of extradural synovial cysts appearing in the cervicothoracic junction and 20 cases occurring between T10 and T12 [7, 8]. Other risk factors for the formation of juxtafacet synovial cysts include rheumatoid arthritis, osteoarthritis, and posttraumatic instability [3]. Giovannini et al. identified 43 cases of thoracic juxtafacet synovial cysts. Only 5 of the 43 cases occurred between T1 and T7, which can be attributed to the anatomical characteristics of the thoracic spine leading to decreased mobility [3, 8, 9].

Patients are typically treated conservatively initially with analgesics, immobilization, and occasionally CT-guided aspiration with, or without, steroid injection [8, 10]. Graham et al. determined the use of CT-guided aspiration as a good option for temporary symptomatic relief. On the other hand, Shah et al. evaluated 10 patients with radiculopathy that were initially treated conservatively and reported that nonsurgical management is not successful and surgery should be recommended for a zero rate of recurrence [10, 11]. In the event a patient develops ambulatory dysfunction, urgent surgical decompression should be completed once an etiology for the dysfunction is identified [12]. Multiple surgical options have been studied and found to be acceptable with laminectomy with, or without, fusion being most commonly used [3, 10, 13–17]. In this case, we opted to perform facetectomies and fusion in addition to decompressive laminectomy to eliminate the pathologic zygapophyseal joints and the associated motion in order to prevent recurrence.

4. Conclusion

Juxtafacet synovial cysts are rare, but the rate of diagnosis has increased due to the use of MRI. This pathology is exceedingly rare in the thoracic spine, and upper thoracic presentation is even more infrequent. In patients who develop ambulatory dysfunction, a thorough workup for thoracic pathology should be conducted even in the absence of thoracic pain. The presence of a synovial cyst should prompt continued evaluation as the cyst can increase in size leading to progressive myelopathy. Synovial cysts do not necessarily illicit axial back pain. In the case presented, it is hypothesized that the minor trauma the patient experienced caused inflammation that may have lead to the synovial cyst expansion. Nonsurgical management has been described; however, surgical excision is recommended as symptoms commonly persist with nonoperative management. This patient had an incomplete Brown-Sequard presentation, which typically have a good clinical prognosis. Facetectomy with posterior spinal fusion after cyst excision should be determined on a case by case basis but should be considered to help prevent cyst recurrence. When ambulatory dysfunction is present, operative intervention should be urgently completed to optimize patients' chance of improvement.

References

[1] R. Almefty, K. I. Arnautović, and B. L. Webber, "Multilevel bilateral calcified thoracic spinal synovial cysts," *Journal of Neurosurgery: Spine*, vol. 8, no. 5, 2008.

[2] R. N. Holtzman, R. Dubin, W. C. Yang, E. Rorat, H. M. Liu, and N. E. Leeds, "Bilateral symptomatic intraspinal TL2-11 synovial cysts," *Surgical Neurology*, vol. 28, no. 3, pp. 225–230, 1987.

[3] M. Merkle, T. Psaras, M. Tatagiba, S. Danz, and F. Schmidt, "Synovial cyst of the thoracic spine causing myelopathy," *Spine*, vol. 34, no. 5, 2009.

[4] Z. Zhenbo, L. Huanting, W. Jin, G. Haifeng, F. Yuan, and L. Ming, "Hemilaminoplasty for the treatment of lumbar intraspinal synovial cysts (LISCs) and literature review," *European Spine Journal*, vol. 25, no. 11, pp. 3393–3402, 2016.

[5] E. F. Bisson, J. C. Sauri-Barraza, T. Niazi, and M. H. Schmidt, "Synovial cysts of the cervicothoracic junction causing myelopathy: report of 3 cases and review of the literature," *Neurosurgical Focus*, vol. 35, no. 1, p. E3, 2013.

[6] M. Sundskaro and S. Gaini, "Thoracic synovial cyst at the Th2-3 level causing myelopathy," *Case Reports in Neurological Medicine*, vol. 2017, Article ID 6257294, 2 pages, 2017.

[7] A. A. Cohen-Gadol, J. B. White, J. J. Lynch, G. M. Miller, and W. E. Krauss, "Synovial cysts of the thoracic spine," *Journal of Neurosurgery*, vol. 1, no. 1, pp. 52–57, 2004.

[8] S. J. M. Giovannini, H. Pinto, P. Marino, and A. Cervio, "Bilateral synovial cyst of the thoracic spine causing paraparesis," *Neuro-Chirurgie*, vol. 65, no. 2-3, pp. 89–92, 2019.

[9] D. Daentzer and D. Stüder, "Thoracic juxtafacet cyst (JFC) as a rare cause of myelopathy - an additional reference to support the instability theory," *Joint Bone Spine*, vol. 77, no. 2, pp. 178–180, 2010.

[10] E. Graham, L. G. Lenke, D. Hannallah, and C. Lauryssen, "Myelopathy induced by a thoracic intraspinal synovial cyst: case report and review of the literature," *Spine*, vol. 26, no. 17, pp. E392–E394, 2001.

[11] R. V. Shah and G. E. Lutz, "Lumbar intraspinal synovial cysts: conservative management and review of the world's literature," *The Spine Journal*, vol. 3, no. 6, pp. 479–488, 2003.

[12] P. F. Doherty, S. C. Stein, and R. White, "Bilateral synovial cysts of the thoracic spine: a case report," *Surgical Neurology*, vol. 39, no. 4, pp. 279–281, 1993.

[13] E. F. Bashir and O. Ajani, "Management of lumbar spine juxtafacet cysts," *World Neurosurgery*, vol. 77, no. 1, pp. 141–146, 2012.

[14] E. J. Boviatsis, L. C. Staurinou, A. T. Kouyialis et al., "Spinal synovial cysts: pathogenesis, diagnosis and surgical treatment in a series of seven cases and literature review," *European Spine Journal*, vol. 17, no. 6, pp. 831–837, 2008.

[15] R. Gazzeri, M. Galarza, L. Gorgoglione, M. Bisceglia, and V. D'Angelo, "Cervical cyst of the ligamentum flavum and C7-T1 subluxation: case report," *European Spine Journal*, vol. 14, no. 8, pp. 807–809, 2005.

[16] C. Scholz, U. Hubbe, E. Kogias, R. Roelz, and J. H. Klingler, "Microsurgical resection of juxtafacet cysts without concomitant fusion—long-term follow-up of 74 patients," *Clinical Neurology and Neurosurgery*, vol. 153, pp. 35–40, 2017.

[17] A. Yurt, M. Seçer, M. Aydin et al., "Surgical management of juxtafacet cysts in the lumbar spine," *International Journal of Surgery*, vol. 29, pp. 9–11, 2016.

14

Spina Bifida Occulta with Bilateral Spondylolysis at the Thoracolumbar Junction Presenting Cauda Equina Syndrome

Kentaro Mataki, Masao Koda, Yosuke Shibao, Hiroshi Kumagai, Katsuya Nagashima, Kousei Miura, Hiroshi Noguchi, Toru Funayama, Tetsuya Abe, and Masashi Yamazaki

Department of Orthopedic Surgery, Faculty of Medicine, University of Tsukuba, 1-1-1 Tennodai, Tsukuba, Ibaraki 305-8575, Japan

Correspondence should be addressed to Kentaro Mataki; kentaromataki@yahoo.co.jp

Academic Editor: Sigita Burneikiene

Several reports have described the coexistence of spina bifida occulta (SBO) and spondylolysis, but the majority of defects occur at L5. No report has described the coexistence of SBO and spondylolysis at the thoracolumbar junction. We report a case of SBO with spondylolysis at L1, presenting cauda equine syndrome. A 37-year-old man presented with a gait disorder as a result of bilateral motor weakness of the lower extremities. A plain radiograph showed local kyphosis at L1-2 as a result of severe degenerative change and wedging of the vertebral body at L1. Magnetic resonance imaging (MRI) revealed degenerative disc changes and severe canal stenosis at L1-2. Computed tomography (CT) revealed SBO and spondylolysis at L1. He was diagnosed with cauda equina syndrome related to SBO and spondylolysis at L1. Posterior interbody fusion and decompression at L1-2 were performed. After surgery, his muscle power recovered to normal strength. The possible mechanisms in this case are the strain on anterior elements as a result of disruption of the posterior elements due to SBO and spondylolysis. The coexistence of SBO and spondylolysis at the thoracolumbar junction might induce at risk status of increased strain to the anterior elements that may cause cauda equina syndrome.

1. Introduction

Spina bifida occulta (SBO) is a common malformation of the lamina of the spine, most commonly occurring in the sacrum or lower lumbar spine [1, 2]. Spondylolysis is a common etiology of back pain in children and adolescents. SBO is associated with spondylolysis of the lumbar spine in 11.8-35% of patients [3, 4]. There are several reports of the coexistence of SBO and spondylolysis; the majority occur at L5 [2, 5]. However, no report has described the coexistence of SBO and spondylolysis at the thoracolumbar junction.

The aim of this paper is to describe a clinical example of treatment for cauda equina syndrome as a result of the coexistence of SBO and spondylolysis at the thoracolumbar junction.

2. Case Report

A 37-year-old man presented with progressive limitation of activities as a result of bilateral motor weakness of the lower extremities for several weeks. He had no history of strenuous sporting activity or low back pain. Neurological examination revealed motor weakness in iliopsoas and quadriceps muscles, and muscle power was rated at a manual muscle testing level of 2. He had no urinary dysfunction or lower extremity sensory dysfunction.

A plain radiograph showed local kyphosis at L1-L2 as a result of severe degenerative change at the L1-2 disc level and wedging of the vertebral body at L1 (Figures 1(a) and 1(b)). Magnetic resonance imaging (MRI) revealed severe degenerative disc change and severe canal stenosis at L1-2 (Figures 1(c) and 1(d)). Computed tomography (CT) revealed SBO and spondylolysis at L1 and no other malformations (Figures 2(a)–2(c)).

He was diagnosed with cauda equina syndrome at the L1-2 level related to SBO and spondylolysis at L1. Posterior lumbar interbody fusion at L1-2 was performed (Figure 3). After surgery, his symptoms improved promptly, and he was able to walk with a cane on his discharge.

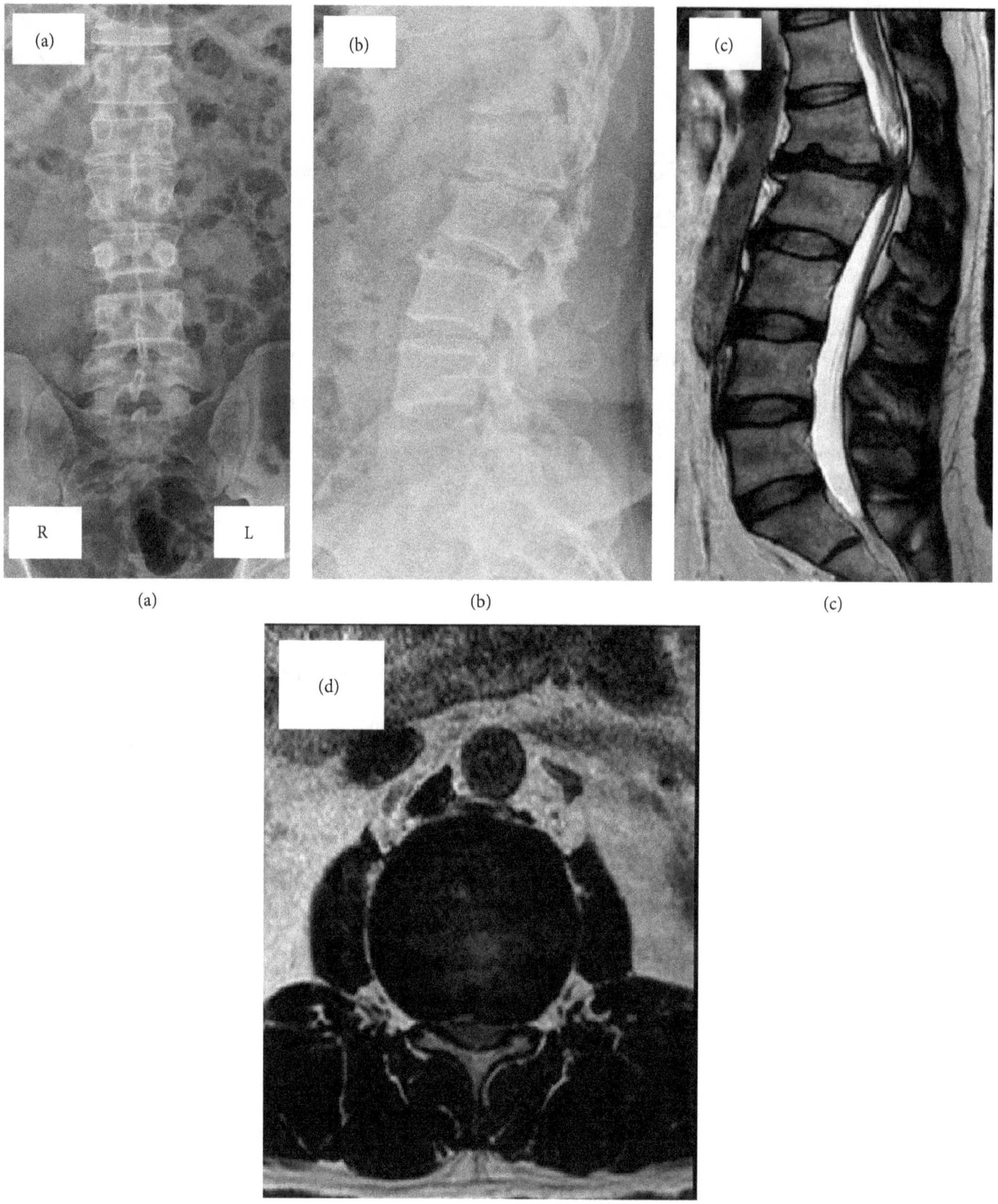

(a) (b) (c) (d)

FIGURE 1: Anterior-posterior radiograph (a) and lateral radiographs (b) of the lumbar spine showing severe degenerative change at L1-2 and compression of the L1 vertebral body. Sagittal (c) and axial (d) T2-weighted magnetic resonance images showing degeneration of the disc and severe canal stenosis at the L1-2 level. R indicates right side; L, left side.

3. Discussion

SBO is caused by failure of fusion between posterior vertebral elements without affecting the spinal cord or meninges. It is usually observed at L5 and/or at the upper one or lower two sacral vertebrae [1, 2]. Goto et al. reported a case of SBO at the thoracolumbar junction and estimated the incidence as <5% within all SBO patients [6, 7]. SBO is associated with spondylolysis and spondylolisthesis of the lumbar spine [4, 8]. SBO occurs with spondylolysis of the lumbar spine in 11.8-35% of patients [3], and in one-third of patients with the isthmic type of spondylolisthesis [8].

The presence of dysplastic or disrupted posterior elements in SBO may increase load on the pars interarticularis. Sakai et al. reported that the incidence of spondylolysis

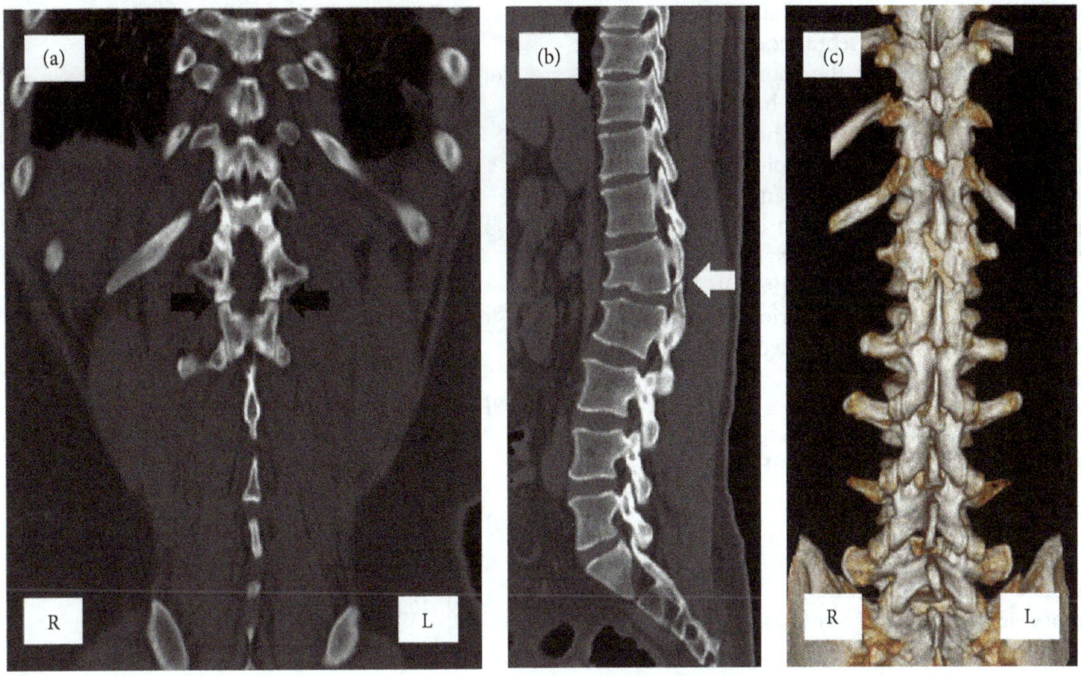

(a) (b) (c)

FIGURE 2: Computed tomographic (CT) scan. Coronal view (a) revealed bilateral spondylolysis (black arrow) and a bony defect of the lamina at L1. A sagittal view (b) revealed spondylolysis (white arrow) at L1. Three-dimensional reconstruction of the computed tomography scan (c) showing the coexistence of spina bifida and spondylolysis at L1. R indicates right side; L, left side.

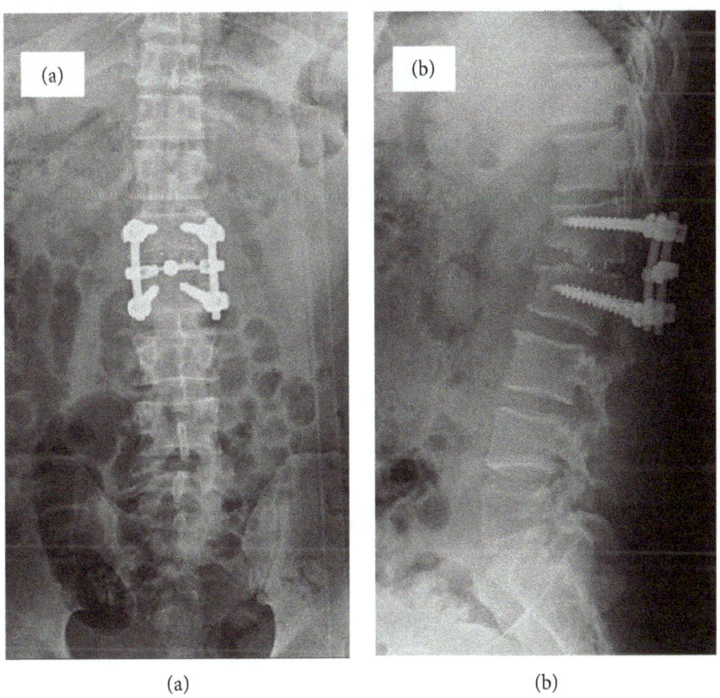

(a) (b)

FIGURE 3: Postsurgery radiographs. Anteroposterior (a) and lateral (b) views, showing instrumented posterolateral interbody fusion at L1-2.

was significantly higher in patients with SBO than in those without SBO (odds ratio = 3.7) [4].

The coexistence of SBO and spondylolysis occurs at L5 in the majority of cases [2, 5]. To our knowledge, no report has described the coexistence of SBO and spondylolysis at the thoracolumbar junction.

We hypothesize that the possible mechanism for this is that the disruption of the posterior elements caused by SBO and spondylolysis increases strain on the anterior elements, such as the L1-2 disc and L1 vertebral body.

In our case, the etiology of the spondylolysis remains unclear because lumbar spondylolysis had not been diagnosed until the patient's first visit to our hospital. The patient had no history of low back pain as an adolescent. This patient required immediate decompression and fusion surgery because of neurological deficits due to cauda equina syndrome. Several cases of cauda equina syndrome caused by L1-2 disc hernia have been reported [9, 10]. In this case, because of the disruption of the posterior elements caused by SBO and spondylolysis, we performed posterior lumbar interbody fusion at L1-2.

Kumar et al. reported that there is a significant risk of nerve root damage during surgical exposure due to defects of the posterior elements in patients with such a coexistent lesion. Therefore, it is mandatory to be examined prior to surgery by pelvic outlet views using CT [5]. With preoperative images including MRI and CT, we were aware of the coexistence of SBO and spondylolysis at the thoracolumbar junction before surgery in the present case.

4. Conclusion

The coexistence of SBO and spondylolysis at the thoracolumbar junction might induce at-risk status of increased strain to the anterior elements of the spine that may cause cauda equina syndrome.

Additional Points

Highlights. Spina bifida occulta (SBO) is associated with spondylolysis of the lumbar spine. The coexistence of SBO and spondylolysis often occurs at L5. No report has described those disruptions at L1 presenting cauda equina syndrome. Defects of the posterior elements might increase the strain on the anterior aspect. The coexistence of SBO and spondylolysis may cause cauda equina syndrome.

References

[1] T. Sakai, Y. Goda, F. Tezuka et al., "Clinical features of patients with pars defects identified in adulthood," *European Journal of Orthopaedic Surgery and Traumatology*, vol. 26, no. 3, pp. 259–262, 2016.

[2] L. Babbi, S. Terzi, S. Bandiera, and G. Barbanti Brodano, "Spina bifida occulta in high grade spondylolisthesis," *European Review for Medical and Pharmacological Sciences*, vol. 18, Supplement 1, pp. 8–14, 2014.

[3] J. E. Lonstein, "Spondylolisthesis in children: cause, natural history, and management," *Spine*, vol. 24, no. 24, pp. 2640–2648, 1999.

[4] T. Sakai, K. Sairyo, S. Takao, H. Nishitani, and N. Yasui, "Incidence of lumbar spondylolysis in the general population in Japan based on multidetector computed tomography scans from two thousand subjects," *Spine*, vol. 34, no. 21, pp. 2346–2350, 2009.

[5] R. Kumar, D. Niall, A. Walsh, K. Khalihullah, and D. McCormack, "Spina bifida occulta in isthmic spondylolisthesis: a surgical trap," *European Spine Journal*, vol. 11, no. 2, pp. 159–161, 2002.

[6] T. Goto, T. Sakai, N. Sato, S. Katoh, and K. Sairyo, "An adolescent athlete with low back pain associated with spina bifida occulta at the thoracolumbar junction: a case report," *The Journal of Medical Investigation*, vol. 66, no. 1.2, pp. 199-200, 2019.

[7] T. R. Yochum and L. J. Rowe, *Essentials of Skeltal Radiology*, Lippincott Williams & Wilkins, Philadelphia, 3rd edition, 2005.

[8] R. Wynne-Davies and J. H. Scott, "Inheritance and spondylolisthesis: a radiographic family survey," *The Journal of Bone and Joint Surgery*, vol. 61-B, no. 3, pp. 301–305, 1979.

[9] M. Gallo, G. Caggiari, L. Puddu, E. Ciurlia, G. R. Mosele, and C. Doria, "Intradural lumbar disc herniations associated with cauda equina syndrome: report of two cases and review of literature," *Chirugia*, vol. 30, no. 5, pp. 167–172, 2017.

[10] R. M. Aprígio, R. L. Caramanti, F. O. R. Santos et al., "Intradural disc herniation at the L1-L2 level: a case report and literature review," *Surgical Neurology International*, vol. 10, p. 196, 2019.

15

Humeral Avulsion of the Lateral Collateral Ligament of the Elbow Concomitant with the Medial Epicondyle Fracture of a Child with General Joint Laxity

Toru Morimoto, Masashi Izumi, Hiroaki Ueba, and Masahiko Ikeuchi

Department of Orthopaedic Surgery, Kochi University, Kochi Medical School, Kohasu, Oko-cho, Nankoku 783-8505, Japan

Correspondence should be addressed to Masashi Izumi; izumim@kochi-u.ac.jp

Academic Editor: Federico Canavese

Medial epicondyle fracture is a common elbow injury for children, and it was reported that 30-50% of this fracture was associated with elbow dislocation. However, dysfunction of the lateral collateral ligament (LCL) complex accompanied with the medial epicondyle fracture has rarely been reported. In this report, a 13-year-old girl who had a humeral avulsion of the LCL concomitant with a displaced medial epicondyle fracture was presented. Since her general joint laxity had been recognized from past medical history and the humeral avulsion of the LCL was clearly confirmed by ultrasonography, simultaneous surgical repair for the LCL avulsion and medial epicondyle fracture was conducted and satisfactory outcome was achieved. Although general joint laxity does not tend to receive attention in trauma as much as chronic conditions, it should be borne in mind to prevent overlooking important soft tissue damage coexisting with apparent fractures.

1. Introduction

Medial epicondyle fracture is the most common avulsion injury of the elbow and accounts for 11-20% of all pediatric elbow fractures [1–3]. It occurs most frequently between the ages of 9 and 14 and is four times more common in boys [4]. Reviews of previous literatures described that medial epicondyle fractures were associated with elbow dislocation in 30-50% of children [5]; however, there were very few reports highlighting possible concurrent elbow injury such as coronoid fracture, radial head fracture, and lateral collateral ligament avulsion. In this report, we present a rare case of humeral avulsion of the lateral collateral ligament (LCL) concomitant with the medial epicondyle fracture of a young girl, which was presumably associated with her general joint laxity.

2. Case Report

A 13-year-old right hand-dominant girl had fallen on her hand and injured the right elbow during her way to school and visited our clinic soon after. Her chief complaint was a severe pain of the right elbow that was apparently swollen. Active and passive motion of the elbow was not possible due to pain, but no neurovascular deficits were observed in her left arm. She had a history of dwarfism and had been undergoing growth hormone replacement therapy since she was 7 years old at our hospital. She also had a history of developmental dysplasia of the left hip and a habitual patellar dislocation of the right knee. For the patellar dislocation, she underwent reconstructive surgery of the medial patellofemoral ligament when she was 12 years old, and at that time, her general joint laxity was diagnosed with the Beighton score of 6 points.

In plain X-ray and CT scan of the elbow, apparent displaced medial epicondyle fracture (Watson-Jones classification type 2) together with an avulsed thin fragment of the lateral epicondyle was detected; however, no proximal radial fracture or a coronoid fracture was observed (Figure 1). She could not undergo MRI because of her panic disorder and claustrophobia.

The next day after the injury, her surgery was performed under general anesthesia. Prior to skin incision, ultrasonography and stress X-rays of the elbow were evaluated.

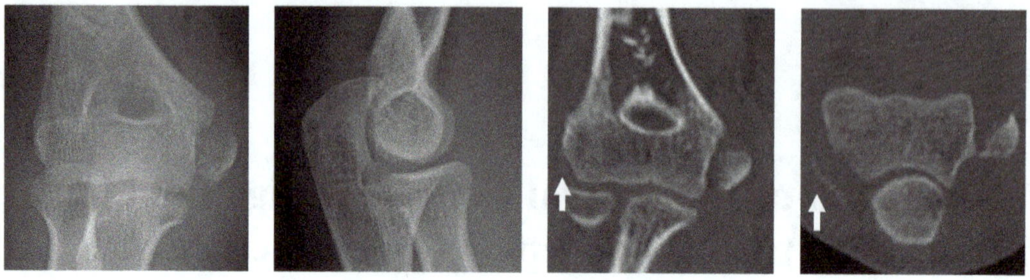

(a) (b) (c) (d)

Figure 1: Preoperative X-ray (a, b) and CT (c, d) of the right elbow. (a) AP view. (b) Lateral view. (c) Coronal plane. (d) Axial plane. Thin bony fragment of the lateral epicondyle (arrow) was observed in (c) and (d).

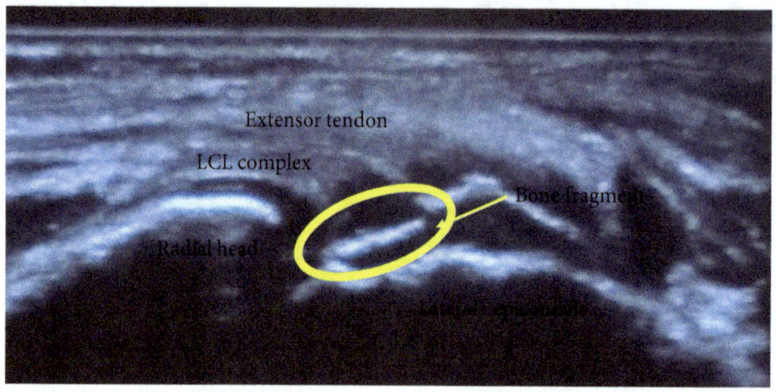

Figure 2: Preoperative ultrasonography of the right elbow. Humeral avulsion of the LCL was clearly confirmed.

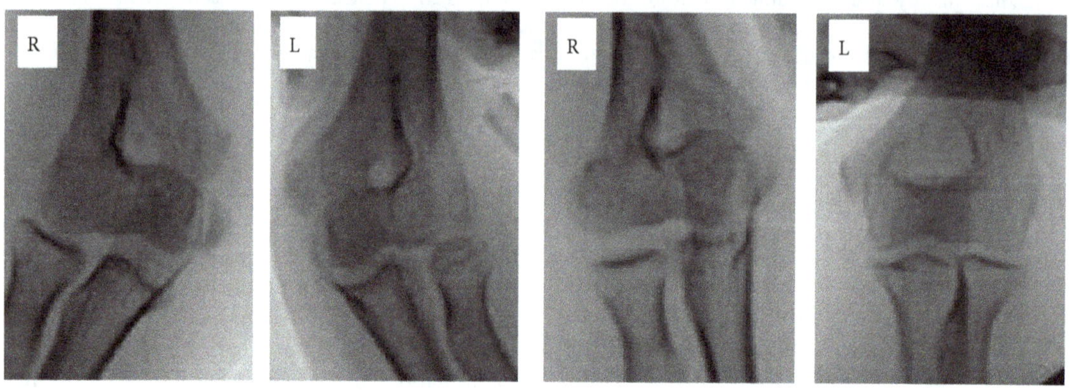

(a) (b)

Figure 3: Preoperative stress X-ray of the bilateral elbow evaluated under anesthesia. (a) Valgus. (b) Varus. (R: right elbow, L: left elbow.) The side-to-side differences of the joint space widening were significantly worse in the right elbow.

Proximal avulsion of LCL from the epicondyle was clearly seen in the ultrasonography (Figure 2). Valgus and varus stress tests were performed bilaterally with her elbows at a 20-degree flexed position. The side-to-side differences of the joint space widening were 8 mm in the valgus stress and 3 mm in the varus stress, which were significantly worse in the right elbow (Figure 3).

For the medial epicondyle fracture, conventional open reduction and internal fixation was performed using tension band wiring technique. Then, the lateral epicondyle was exposed and there was a complete avulsion of the LCL complex but the conjoined extensor tendon was not involved. After refreshing the stump of the ligament and footprint, 3 suture anchors (φ1.4 mm JuggerKnot®, Zimmer Biomet, Warsaw, IN, US) were inserted into the footprint and LCL complex was sutured by double row fixation technique (Figure 4).

Postoperatively, her elbow was immobilized with a plastic cast for 3 weeks and then was allowed active and passive motion with a soft brace. She was able to return to her preinjury daily activities 2 months after the surgery. The wires were removed 4 months after the primary surgery. At that time, the medial epicondyle fracture was united, and side-to-side differences of the joint space widening were 2 mm in the valgus stress and 1 mm in the varus stress, which had significantly improved compared with the previous findings

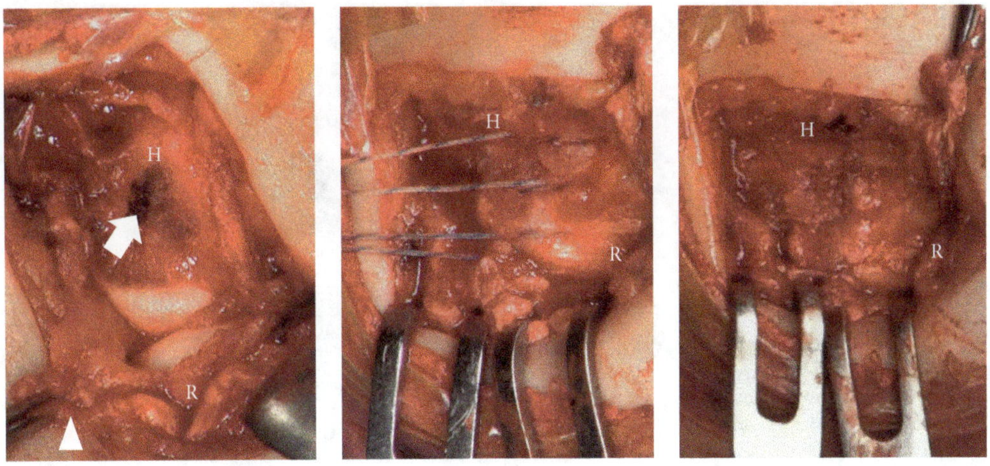

(a) (b) (c)

FIGURE 4: Intraoperative photos. Upper: cranial, lower: caudal. H: humerus; R: radius. (a) Humeral avulsion of the LCL (arrow: foot print, arrow head: LCL complex). (b) Suture preparation. (c) After repair.

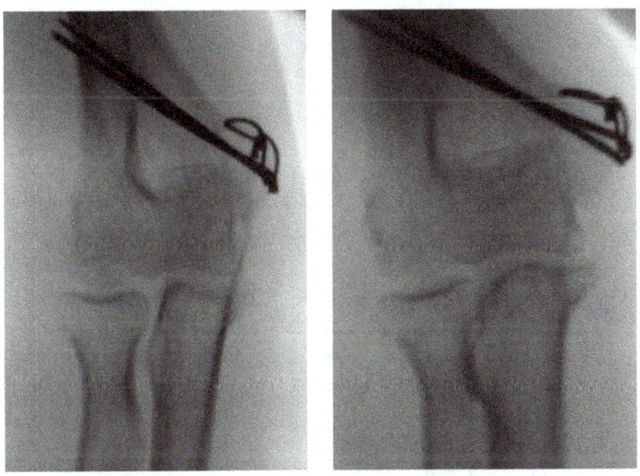

(a) (b)

FIGURE 5: Postoperative stress X-ray of the right elbow evaluated under anesthesia (4 months after the primary surgery). There was no difference of the instability.

(Figure 5). Her follow-up was completed 7 months after the primary surgery, with no pain, no limitation of ROM, and no functional deficits due to the elbow injury.

3. Discussion

A rare child case of elbow injury was successfully treated with simultaneous surgical repair for LCL avulsion and medial epicondyle fracture. In this case, general joint laxity was certainly a key of diagnosis and treatment (Figure 6). Basically, the general joint laxity is essential information for diagnosing and determining treatment plan of instability-associated chronic joint disorders such as recurrent dislocation of the shoulder and patella [6–8], so experienced orthopedic surgeons usually keep in mind when they see a juvenile patient with joint instability. However, it does not tend to receive attention in trauma as much as chronic conditions, especially in cases with apparent and typical fracture, and is often overlooked by important soft tissue injury. In our case, her general joint laxity had been recognized from the past medical history, which provided more suitable assessments particularly regarding LCL injury and subsequent optimal treatment.

As mentioned, half of pediatric medial epicondyle fractures is associated with elbow dislocation [5]. According to cadaveric biomechanical studies, rotatory forces accompanied with valgus or varus stress are essential to the elbow dislocation mechanism, which typically results in medial and lateral collateral ligament avulsion at the humeral insertion [9]. In our case, it was unclear whether dislocation had occurred or not and whether it had naturally reduced before visiting the hospital because typical dislocation-associated fractures such as coronoid fracture and proximal radius fracture were not observed. However, humeral avulsion of the LCL concomitant with medial epicondyle fracture strongly suggested that abnormal varus and valgus forces were applied at the time of injury, which was possibly exaggerated by her original joint laxity. Though most of medial epicondyle fractures will have some ligament damages and not every case needs to fix the LCL complex, it would be beneficial to mind the possibility of severe LCL injury especially in cases with general joint laxity.

It should be discussed that treatment option of LCL avulsion, i.e., nonsurgical treatment with elbow immobilization following the repair of medial epicondyle fracture, might be a reasonable management for this injury. However, in our case, simultaneous surgical repair of the LCL was recommended because of the following reasons: (1) she had originally lax ligaments around her joints, (2) humeral LCL avulsion was strongly suspected from the preoperative CT and clearly confirmed by the ultrasonography, and (3) significant side-to-side difference of lateral instability was documented from the stress X-rays evaluated under anesthesia. It has been well known that posterolateral rotatory instability of the elbow after dislocation is one of the most significant causes of terrible dysfunction in daily and sports activities [9, 10], and a primary repair of the LCL complex could

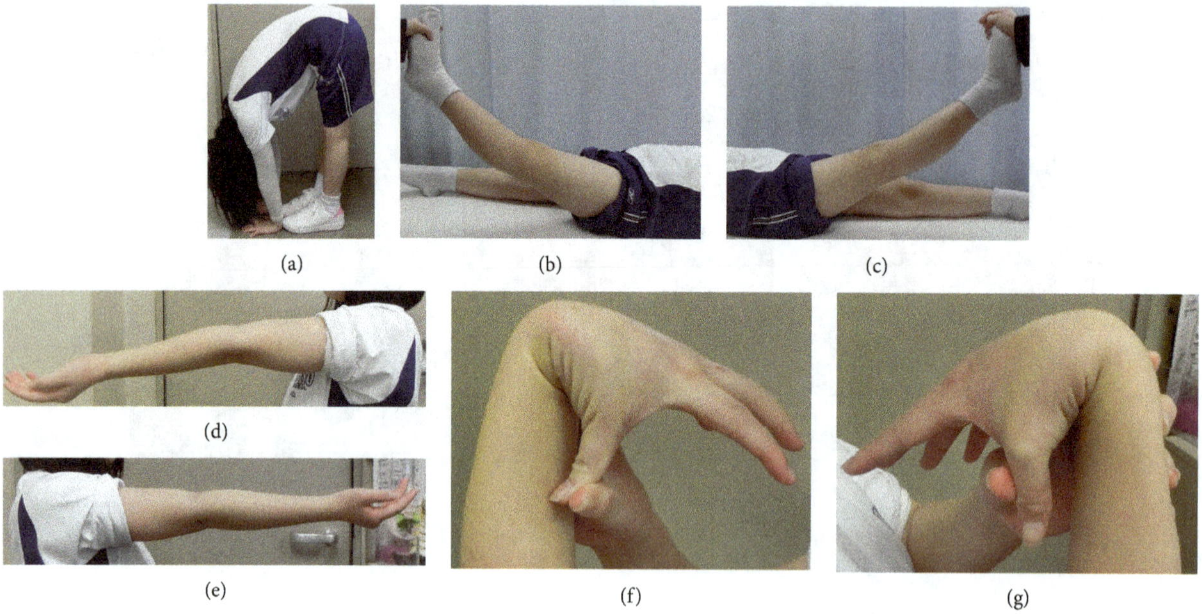

FIGURE 6: Her general joint laxity. (a) Spine. (b) Left knee. (c) Right knee. (d) Left elbow. (e) Right elbow. (f) Left wrist. (g) Right wrist. All photos were taken at the point of final follow-up so that the right knee (c) and the right elbow (e) did not show hyperextension due to surgical intervention.

possibly reduce risk for developing residual instability [11]. Though the follow-up period was relatively short in this report, our case showed satisfactory clinical and radiological results after the simultaneous surgical repair.

MRI should be a gold standard to assess ligament injury; however, ultrasonography is a good alternative that can provide both static and dynamic evaluations specifically for a site of ligament avulsion. In our case, it was hard to carry out a MRI because of her panic disorder and claustrophobia; nevertheless, avulsed LCL complex combined with unstable thin bony fragment was clearly confirmed by the ultrasonography before the skin incision, which encouraged us for determining the treatment plan. In addition, displaced medial epicondyle fracture did not cause any disturbance for the evaluation of the LCL complex. Of course, not every medial epicondyle fracture case needs ultrasonography, but it seems to be the most suitable evaluation to prevent overlooking important soft tissue damage coexisting with apparent elbow fractures in children.

References

[1] K. E. Wilkins, "Fractures involving the medial epicondylar apophysis," in *Fractures in Children*, C. A. Rockwood Jr., K. E. Wilkins, and R. E. King, Eds., JB Lippincott, Philadelphia, PA, USA, 3 edition, 1991.

[2] J. V. Fowles, N. Slimane, and M. T. Kassab, "Elbow dislocation with avulsion of the medial humeral epicondyle," *The Journal of Bone and Joint Surgery. British volume*, vol. 72-B, no. 1, pp. 102–104, 1990.

[3] H. H. Lee, H. C. Shen, J. H. Chang, C. H. Lee, and S. S. Wu, "Operative treatment of displaced medial epicondyle fractures in children and adolescents," *Journal of Shoulder and Elbow Surgery*, vol. 14, no. 2, pp. 178–185, 2005.

[4] A. F. Kamath, S. R. Cody, and H. S. Hosalkar, "Open reduction of medial epicondyle fractures: operative tips for technical ease," *Journal of Children's Orthopaedics*, vol. 3, no. 4, pp. 331–336, 2009.

[5] N. I. Wilson, R. Ingram, L. Rymaszewski, and J. H. Miller, "Treatment of fractures of the medial epicondyle of the humerus," *Injury*, vol. 19, no. 5, pp. 342–344, 1988.

[6] K. L. Camereon, M. L. Duffey, and T. M. DeBeradino, "Association of generalized joint hypermobility with a history of glenohumeral joint instability," *Journal of Athletic Training*, vol. 45, no. 3, pp. 253–258, 2010.

[7] J. M. Wolf, K. L. Camelon, and B. D. Owens, "Impact of joint laxity and hypermobility on the musukloskeletal system," *Journal of the American Academy of Orthopaedic Surgeons*, vol. 19, no. 8, pp. 463–471, 2011.

[8] G. Gurer, G. T. Bozbas, and T. Tuncer, "Frequency of joint hypermobility in Turkish patients with knee osteoarthritis: a cross sectional multicenter study," *International Journal of Rheumatic Diseases*, vol. 21, no. 10, pp. 1787–1792, 2016.

[9] S. Shemesh, M. I. Loebenberg, Y. Kosasahvilli, E. Sidon, S. Velkes, and S. D. Iordache, "Posterolateral rotatory instability of the elbow," *Harefuah*, vol. 153, no. 5, pp. 261–265, 2014.

[10] M. Hackl, T. Leschinger, L. P. Muller, and K. Wegmann, "Chronische Bandinstabilitäten des Ellenbogengelenks," *Der Orthopäde*, vol. 45, no. 10, pp. 809–821, 2016.

[11] B. S. Kim, K. H. Park, H. S. Song, and S. Y. Park, "Ligamentous repair of acute lateral collateral ligament rupture of the elbow," *Journal of Shoulder and Elbow Surgery*, vol. 22, no. 11, pp. 1469–1473, 2013.

16

Traumatic Craniocervical Dissociation in Patients with Congenital Assimilation of the Atlas to the Occiput

Celeste Tavolaro, Hector Pulido, Richard Bransford, and Carlo Bellabarba

Department of Orthopaedics & Sport Medicine, Harborview Medical Center, 325 Ninth Avenue Seattle, WA 98104, USA

Correspondence should be addressed to Richard Bransford; rbransfo@uw.edu

Academic Editor: Akio Sakamoto

Traumatic atlantooccipital dissociation (AOD) is a severe and usually fatal injury. Patients with assimilation of the atlas to the skull are exposed to a higher risk of injury and delay diagnosis due to the abnormal anatomy. We report two cases of acute traumatic craniocervical dislocation in patients with baseline congenital assimilation of the atlas to the skull. Computer tomography (CT) was used to identify the injury. Computer tomography angiography (CTA) showed variations of the vertebral arteries' location on both patients. Assimilation of the atlas was complete in patient one and partial in patient two. Emergent surgical instrumentation and fusion were performed with a very careful and meticulous posterior dissection. As general rule, most of the patients with CCD will undergo occiput to C2 posterior segmental instrumentation and fusion. In the presented cases, a more extensive fusion was necessary based on the type and severity of the CCJ injury and the anatomical anomalies associated. Postoperatively, patient one remained neurologically intact and patient two died. Alternative fixation techniques should be used to minimize risk of VA injury during the surgical procedures.

1. Introduction

Traumatic atlantooccipital dissociation (AOD) is a severe injury of the osseous and ligamentous complex that stabilizes the skull base to C1. The most common mechanism of injury is a high-energy trauma. AOD is associated with brainstem injury, neurogenic shock, and respiratory failure. Diagnosis delay is associated with higher rates of morbidity and mortality [1–4].

Congenital assimilation of the atlas is caused by failure of segmentation between the last occipital and first cervical sclerotome during the early fetal development with a reported incidence of 0.75%-3% [5, 6]. Due to the anomalous craniocervical anatomy, these patients are exposed to a higher risk for delay of injury recognition. A number of anatomical variants are associated with occipitalization of the atlas to the skull such as abnormal location of the vertebral arteries. Treatment options may vary depending on the type and severity of the AOD injury and the anatomical anomalies associated.

We describe two cases of traumatic craniocervical dislocation in patients with baseline congenital assimilation of the atlas to the skull. Our purpose is to highlight the surgical relevance and implications of these traumatic unstable injuries on patients with this abnormal anatomy.

2. Case 1

A 53-year-old male was involved in a mountain bike accident. Initial vital signs and neurological examination were normal, but he reported pain and tenderness on the upper part of his neck.

Cervical computed tomography (CT) revealed evidence of prior C5-C7 ACDF, as well as a complete congenital assimilation between the occiput and the atlas (C1), and also a congenital fusion through the disc space of the C2 and C3 (Klippel Feil syndrome). Imaging demonstrated a comminuted fracture of the anterior arch of C1 extending into the bilateral lateral mases of C1 as well as a fracture extending into the right atlantooccipital fusion mass. There was also

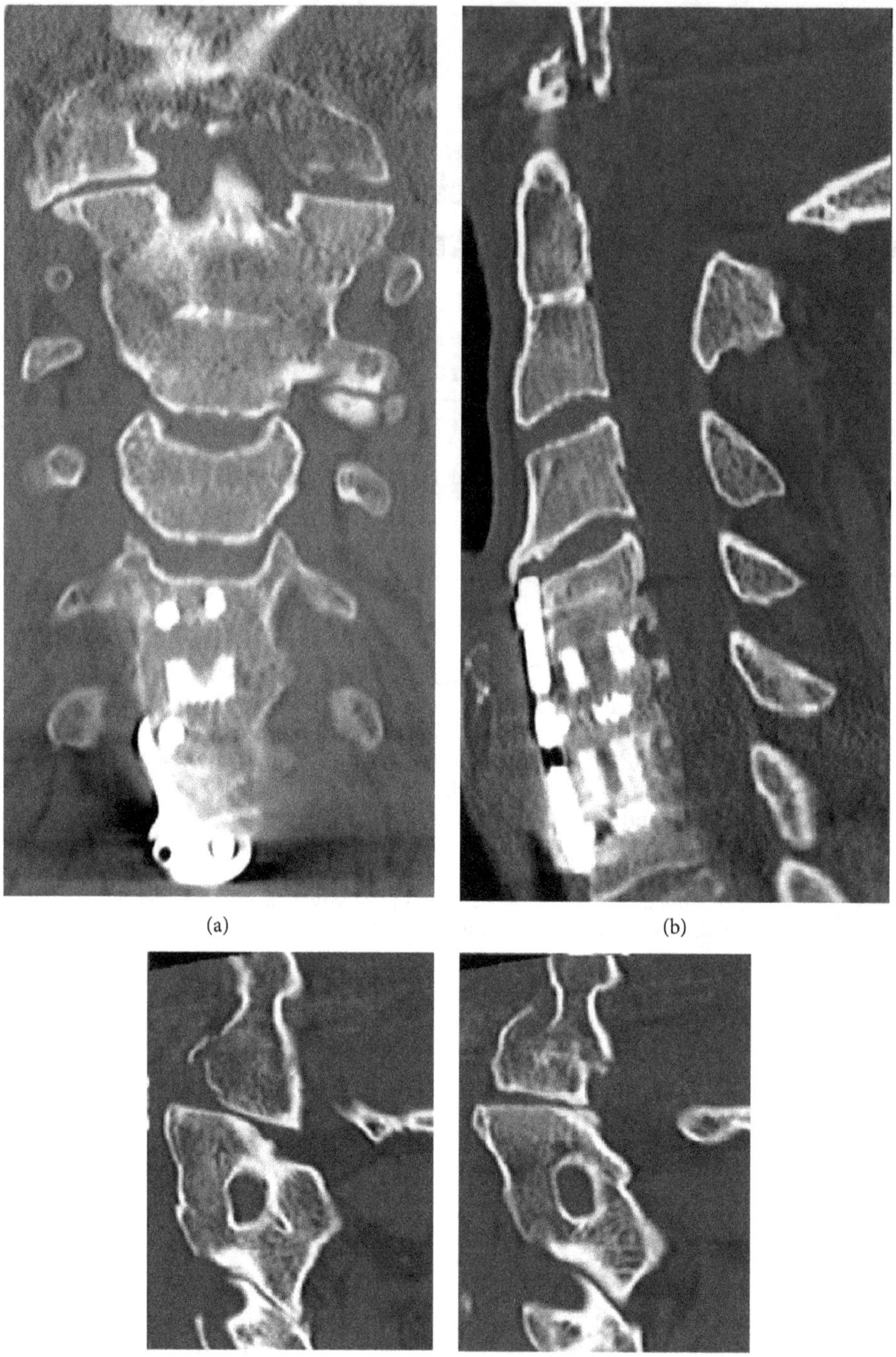

(a) (b) (c) (d)

Figure 1: Case 1: cervical CT. (a) Complete C1 assimilation, C2-C3 congenital fusion block. (b) Previous C5-C7 ACDF. The C1 anterior ring is fracture displaced and positioned anterior to the clivus. The C1 posterior arch is fused to the occiput. (c) Left atlantoaxial subluxation. (d) Right condyle C1 lateral mass fracture dislocation.

distraction on the left side between the atlantoaxial joint (Figure 1). Cervical computed tomography angiography (CTA) showed in the right vertebral artery, as it courses through the fracture occipito-C1 posterior arch assimilation, a focal luminal narrowing of 50% approximately (Biffl type 2) caused by blunt trauma mechanism.

Due to the complexity of the case, the patient was transported to our hospital's level 1 trauma center. After obtaining baseline electrodiagnostic signals, Mayfield tongs were applied and the patient was transferred to the Jackson table and rotated into a prone position. A cervical spine lateral fluoroscopic image was performed to evaluate the patient's craniocervical alignment. Electrodiagnostic signals remained stable after positioning. A midline posterior cervical incision and meticulous subperiosteal dissection were performed of the occiput to the level of C6. Open reduction of his craniocervical dissociation and occiput to C6 posterior segmental arthrodesis with placement of cortical screws in the occiput,

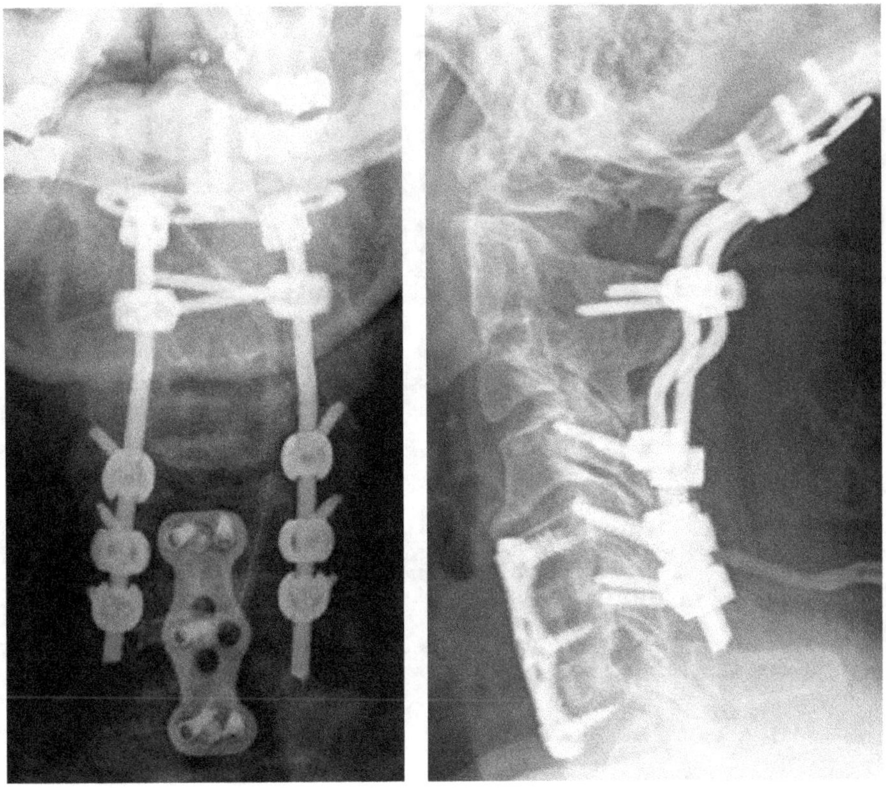

FIGURE 2: Case 1: postoperative X-ray. Occipito-C6 PSIF.

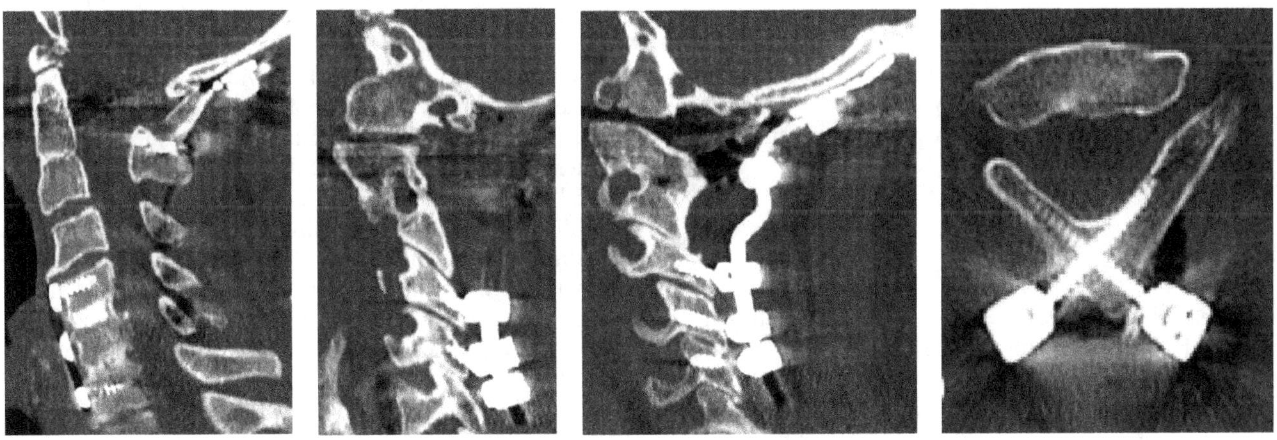

(a) (b) (c) (d)

FIGURE 3: Case 1: postoperative CT. (a) The reduction of the cortical step-off between the anterior arch of C1 and the clivus with partial reduction of the odontoid. (b) Right and (c) left. C1 screws were not placed. The vertebral arteries course bilaterally below the C1 ring. Lateral mass screw placed bilaterally at C4, C5, and C6. (d) Fixation to C2-C3 vertebrae block was obtained by placing laminar screws bilaterally at C2.

laminar screws bilaterally at C2, and lateral mass screws bilaterally at C4, C5, and C6 (Figure 2) were performed. Given the fact that the patient had a congenital fusion down to C3 as well as degenerative changes at C3-C4 and C4-C5, and previous ACDF at C5-C6 and C6-C7, his posterior cervical fixation was performed down into his subaxial cervical fusion in order to avoid short-term adjacent segment degeneration at C3-4 and C4-5 (Figure 3). Intraoperative, extensive instability and hypermobility at the C1-C2 levels as well as the C3 to C5 levels were noticeable. The vertebral arteries were identified coursing bilaterally below the C1 ring, given that the posterior ring of C1 was completely coalesced to the occiput. Due to these anatomical findings associated with the right atlantooccipital fracture dislocation, the C1 lateral mass screws were not placed. Atricortical structural iliac crest allograft was applied from the occiput to the C2 spinous

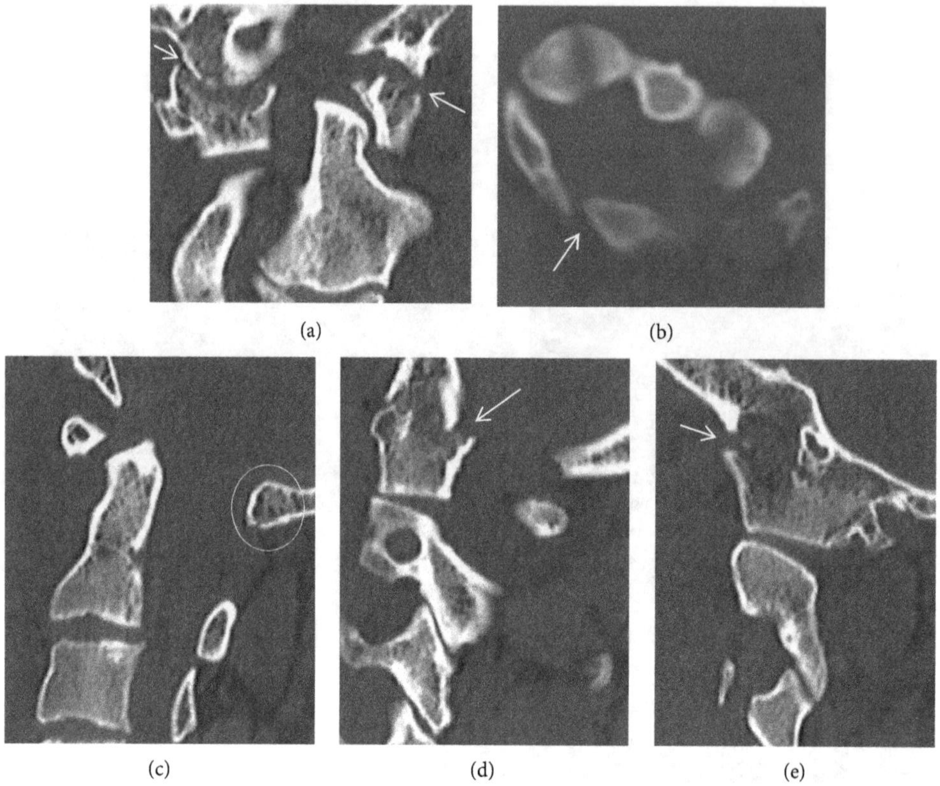

FIGURE 4: Case 2: cervical CT. C1 congenital partial assimilation to the skull base. (a) The right C1 lateral mass is partially fused with the right occipital condyle. The left C1 lateral mass is completely fused to the left condyle. The tip of the dens is dysplastic and asymmetrically positioned towards the left lateral mass. (b) The rachischisis of the C1 posterior arch. (d, e) Acute fracture dislocation of the previously right and left lateral mass assimilation, respectively.

process, and locally harvested autologous bone graft, allograft, and tricalcium phosphate bone graft substitutes were placed locally after decorticated the posterior occipitocervical spine.

3. Case 2

A 35-year-old male was a restrained driver involved in a head-on high-speed motor vehicle collision. He was unresponsive at the scene, intubated, and transferred to our hospital. On arrival to the emergency room, the patient received a high mechanism work-up which was negative for thoracic, abdominal, or pelvic injuries but did reveal an open right ulna fracture.

Head CT showed a left frontal subdural hematoma and epidural hematoma in the upper cervical region anterior to the cord which extended to the C4 level. Cervical CT revealed a congenital partial fusion of C1 to the occiput, involving complete fusion of the left lateral mass with the occipital condyle and partial fusion of the right lateral mass with the right occipital condyle. Posteriorly, the lamina was fused to the occiput on the left side. Craniocervical dissociation due to an acute fracture with distraction through the fused left occipital condyle-C1 lateral mass was recognized. The right C1 lateral mass was laterally subluxated in relation to the C2 lateral mass. The dysplastic tip of the dens showed an asymmetric mild widening on the right side in relation to the C1 lateral mass (Figure 4). Cervical computed tomography angiography (CTA) did not reveal any vascular injury.

Magnetic resonance imaging (T2 sequence) revealed a posterior longitudinal ligament disruption along with the apical, right alar, and right transverse ligaments as well as the disruption of the interspinous ligament at C1-C2 and the ligamenta nuchae. Posterior to the dens, an epidural hematoma that compressed the spinal cord was identified without evidence of spinal cord signal change. Also, a prevertebral hematoma extending from the CCJ to the C6 level was found.

Initially, the patient underwent a left-sided decompressive craniectomy. Once he was clear for spine surgery, baseline electrodiagnostic signals were obtained. Mayfield tongs were applied, and the patient was transferred to the Jackson table and rotated into a prone position. A cervical spine lateral fluoroscopic image was performed to evaluate the patient's craniocervical alignment. Electrodiagnostic signals remained stable after positioning. A midline posterior cervical incision and dissection were performed from the occiput to C3. Open reduction of the craniocervical dislocation and occiput to C3 posterior segmental arthrodesis was performed. C1 and C3 bilateral lateral mass screws and bilateral C2 pars screws were placed. Intraoperatively, significant instability between the occipital to C2 region was noticed as well as an abnormal vertebral artery (Figure 5). On the left side, the vertebral artery traversed underneath the fused occiput-C1 ring, whereas, on the right side, the C1 posterior

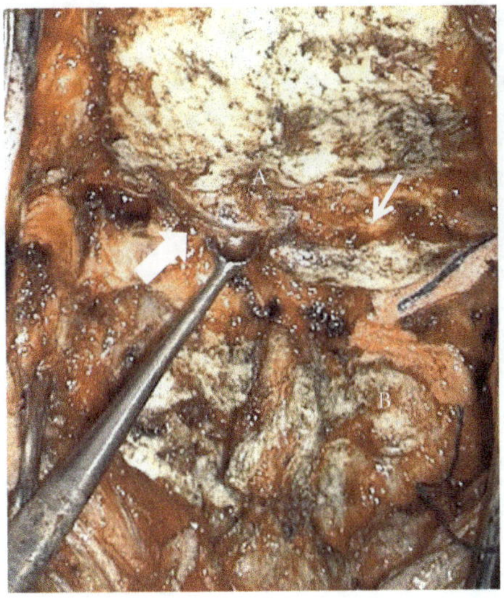

FIGURE 5: Case 2: intraoperative image. (A) Occiput. (B) C2 vertebra. (Upper arrow) left VA coursing above the free C1 posterior ring. (Thick arrow) right VA fused C1 posterior ring assimilated to the occiput.

arch was free of the occiput and the vertebral artery traversed above this (Figures 6 and 7). Atricortical structural iliac crest allograft was applied from the occiput to the C2 spinous process, and locally harvested autologous bone graft, allograft, and tricalcium phosphate bone graft substitutes were placed locally after decorticated the posterior occipitocervical spine.

During the postoperative hospital stay, the patient had a complication related to his severe traumatic brain injury which led to death.

4. Discussion

Traumatic atlantooccipital dissociation is a rarely observed but potentially severe injury of the osseous and ligamentous complex that stabilizes the skull base to the spine. The most common mechanism of injury is a high-energy trauma. The delay of injury recognition is associated with higher rates of morbidity and mortality [1–4]. In our patients, the atlantooccipital injury was recognized with index CT imaging.

Congenital assimilation of the atlas is caused by failure of segmentation between the last occipital and first cervical sclerotome during the early fetal development [5, 6]. It is described in the literature as the most common anomaly of the craniocervical junction with an incidence of 0.75%-3% and a male to female ratio of 5 : 1 [7–9]. Complete and partial assimilation have been described. Kim et al. [10] classified the assimilation of the atlas in zones depending on the location of the bony fusion between the atlas and the occiput. Zone 1 fusion involves the anterior arch of the atlas in front of the lateral masses; zone 2 fusion primarily involves the lateral processes; zone 3 fusion involves the posterior arch of the atlas behind the lateral masses; and zone 4 involves a combination of zones. According to this classification, the type of assimilation in both our patients included a combination of zones or zone 4. In case 1, the patient presents a complete assimilation of the atlas to the occiput, including the fusion of the bilateral lateral masses plus the anterior and posterior arch to the occiput. In case 2, the assimilation of the atlas was partial, including the complete fusion of the left lateral mass and the left side of the posterior arch of C1 to the skull and a partial fusion of the right lateral mass with the right occipital condyle.

There are a number of anatomical variants associated with occipitalization of the atlas to the occiput which are essential to know to make a correct diagnosis and surgical decision in the setting of trauma to the craniocervical junction (CCJ). Some of these anatomical variants can mimic fractures and should not be misinterpreted in patients with craniocervical injuries. Condylus tertius and calcification of the alar ligament may mimic an avulsion fracture of the occipital condyle. The posterior or/and anterior atlas rachischisis could be confuse with a C1 ring fracture. The ossiculum terminale may mimic a type 1 dens fracture and the Os odontoideum, a type 3 dens fracture [5]. The patient in case 2 presented a partial posterior ring assimilation associated to a posterior ring rachischisis, as well as a dysplastic C2 dens.

Furthermore, the assimilation of the atlas has been associated with other craniovertebral anomalies such as basilar invagination, atlantoaxial subluxation, variations of the vertebral arteries' (VAs') location, and cervical vertebral fusions [11]. The presence of blocked vertebrae between the skull and the atlas may accelerate the development of atlantoaxial instability, due to compensatory motion at the atlantoaxial joint. Both cases did not show any signs of basilar invagination or atlantoaxial subluxation. However, as can occur in up to 70% of the cases with assimilation of the atlas [8], the patient in case 1 presented a fusion block of the second and third cervical vertebrae (Klippel Feil syndrome).

In patients without anatomical variants of the craniocervical junction, the path of the vertebral artery (VA) is described in four segments: the first segment originates from the subclavical artery and enters the C6 transverse process, the second segment courses from C6 to C2 transverse process, the third from C2 to the foramen magnum, and the fourth segment enters the cranium to attend the basilar artery [12]. Patients with assimilation of the atlas may demonstrate an abnormal course of VA at the third segment, due to the osseous fusion between the atlas and occiput. Four types of VA courses were described in patients with assimilation of the atlas [13]. Type I VA is wherein the vessel enters the spinal canal below the C1 posterior arc and courses below the occipitalized C1 lateral mass; type II wherein the VA courses on the posterior surface of the occipitalized C1 lateral mass or makes a curve on it; type III in which the VA ascends laterally after leaving the axis transverse foramen, enters an osseous foramen created between the atlas and occipital bone, then reaches the cranium; and type IV wherein the VA is absent.

Both of our patients proved to have an abnormal course of the VA at the third segment. In case 1, the VA was identified as coursing bilaterally below the C1 ring, given that the posterior ring of C1 was completely coalesced to the occiput, corresponding to type I of the VA course classification described above. In case 2, on the left side, where a partial fusion of C1 was present, the VA coursed below the

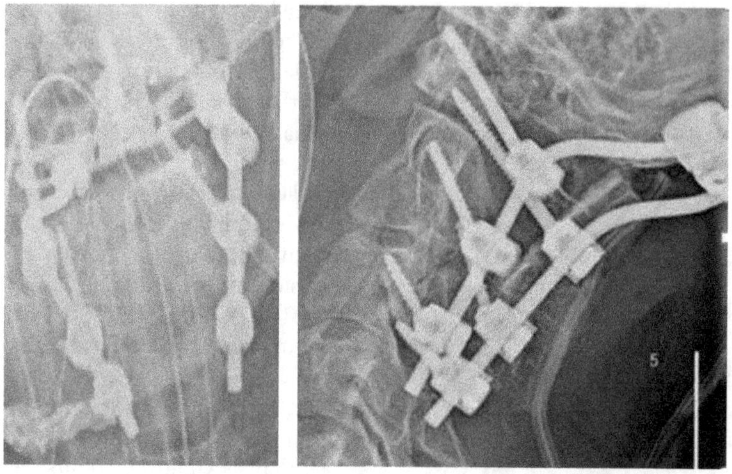

FIGURE 6: Case 2: postoperative X-ray. Occipito-C6 PSIF.

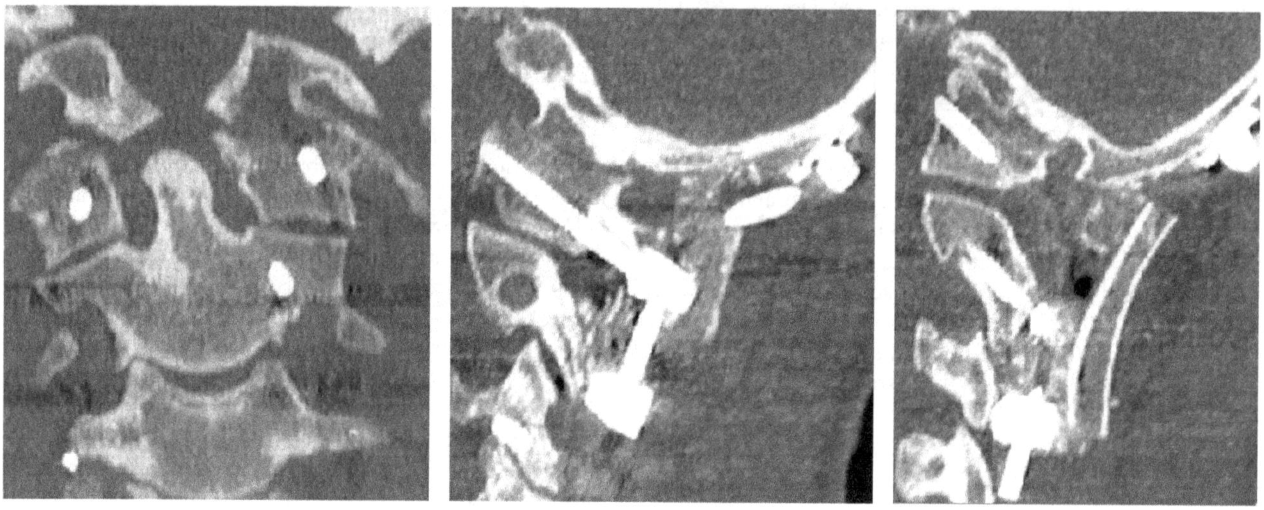

FIGURE 7: Case 2: CT postoperative. Anatomic alignment with reduction of the atlantooccipital fracture dislocation with bilateral C1, C2, and C3 lateral mass screws.

assimilated C1, and on the right side, where the C1 ring was free, the VA had a normal course. In this patient, there was no correlation with any of the VA course classifications.

As general rule, most of the patients with CCD will undergo at least an occiput to C2 posterior segmental instrumentation and fusion. Treatment options may vary depending on the type and severity of the CCJ injury and the anatomical anomalies associated. A detailed CT and CTA review should be performed in order to have a better understanding of the injury and the potential anatomical variations, especially to determine the course of the vertebral arteries. A very careful and meticulous posterior dissection should be performed in all the cases with CCD but especially in those with bony assimilations and VA abnormalities, in order to decrease the risk of VA injury during the surgical approach [11]. When the VA courses above the posterior C1 arch, the placement of lateral mass screws at C1 is relatively safe. However, the risk may increase significantly with any anomalous coursing of the VA, and other techniques of internal fixation may be safer options [10].

In both cases presented in this study, given the instability, the treatment of choice was open reduction and occipitocervical fusion. However, in case 1, it was not possible to place the C1 lateral mass screws due to the anomalous path of the VA, along with the fracture of the hypoplastic C1 lateral mass-condyle. The C2-C3 block vertebrae associated with an anomalous lateral mass did not allow the placement of lateral mass screws at these levels, and thus the fixation was obtained by the placement of C2 bilateral laminar screws. Finally, due to the previous C5-C7 ACDF associated with intraoperative findings of extensive instability and hypermobility at C3-C4 and C4-C5 levels, the extension of the instrumentation was performed down to the C6 level. In case 2, intraoperative, the dislocation between the occipital and C2 was noticed. On the right side where the C1 posterior arch was not assimilated to the occiput, the VA traversed above this, allowing for safe placement of the C1 lateral mass screw. On the left side, the VA was below and well protected by the ring attached to the occiput, allowing the placement of the C1 lateral mass. The patients had smaller size of C2 pedicles, particularly on the right side for screw placement. Ji et al. [14] describe in their study that the C2 pars/pedicle architectures are significantly smaller in patients with assimilation of the atlas than in the normal population. They suggested that translaminar screw is the more viable option in comparison with pedicle screw for C2. In our case, short screws were placed at C2 level but we do not consider that it had sufficient stability given the injury, and thus, we decided to extend to the fixation down to the C3 level with lateral mass screws.

5. Conclusion

(i) High clinical suspicion, early recognition, and treatment of traumatic craniocervical dissociation are associated with better outcomes and a higher survival rate

(ii) Patients with assimilation of the atlas to the skull frequently have other associated craniocervical malformations, such as variations of the vertebral arteries' location and other cervical vertebral fusions

(iii) The identification of an abnormal path of the vertebral artery, under the posterior ring of C1, along a C1 lateral mass hypoplastic and fracture, made the C1 lateral mass screw placement difficult and dangerous. Alternative fixation techniques should be used to minimize risk of VA injury during the surgical procedures

(iv) The association of cranial cervical assimilations with other subaxial congenital fusions may require a more extensive instrumentation and fusion than what is normally performed in cases without assimilation of the atlas to the occiput

References

[1] A. Reis, R. Bransford, T. Penoyar, J. R. Chapman, and C. Bellabarba, "Diagnosis and treatment of craniocervical dissociation in 48 consecutive survivors," *Evidence-Based Spine-Care Journal*, vol. 1, no. 2, pp. 69-70, 2010.

[2] C. Bellabarba, S. K. Mirza, G. A. West et al., "Diagnosis and treatment of craniocervical dislocation in a series of 17 consecutive survivors during an 8-year period," *Journal of Neurosurgery: Spine*, vol. 4, no. 6, pp. 429–440, 2006.

[3] J. B. Shatsky, T. B. Alton, C. Bellabarba, and R. J. Bransford, "Occult cranial cervical dislocation: a case report and brief literature review," *Case Reports in Orthopedics*, vol. 2016, Article ID 4930285, 6 pages, 2016.

[4] C. Tavolaro, R. Bransford, A. Yerrapragada, C. Bellabarba, and H. Zhou, "Occipitocervical dislocation in low-energy trauma," *Case Reports in Orthopedics*, vol. 2018, no. 20, 5 pages, 2018.

[5] C. E. Offiah and E. Day, "The craniocervical junction: embryology, anatomy, biomechanics and imaging in blunt trauma," *Insights Imaging*, vol. 8, no. 1, pp. 29–47, 2017.

[6] D. K. Sharma, D. Sharma, and V. Sharma, "Atlantooccipital fusion: prevalence and its developmental and clinical correlation," *Journal of Clinical and Diagnostic Research: JCDR*, vol. 11, no. 6, 2017.

[6] D. K. Sharma, D. Sharma, and V. Sharma, "Atlantooccipital fusion: prevalence and its developmental and clinical correlation," *Journal of Clinical and Diagnostic Research: JCDR*, vol. 11, no. 6, 2017.

[7] S. M. Burke, T. A. Huhta, C. E. Mackel, and R. I. Riesenburger, "Occipital condyle fracture in a patient with occipitalisation of the atlas," *BML Case Reports*, vol. 2015, no. may14 1, 2015.

[8] P. Soni, V. Sharma, and J. Sengupta, "Cervical vertebrae anomalies - incidental findings on lateral cephalograms," *The Angle Orthodontist*, vol. 78, no. 1, pp. 176–180, 2008.

[9] K. Khamanarong, W. Woraputtaporn, S. Ratanasuwan, M. Namking, W. Chaijaroonkhanarak, and S. Sae-Jung, "Occipitalization of the atlas: its incidence and clinical implications," *Acta Medica Academica*, vol. 42, no. 1, pp. 41–45, 2013.

[10] M. S. Kim, "Anatomical variant of atlas: arcuate foramen, occpitalization of atlas, and defect of posterior arch of atlas," *Journal of Korean Neurosurgical Association*, vol. 58, no. 6, pp. 528–533, 2015.

[11] Y. Tatara, T. Shimizu, K. Fueki et al., "Clinical and anatomical features as well as pathological conditions of surgically treated adult patients with occipitalization of the atlas," *International Journal of Spine Surgery*, vol. 10, 2016.

[12] T. Gupta, "Quantitative anatomy of vertebral artery groove on the posterior arch of atlas in relation to spinal surgical procedures," *Surgical and Radiologic Anatomy*, vol. 30, no. 3, pp. 239–242, 2008.

[13] S. Wang, C. Wang, Y. Liu, M. Yan, and H. Zhou, "Anomalous vertebral artery in craniovertebral junction with occipitalization of the atlas," *Spine (Phila Pa 1976)*, vol. 34, no. 26, pp. 2838–2842, 2009.

[14] W. Ji, X. Liu, W. Huang et al., "Feasibility of C2 vertebra screws placement in patient with occipitalization of atlas: a tomographic study," *Medicine*, vol. 94, no. 37, p. e1492, 2015.

17

Impact of Jiggling Exercise as Conservative Treatment for Hip Osteoarthritis: A Report of Two Cases

Yohei Teramoto,[1] Kensuke Fukushima,[1] Tomohisa Koyama,[1] Yoshihisa Ohashi,[1] Katsufumi Uchiyama,[1] Naonobu Takahira,[2] and Masashi Takaso[1]

[1]*Department of Orthopaedic Surgery, Kitasato University School of Medicine, 1-15-1 Kitasato, Minami-ku, Sagamihara, Kanagawa 252-0374, Japan*
[2]*Department of Rehabilitation, Kitasato University School of Allied Health Sciences, Japan*

Correspondence should be addressed to Kensuke Fukushima; kenfu@r4.dion.ne.jp

Academic Editor: Werner Kolb

Total hip arthroplasty has been recognized as a feasible treatment for hip osteoarthritis, especially in advanced and terminal stages, but whether it is the best treatment for patients who are younger, have comorbidities, and/or are likely to have low compliance to medical treatment is unknown. Jiggling exercise, which involves the continuous shaking of the foot and leg in small steps, has been reported to be the easiest and a less invasive exercise for patients with hip osteoarthritis. We herein report two patients who performed jiggling exercise as conservative treatment and had successful outcomes. The first case was a 28-year-old woman with advanced-stage hip osteoarthritis that could not be treated with hip preservation surgery; furthermore, the patient refused to undergo total hip arthroplasty because of her young age. The second case was a 74-year-old woman with terminal-stage hip osteoarthritis in whom total hip arthroplasty was deemed not feasible because of possible low compliance due to mental disorder. One year after the initiation of the jiggling exercise, both patients had remarkable clinical improvement. Three years later, remarkable joint remodelling was also revealed in plain radiographs. Jiggling exercise might be a feasible conservative treatment option for joint preservation.

1. Introduction

Hip disorders such as hip osteoarthritis (OA) directly affect patients' activities of daily living (ADLs). Advanced- and terminal-stage hip OA causes severe restriction of hip range of motion (ROM) and hip pain. Total hip arthroplasty (THA) has been recognized as a feasible treatment for hip OA especially in advanced and terminal stages. THA has a great advantage in terms of early rehabilitation and recovery of ADL [1] as well as successful longevity [2, 3]. However, disadvantages and complications after THA, such as lack of durability and dislocation, have also been reported [4]. In addition, the question remains whether THA is the best treatment solution for patients who are younger, have comorbidities, and/or are likely to have low compliance to medical treatment [5].

Jiggling exercise, which involves the continuous shaking of the foot and leg in small steps (Figure 1), has been reported to be the easiest and a less invasive exercise for patients with advanced- and terminal-stage hip OA [6]. Some case reports describing the efficacy of jiggling exercise for hip OA based on clinical and radiographic results have been published only in Japanese [7–9].

We have attempted jiggling exercise as conservative treatment for patients with advanced- and terminal-stage hip OA and patients who note OA progression after performing joint preservation surgery such as hip osteotomy and hip arthroscopy. We believe that patients who refuse to undergo THA or have contraindication(s) to THA (e.g., relatively young age, presence of comorbidities, and low compliance to medical treatments) might be good candidates for jiggling exercise. Patients are instructed to shake their foot and legs continuously in small steps whilst sitting on a chair for at least 30 minutes a day and for two sets, or for as long as the patients can tolerate the exercise. We also coadminister medications

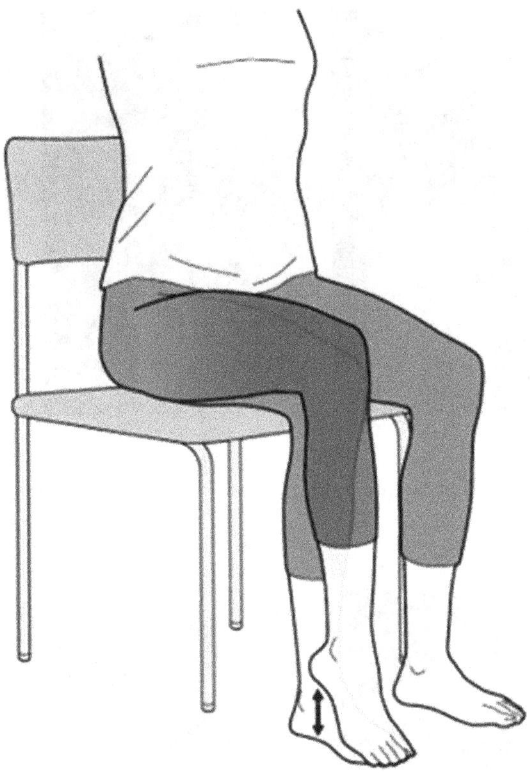

Figure 1: Jiggling exercise method. The patient continuously shakes his or her foot and leg in small steps whilst sitting on a chair for at least 30 minutes a day.

such as nonsteroidal anti-inflammatory drugs (NSAIDs) to the patients especially during the initial application of the exercise.

Our aim is to report typical cases of our two patients who were successfully treated with jiggling exercise. Both patients provided written consent for the publication of the case reports, including patient information and accompanying images.

2. Case Presentation

2.1. Case 1. A 28-year-old woman complained of severe left hip pain and difficulty walking. The pain started to develop when she was in her early twenties, with the intensity increasing with the intensity of physical work. She consulted a nearby orthopaedic department. The attending physician diagnosed her as having hip OA and referred her to our hospital for advanced examination and treatment. The patient was a nurse. She had no clinical history of treatment for hip disorders such as developmental dysplasia of the hip in childhood. With regard to her hip pain, she reported that the pain was present both at rest and during walking. Regarding her left hip, she additionally had tenderness at the femoral triangle of Scarpa, and both Patrick's test and anterior impingement test had positive results. The ROMs of her left hip were 130° in flexion, 20° in abduction, 30° in adduction, 30° in external rotation, and 10° in internal rotation, whereas ROMs of her right hip were limited especially in abduction and internal rotation, and she reported groin pain at the end of the motion. Her Japanese Orthopaedic Association (JOA) hip score was 57/100. Her left hip radiograph showed degenerative arthritis categorised as Tönnis grade 2, and bone cysts were noted on the femoral heads (Figure 2(a)).

Since improvements of joint congruity and space width were not investigated in hip abduction and adduction radiographs, we concluded that joint preservation surgeries such as periacetabular osteotomy could not be indicated for this patient. Moreover, she refused to undergo THA because of her young age. She was treated with NSAIDs and was instructed to perform general muscle and ROM exercises around the hip joint for 6 months. However, her hip pain did not improve, and repeat radiographs revealed OA progression. Hence, we recommended intensive jiggling exercise combined with medication.

One year after the initiation of jiggling exercise, the patient's hip pain notably improved, despite the absence of changes in the hip radiographs (Figure 2(b)). She was able to interrupt NSAID treatment. Three years later, the patient's hip pain remarkably improved and the radiographs of the hip joint showed notable improvement in terms of congruity and space width (Figure 2(c)). At the last follow-up, 4 years after the indication of the jiggling exercise, radiography revealed improved joint remodelling (Figure 2(d)). The ROMs of her left hip were slightly increased as 130° in flexion, 30° in abduction, 30° in adduction, 40° in external rotation, and 10° in internal rotation. Additionally, the JOA hip score was 84/100, which was assessed to be clinically effective.

2.2. Case 2. A 74-year-old woman was referred to our department for examination and treatment of severe left hip pain. The patient underwent surgical intervention for breast cancer 10 years before. In addition, she has been treated for schizophrenia for more than 30 years, and her communication skills were hindered by her mental disorder. Although she could perform her main ADLs whilst using a wheelchair, she complained of severe hip pain on sitting and when transferring to a wheelchair and thus required a high level of assistance.

She presented with tenderness at the femoral triangle of Scarpa on her left hip, and both the Patrick's test and anterior impingement test had positive results. The ROMs of her left hip were 60° in flexion, -20° in extension, 10° in abduction, 10° in adduction, 20° in external rotation, and 10° in internal rotation, which were severely limited. The radiograph on her left hip showed degenerative arthritis categorised as Tönnis grade 3, terminal OA (Figure 3(a)).

Considering her comorbidities and ADLs, THA was concluded to be too invasive for the patient. Since she could follow simple instructions, we prescribed an intensive jiggling exercise without additional medication. One year after the initiation of jiggling exercise, the patient's hip pain and ROM remarkably improved, and the plain radiograph of the hip revealed some improvement of joint congruity (Figure 3(b)). After 2 years, she could walk indoors with a cane. The radiographs of the hip joint showed remarkable improvement of joint congruity and space width (Figure 3(c)). After 3 years, at the last follow-up, her pain had already disappeared. The ROMs of her left hip were 120° in flexion, 40° in abduction,

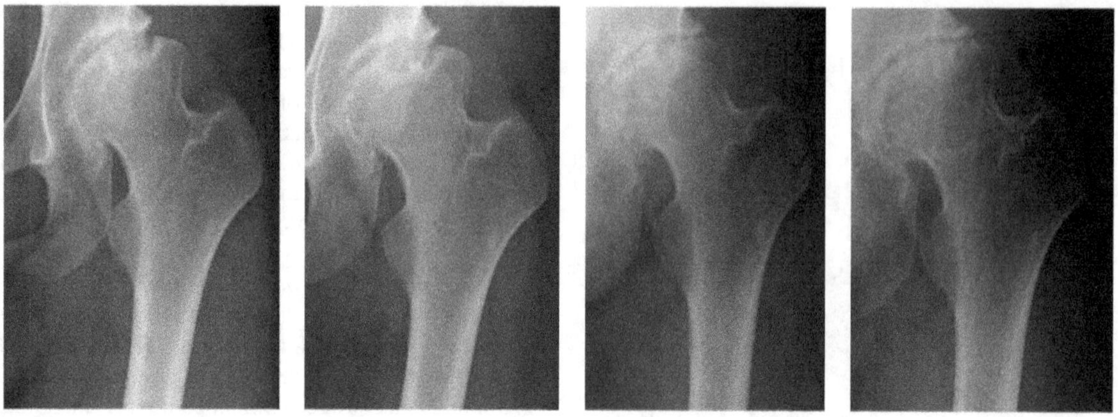

(a) (b) (c) (d)

FIGURE 2: Plain radiograph for case 1, showing the hips at (a) first admission and at (b) 1 year, (c) 3 years, and (d) 4 years after the initiation of jiggling exercise.

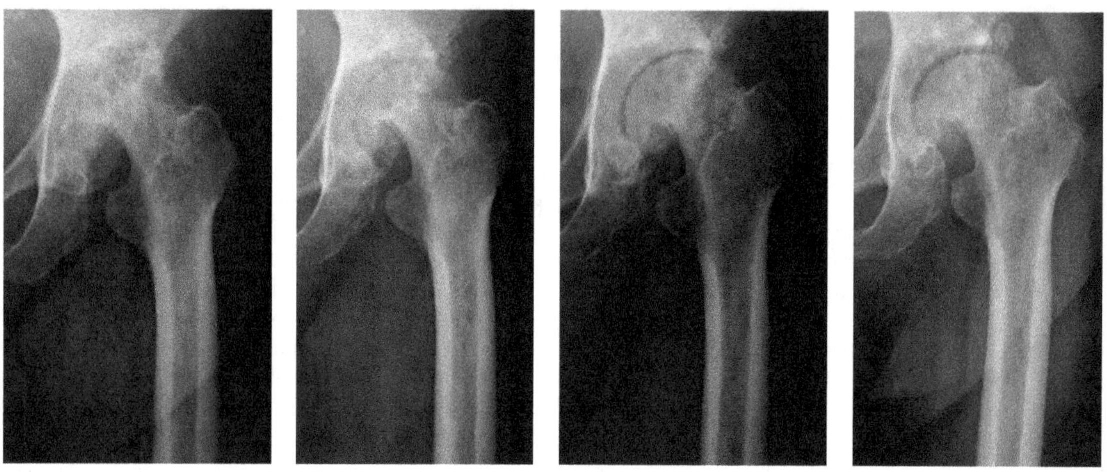

(a) (b) (c) (d)

FIGURE 3: Plain radiograph for case 2, showing the hips at (a) first admission and at (b) 1 year, (c) 2 years, and (d) 3 years after the initiation of jiggling exercise.

30° in adduction, 50° in external rotation, and 20° in internal rotation, which were remarkably improved. Furthermore, plain radiographs revealed improving joint remodelling (Figure 3(d)).

3. Discussion

Conservative treatment for patients with advanced- and terminal-stage hip OA and patients with OA progression after joint preservation surgery is quite limited. Many guidelines for OA management recommend low-impact exercise such as ROM/flexibility, quadriceps strengthening, and aerobic exercises (land or water based) [10]. Teirlinck et al. [11] reported the results of a multicentre, pragmatic randomised controlled trial for patients with hip OA who underwent physical therapy, and they observed a difference in function at the 3-month follow-up, but there was no difference at the 12-month follow-up. In addition, performing exercise for patients with advanced- and terminal-stage hip OA might increase hip joint pain.

With regard to treatment using medications, many guidelines consistently recommend acetaminophen as first-line pharmacologic management of OA [10]. However, acetaminophen treatment might not affect the pathological mechanism of OA. Thus, its effectiveness might be temporary for patients with advanced- and terminal-stage hip OA. NSAIDs are also generally used in the treatment of OA. The Coxib and Traditional NSAID Trialists' Collaboration [12] reported on the side effects of NSAIDs, including selective COX-2 inhibitors and traditional NSAIDs, based on the results of a meta-analysis and stated that all NSAID regimens increased upper gastrointestinal complications compared to placebo. Emkey et al. [13] reported that the rate of pain relief was significantly lower for participants treated with tramadol/acetaminophen in combination with COX-2 inhibitors compared with participants treated with placebo and a COX-2 NSAID. However, in this multicentre, placebo-controlled study intended for patients with OA, tramadol recipients frequently had central nervous system complications [14]. Since hip OA is a chronic and degenerative disorder, longitudinal administration of drugs might increase the risks of side effects. We believe that easy administration and increasing the dose of the medicine should be avoided as much as possible.

THA is advantageous in terms of early postoperative pain relief and rehabilitation for patients with advanced- and terminal-stage hip OA. However, there is a risk of complications such as aseptic loosening and/or dislocation especially in relatively younger, active, and nonadherent patients [15]. Furthermore, we should consider the management for patients who cannot undergo THA because of physical and/or social constraints or those who refuse to undergo THA.

Jiggling exercise was first described as a conservative treatment for patients with OA progression following hip osteotomy by Hiromatsu and Inoue [6]. The concept of the exercise was developed as a form of continuous passive motion (CPM) exercise, which was described by Salter et al. [16, 17] who investigated the biological effect of CPM on the healing of full-thickness articular cartilage using rabbit model. Many studies have followed the study of Salter et al., and CPM has been described to contribute to the improvement of joint health by preventing joint stiffness, preserving normal articular tissue with better histologic and biologic properties and improving the ROM, compared with joint immobilisation and intermittent active motion [18]. Since jiggling exercise was designed to be much simpler and easier than CPM, it could be more feasible for patients to perform and continue as home exercise. Although we did not assess the effectiveness of joint remodelling, we think that the medications for pain control should be combined to perform and continue the exercise.

In the present report, our two patients who performed jiggling exercise were observed radiographically to have remarkable joint remodelling. Similar remodelling has been noted after femoral valgus osteotomy for patients with advanced- and terminal-stage hip OA [19]. Furthermore, a study reported the effectiveness of muscle-release operation for patients with advanced- and terminal-stage hip OA [20]. Maniwa et al. [9] have investigated the tension of the muscle around the hip joint before and after jiggling exercise. They reported that the tension of the muscle around the hip joint in patients with hip OA significantly decreased after performing jiggling exercise. Changes in mechanical environment of the joint might induce the body's inherent self-repair ability and promote natural healing of the hip joint. We believe that jiggling exercise has effects not only on pain relief and improving range of motion but also on promoting natural healing and joint preservation of the hip joint.

We have indicated jiggling exercise mainly for patients who show advanced- and terminal-stage hip OA and cannot undergo THA for some reason. The cases that we have treated with jiggling exercise have been very few to date. In addition, to confirm the clinical effectiveness of jiggling exercise, a relatively longer observation time compared with other treatments might be needed. The effectiveness of jiggling exercise for the patients with early-stage OA and other hip disorders such as labral tear, femoroacetabular impingement (FAI), and osteonecrosis of femoral head (ONFH) remains unclear. Further case-control and prospective randomised control studies with a sufficient number of patients are needed to clarify the effectiveness and limitations of jiggling exercise.

4. Conclusion

We have described two typical cases of patients with advanced-stage hip OA who were successfully treated with jiggling exercises. Although radiographic joint remodelling took a relatively longer time, the two patients who performed jiggling exercise as conservative treatment showed remarkable clinical improvement. Jiggling exercise might be a feasible conservative treatment option for hip OA.

References

[1] R. Pivec, A. J. Johnson, S. C. Mears, and M. A. Mont, "Hip arthroplasty," *Lancet*, vol. 380, no. 9855, pp. 1768–1777, 2012.

[2] J. J. Callaghan, P. Bracha, S. S. Liu, S. Piyaworakhun, D. D. Goetz, and R. C. Johnston, "Survivorship of a Charnley total hip arthroplasty. A concise follow-up, at a minimum of thirty-five years, of previous reports," *The Journal of Bone & Joint Surgery*, vol. 91, no. 11, pp. 2617–2621, 2009.

[3] H. S. Khanuja, J. J. Vakil, M. S. Goddard, and M. A. Mont, "Cementless femoral fixation in total hip arthroplasty," *The Journal of Bone & Joint Surgery*, vol. 93, no. 5, pp. 500–509, 2011.

[4] K. J. Bozic, S. M. Kurtz, E. Lau, K. Ong, T. P. Vail, and D. J. Berry, "The epidemiology of revision total hip arthroplasty in the United States," *The Journal of Bone and Joint Surgery. American Volume*, vol. 91, no. 1, pp. 128–133, 2009.

[5] M. G. J. Gademan, S. N. Hofstede, T. P. M. Vliet Vlieland, R. G. H. H. Nelissen, and P. J. Marang-van de Mheen, "Indication criteria for total hip or knee arthroplasty in osteoarthritis: a state-of-the-science overview," *BMC Musculoskeletal Disorders*, vol. 17, no. 1, 2016.

[6] M. Hiromatsu and A. Inoue, "Is leg jiggling effective for articular cartilage regeneration of osteoarthritis of the hip?," *Bone Joint Nerve.*, vol. 3, pp. 475–482, 2013, (in Japanese).

[7] M. Sakaino, H. Kinoshita, T. Isayama, and A. Inoue, "Treatment for the unsuccessful cases after rotational acetabular osteotomy for secondary hip osteoarthritis," *Orthopaedics and Traumatology*, vol. 62, pp. 124–130, 2013, (in Japanese).

[8] M. Hiromatsu, H. Kinoshita, and A. Inoue, "Impact of jiggling exercise to hip osteoarthritis after hip preservation surgery," *Orthopaedics and Traumatology*, vol. 65, pp. 389–395, 2016, (in Japanese).

[9] S. Maniwa, T. Tanaka, S. Kadowaki, and Y. Uchio, "Jiggling changes muscle tones around hip joint in the patients with hip osteoarthritis," *Hip Joint.*, vol. 43, pp. 998–1000, 2017, (in Japanese).

[10] A. E. Nelson, K. D. Allen, Y. M. Golightly, A. P. Goode, and J. M. Jordan, "A systematic review of recommendations and guidelines for the management of osteoarthritis: The Chronic Osteoarthritis Management Initiative of the U.S. Bone and Joint Initiative," *Seminars in Arthritis and Rheumatism*, vol. 43, no. 6, pp. 701–712, 2014.

[11] C. H. Teirlinck, P. A. J. Luijsterburg, J. Dekker et al., "Effectiveness of exercise therapy added to general practitioner care in patients with hip osteoarthritis: a pragmatic randomized con-

trolled trial," *Osteoarthritis and Cartilage*, vol. 24, no. 1, pp. 82–90, 2016.

[12] Coxib and traditional NSAID Trialists' (CNT) Collaboration, N. Bhala, J. Emberson et al., "Vascular and upper gastrointestinal effects of non-steroidal anti-inflammatory drugs: meta-analyses of individual participant data from randomised trials," *The Lancet*, vol. 382, no. 9894, pp. 769–779, 2013.

[13] R. Emkey, N. Rosenthal, S. C. Wu, D. Jordan, M. Kamin, and CAPSS-114 Study Group, "Efficacy and safety of tramadol/-acetaminophen tablets (Ultracet) as add-on therapy for osteoarthritis pain in subjects receiving a COX-2 nonsteroidal antiinflammatory drug: a multicenter, randomized, double-blind, placebo-controlled trial," *The Journal of Rheumatology*, vol. 31, no. 1, pp. 150–156, 2004.

[14] H. Malonne, M. Coffiner, B. Sonet, A. Sereno, and F. Vanderbist, "Efficacy and tolerability of sustained-release tramadolin the treatment of symptomatic osteoarthritis of the hip or knee: A multicenter, randomized, double-blind, placebo-controlled study," *Clinical Therapeutics*, vol. 26, no. 11, pp. 1774–1782, 2004.

[15] J. Girard, C. Glorion, F. Bonnomet, D. Fron, and H. Migaud, "Risk factors for revision of hip arthroplasties in patients younger than 30 years," *Clinical Orthopaedics and Related Research*, vol. 469, no. 4, pp. 1141–1147, 2011.

[16] R. B. Salter, D. F. Simmonds, B. W. Malcolm, E. J. Rumble, D. MacMichael, and N. D. Clements, "The biological effect of continuous passive motion on the healing of full-thickness defects in articular cartilage. An experimental investigation in the rabbit," *The Journal of Bone and Joint Surgery. American Volume*, vol. 62, no. 8, pp. 1232–1251, 1980.

[17] R. B. Salter, "The biologic concept of continuous passive motion of synovial Joints," *Clinical Orthopaedics and Related Research*, vol. &NA;, no. 242, pp. 12???25–12???25, 1989.

[18] D. M. Knapik, J. D. Harris, G. Pangrazzi et al., "The basic science of continuous passive motion in promoting knee health: a systematic review of studies in a rabbit model," *Arthroscopy: The Journal of Arthroscopic & Related Surgery*, vol. 29, no. 10, pp. 1722–1731, 2013.

[19] S. Takasaki, K. Uchiyama, N. Takahira, and M. Itoman, "Results and prognostic factors of valgus osteotomy in middle-aged patients with advanced or terminal osteoarthritis of the hip," *Journal of Orthopaedic Science*, vol. 15, no. 1, pp. 20–29, 2010.

[20] C. P. Van Nes, "The significance of the muscle-release operations in the treatment of osteoarthritis of the hip," *Reconstruction Surgery and Traumatology*, vol. 12, pp. 218–229, 1971.

18

Stress Fracture of the Hamate Hook in a Water Polo Player

Hana Ueda, Shunpei Hama, Masataka Yasuda, Kenta Minato, Masahiro Miyashita, and Kishik Shin

Department of Orthopaedic Surgery, Baba Memorial Hospital, 4-244 Nishiku Hamadera Funao-cho Higashi, Sakai, Osaka 592-8555, Japan

Correspondence should be addressed to Hana Ueda; u.hana-osaka@hotmail.co.jp

Academic Editor: John Nyland

Hamate hook fractures are usually caused by direct trauma while using a tennis racket or a baseball bat. We report stress fracture of the hamate hook in a water polo player without any specific trauma. We consider that the stress fracture occurred via indirect mechanisms through the flexor tendons. Strong ulnar deviation of the wrist during ball release and strong grip on a ball with outstretched fingers, which are unique to water polo, were the likely causes of the stress fracture of the hamate hook.

1. Introduction

The hamate hook is an eminence of bone at the hypothenar region and the attachment point for the flexor digiti minimi brevis, abductor digiti minimi, flexor retinaculum, and piso-hamate ligament as well as a pulley for the flexor tendons. Fractures of the hamate hook are usually caused by direct trauma while playing racket sports, baseball, or golf [1]. We report stress fracture of the hamate hook in a 17-year-old water polo player without any direct trauma, likely caused by indirect mechanisms.

2. Case Presentation

A 17-year-old male water polo player presented with pain in the ulnar side of the right wrist for the past 3 months. He is a member of the water polo team at his high school, and his level was high enough to participate in the interscholastic water polo competition. After shooting a goal 1 week ago, his pain increased; however, there was no previous direct trauma to the right wrist. Upon an initial presentation to a private clinic, no specific injury was diagnosed, and he was then referred to our institution.

Upon initial physical examination, he had tenderness on the hypothenar region and ulnar pain when moving the wrist. The grip strength of his right hand was 10 kg, contrasted with 44 kg of the left hand. Radiographs taken in the previous clinic did not show any injury (Figure 1). Tenderness around the pisiform was also noted, and because arthritis of the joint was suspected, triamcinolone acetonide was injected into the pisotriquetral joint region.

One week after the injection, he showed improved tenderness around the pisiform; however, hypothenar pain persisted when he flexed his right wrist. Furthermore, his grip weakness did not improve.

To diagnose the injury, magnetic resonance imaging (MRI; T1-weighted, T2-weighted, T2-weighted STIR) of the affected region was performed. The right wrist showed intensity changes around the hamate hook, suggesting inflammation (Figure 2). A computed tomography scan finally showed fracture of the hamate hook (Figure 3). Upon a careful reexamination, tenderness was observed on the hamate hook.

Three weeks after his initial presentation, we surgically removed the hamate hook fragment. Mild synovitis of the flexor tendon of the small finger was intraoperatively found but not at the site of injury itself. Radiograph taken after the surgery showed that the hamate hook fragment was completely removed (Figure 4).

He was advised not to play water polo for 3 weeks after the surgery, and he did not resume practice until 4 weeks. Three months after the surgery, mild tenderness around the surgical scar was reported; however, his grip strength of the

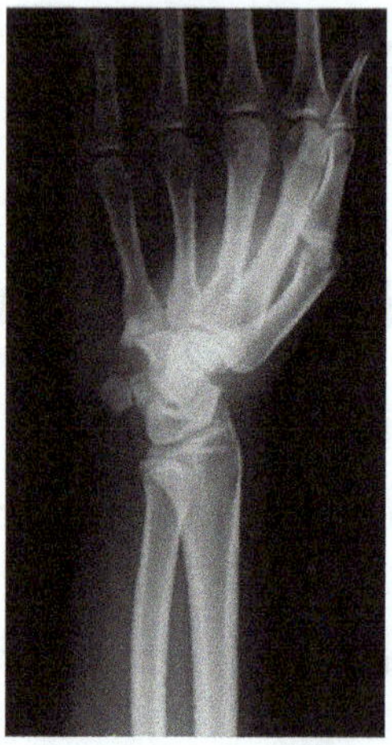

Figure 1: Radiograph taken at the previous clinic in supinated oblique position.

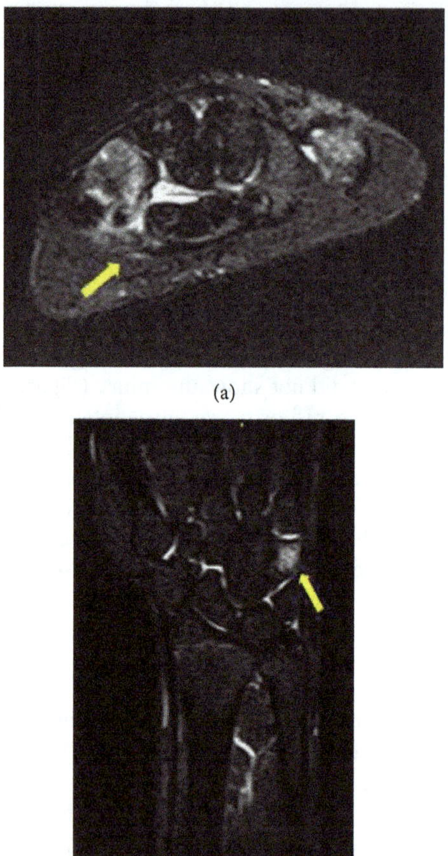

(a)

(b)

Figure 2: Magnetic resonance imaging (MRI) images. (a) Axial T2-weighted STIR image. (b) Coronal T2-weighted STIR image. Intensity changes around the hamate hook suggest inflammation (indicated by arrows).

right hand improved and was measured as 44 kg. One year after the surgery, he was completely pain-free, and the grip strength of his right hand had further improved to 46 kg. He achieved the full range of motion in the wrist (95° extension, 115° flexion) and felt no pain around his right wrist at any time, including while playing water polo. The most recent Disabilities of the Arm, Shoulder and Hand score was 2.6 points.

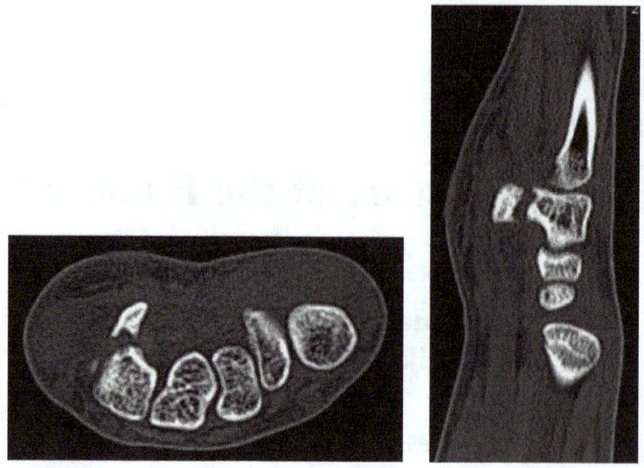

(a) (b)

Figure 3: Computed tomography (CT) images. (a) Axial CT image. (b) Sagittal CT image.

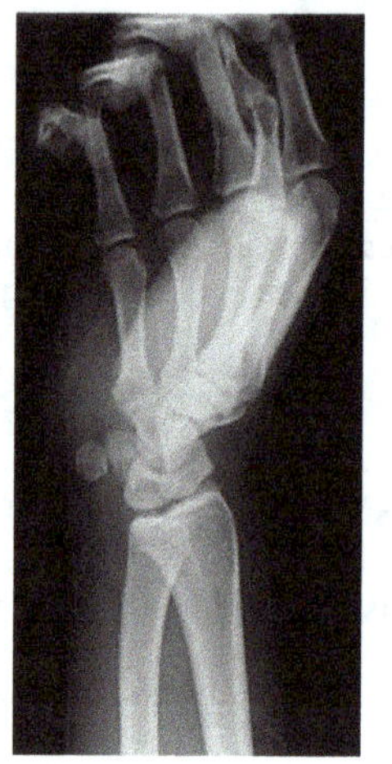

Figure 4: Postoperative radiograph in supinated oblique position.

3. Discussion

Fractures of the hamate account for 2% of all carpal fractures. The most common causes are racket sports, baseball, and golf, and the main mechanism of fracture is the direct injury to the hamate hook [1].

Several reports have indicated fracture of the hamate hook without direct trauma to the hamate hook itself, caused by some other indirect mechanism. How Kit et al. [2] have reported a case of a 23-year-old professional bowler who had gradually increasing hypothenar pain after he changed his bowling technique and ball-drilling layout. He was diagnosed with stress fracture of the hamate hook without previous direct trauma to the wrist. Bowler's wrists were hyperextended, pronated, and deviated to spin the ball because of its weight during the release. It was also noted that changes in the bowling technique and ball-drilling layout produced indirect forces on the hamate hook via the attached ligaments and strain on the flexor tendons. Lutter et al. [3] have reported fractures of the hamate hook in 10 of 12 high-level rock climbers presenting with ulnar wrist pain without any history of direct trauma. Rock climbing does not usually cause direct trauma to the hamate hook; however, it was noted that the side-undercling position that is repetitively used by rock climbers forces the wrists into ulnar deviation and strains the flexor tendon and, thus, may serve as an indirect mechanism of the fracture by compressing the hamate hook. Scheufler et al. [4] have also reported a high incidence of fractures of the hamate hook in underwater rugby players. The flexor digiti minimi brevis and abductor digiti minimi attach to the hamate hook, which works as a pulley for the flexor tendons of the ring and small fingers when the wrist undergoes ulnar deviation or during strong gripping [4, 5]. Because the ball is firmly held with an outstretched hand, strong indirect forces are produced by the muscles and ligaments attached to the hamate hook, as well as the flexor tendons of the ring and small fingers, leading to a high incidence of fractures of the hamate hook in underwater rugby players.

In our case, the fracture of the hamate hook in the water polo player was difficult to detect and diagnose because he had no previous typical direct trauma to his right wrist. However, because the onset of his wrist pain was nonspecific and similar to previous reports of indirect mechanisms, we considered that this may be a case of stress fracture of the hamate hook. In such cases, MRI is useful in diagnosing the fracture.

The following two indirect mechanisms led to stress fracture of the hamate hook in the water polo player. The first mechanism was the indirect forces that resulted from the strong ulnar deviation of the wrist during ball throwing. In water polo, putting snap on the ball is needed to spin the ball while throwing it. Particularly, pushing and knuckling are unique motions used to throw a ball in water polo, which cause strong ulnar deviations of the wrist at ball release, similar to the side-undercling position of rock climbers [3]. Extreme deviation of the wrist likely puts strain on the flexor tendons producing strong forces on the hamate hook. The second mechanism was the indirect forces due to strongly holding the ball with one hand. The ball used in underwater rugby has a circumference of 52–54 cm for males and 49–51 cm for females and adolescents [4], whereas that used in water polo has a much larger circumference of 68–71 cm for males and 65–67 cm for females. Furthermore, water polo players hold the larger ball with one hand in the same manner as underwater rugby players. Thus, it is likely that the indirect forces acting on the hamate hook via the muscles, ligaments, and flexor tendons are greater in water polo players than in underwater rugby players because of the larger ball size. Based on these two mechanisms, the fracture in our case was considered stress fracture of the hamate hook and occurred because of a motion and position of the wrist unique to water polo.

No previous studies relating to stress fractures of the hamate hook in water polo players have been reported. Our patient's range of motion in the bilateral wrists at 1 year after the surgery was wider than normal but cannot be regarded as so-called general joint laxity and may lead to a greater strain on the flexor tendons.

Disclosure

No benefits in any form have been received or will be received related directly or indirectly to the subject of this article.

References

[1] N. Suh, E. T. Ek, and S. W. Wolfe, "Carpal fractures," *The Journal of Hand Surgery*, vol. 39, no. 4, pp. 785–791, 2014.

[2] N. How Kit, M. Malherbe, and C. Hulet, "Hamate hook stress fracture in a professional bowler: case report of an unusual causal sport," *Hand Surgery and Rehabilitation*, vol. 36, no. 1, pp. 62–65, 2017.

[3] C. Lutter, A. Schweizer, T. Hochholzer, T. Bayer, and V. Schöffl, "Pulling harder than the hamate tolerates: evaluation of hamate injuries in rock climbing and bouldering," *Wilderness & Environmental Medicine*, vol. 27, no. 4, pp. 492–499, 2016.

[4] O. Scheufler, P. Kamusella, L. Tadda, S. Radmer, S. G. Russo, and R. Andresen, "High incidence of hamate hook fractures in underwater rugby players: diagnostic and therapeutic implications," *Hand Surgery*, vol. 18, no. 03, pp. 357–363, 2013.

[5] A. T. Bishop and R. D. Beckenbaugh, "Fracture of the hamate hook," *The Journal of Hand Surgery*, vol. 13, no. 1, pp. 135–139, 1988.

19

Nontraumatic Anterior Thigh Pain in a NCAA Lacrosse Athlete: A Case Report and Description of a Rectus Femoris Degloving Injury

Paul A. Krebs,[1] **James R. Borchers**,[2] **and Patrick Brayfield**[3]

[1]*Premier Health, Department of Family Medicine, Wright State University Boonshoft School of Medicine, 2400 Miami Valley Drive Suite 160 Dayton, Ohio 45459, USA*
[2]*The Ohio State University Wexner Medical Center Jameson Crane Sports Medicine Institute, 2835 Fred Taylor Drive, Columbus, Ohio 43202, USA*
[3]*The Ohio State University, Athletic Training Staff, 615 Irving Schottenstein Dr., Columbus, OH 43210, USA*

Correspondence should be addressed to Paul A. Krebs; pakrebs@premierhealth.com

Academic Editor: William B. Rodgers

A 21-year-old female lacrosse player complained of anterior thigh pain with no known mechanism of injury and failed to improve with conservative therapy. An MRI was obtained showing a closed degloving injury of the rectus femoris, an injury only previously reported in a small case series of soccer players. After a brief period of rest, she was progressed conservatively through therapy and did well, with progression back to the level of competition at 56 days. This case highlights a rare injury not previously described in sports outside of soccer and is the first case described in a female athlete. In addition, the discussion of this case focuses on the unique anatomy of the rectus femoris.

1. Introduction

Injuries to the quadriceps muscles are common in athletics. Certain sports such as soccer may show higher rates of adductor injuries compared to quadriceps injuries, but in aggregate studies of all sports, quadriceps injuries appear to be the second most common type of lower extremity muscle injuries behind hamstring injuries [1–4]. Quadriceps injuries include strains, tears, contusions, and hematomas. The purpose of this report is to highlight a case of anterior thigh pain that presented with symptoms similar to a quadriceps strain, and then to discuss closed degloving injuries of the rectus femoris, a rare injury to the quadriceps that may be overlooked in clinics.

The patient was informed that the details of her case would be submitted for print and electronic publication and gave informed consent.

2. Case Presentation

A 21-year-old NCAA Division 1 Lacrosse player presented to the training room with right anterior thigh pain of 4-5 weeks duration. Onset was gradual, occurring in the spring lacrosse season and starting during training and practice. She did not report any new activity or specific mechanism of injury leading to the pain. She had no history of surgery or major injury to the region. She had previously been seen by the athletic trainer at the onset of pain, described initially as a soreness in her anterior thigh of gradual onset at practice, and started on conservative management for a presumed quadriceps strain. This initial management consisted of modified activities at practice, rehabilitation therapy in the training room, NSAIDS, ice, cupping, and needling. Despite some initial improvement with these treatments, symptoms increased with gradual return to lacrosse. The pain was now throbbing, worse after games, occurring at night, waking her up from sleep, and exacerbated when her leg would hang over the edge of the chair. On exam, she had full active and passive range of motion and strength of the hip as well as the knee. She had tenderness over the right anterior mid-proximal thigh, extending over and area of approximately 10 cm. The tenderness was worse medially than laterally with no palpable defect in the muscle, and she had a positive fulcrum and

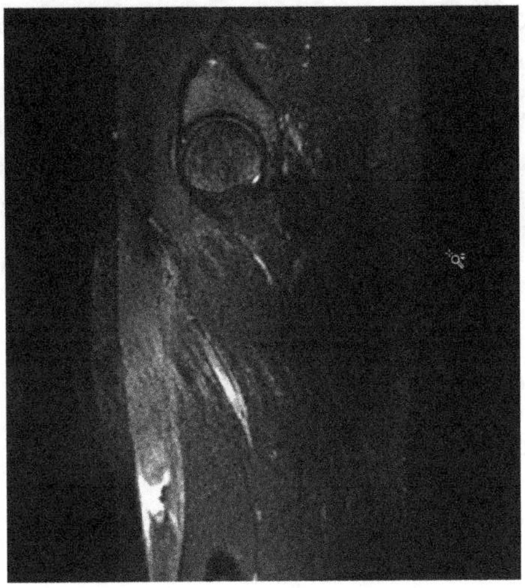

FIGURE 1: T2 STIR sagittal MRI image of the right femur without contrast demonstrating an acute degloving injury of the right rectus femoris.

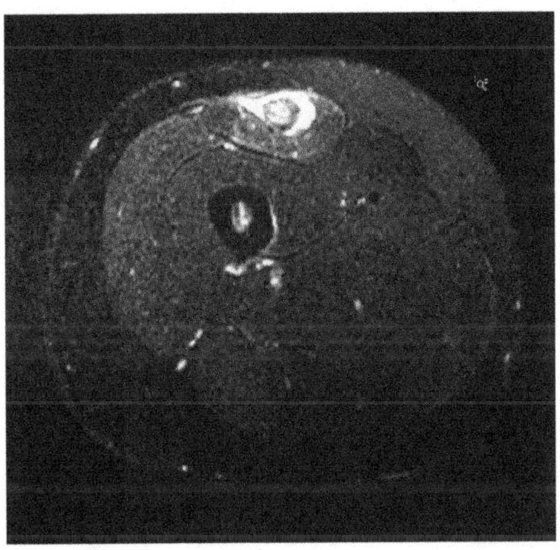

FIGURE 2: TSE T2 axial MRI image of the right femur without contrast demonstrating an acute degloving injury of the right rectus femoris.

hop test. Her neurovascular exam was intact. An X-ray of the femur did not reveal any abnormalities. An MRI was ordered to rule out a stress fracture and to evaluate the quadriceps muscle further. The MRI showed an acute complete disruption of the inner bipennate muscular component of the right rectus femoris from the more superficial unipennate muscular component with retraction of the inner component, consistent with an acute degloving injury. No abnormality was noted in the osseous structure. These findings are highlighted in Figures 1 and 2. Given these findings of a closed degloving injury of the rectus femoris, the decision was made to discontinue all lacrosse activities and start a period of rest. After 2 weeks of rest with only a gentle range of motion exercises, her pain had improved. She progressed through therapy conservatively as the lacrosse season had just ended, starting with isometrics, and then progressing as tolerated to dynamic exercises followed by lacrosse-specific drills and exercise. By six weeks (42 days), she felt great and was cleared for full activity in therapy/progression to sport with estimated return to full competition at eight weeks (56 days) had it not been the offseason. The patient was able to participate in all offseason activities and had no setbacks or recurrence of symptoms the following season, returning fully to the level of play prior to injury.

3. Discussion

Injuries to the quadriceps muscles are common in athletics, with the rates of injury reported to be higher in women and occurring more frequently in competition [1, 5]. Among NCAA athletes, quadriceps strains, the most common type of quadriceps injury, are reported to occur at a rate of 1.07/10,000 athlete exposures (AEs). Examining different sports, women's soccer has the highest overall reported rate at 5.61/10,000 AEs [1]. Of the quadriceps muscles, the rectus femoris is the most commonly injured [6].

The anatomy of the rectus femoris is unique compared to the other quadriceps muscles. In addition to having actions on both the hip and knee joint, the anatomy of the muscle and proximal tendons creates a "muscle within a muscle" [7]. Cadaveric studies and MRI studies demonstrate an intramuscular bipennate structure and central aponeurosis arising from the indirect tendon off the superior acetabular ridge, surrounded by a unipennate superficial portion arising from the direct tendon off the anterior inferior iliac spine [4, 7, 8]. This anatomy creates the possibility for the type of injury highlighted in this case report, termed a closed degloving injury, where the inner bipennate muscle tears and retracts within the outer unipennate muscle [9]. The anatomy of the quadriceps demonstrates two different muscle tendon structures that can be seen in the human body, unipennate and bipennate structures. These terms describe the arrangement of the muscle fibers around the tendon. A unipennate muscle is one where all the fibers originate from one side of the tendon, while a bipennate muscle has muscle fibers originating from two sides of a tendon [4].

Central tendon and muscle injuries have been found to have prolonged recovery when compared to injuries to the periphery [6, 10]. While previous literature describes central tendon and muscle injuries, including proximal tendon injuries leading to "bull's eye injuries" [6, 10], degloving injuries seen on MRI have only been described once, in a case series of 8 male athletes [9]. The case presented is unique in that it is the first reported case in a female and nonsoccer athlete. Additionally, there was no known incident or event precipitating this injury. In the previous case series, the history of 7 of the 8 athletes was described, with all injuries occurring during a soccer practice or game, with the most common mechanism being kicking (4 of 7) [9]. Similar to 4 of the athletes in the previous case series, the athlete in this case report was able to initially continue to play with symptoms. The time until return to competition from diagnosis in the athlete in this case report was 56 days compared to the 38.7 day average in the previous case series [9]. This may be explained by the conservative approach to therapy for the athlete as it was the offseason. Other characteristics of the lesion, including the distance between the acetabular rim and the proximal portion of the injury (17.9 cm vs 15.5 cm (range 11.3-20.3 cm)) and the degree of retraction (1.1 cm vs 1.2 cm (range 0-3.5 cm)) were similar between this case report and the previous case series, respectively [9].

A thorough understanding of the unique anatomy of the rectus femoris first elucidated in the 1990s by Hughes and Hasselman is important to understanding the range of injuries that can occur within the quadriceps muscles [7, 8]. This case report of a female lacrosse player with a degloving injury of the rectus femoris highlights the anatomy of the muscle, the potential for unique injury patterns, and need for further investigation when patient's recovery times are prolonged despite appropriate therapy.

References

[1] T. G. Eckard, Z. Y. Kerr, D. A. Padua, A. Djoko, and T. P. Dompier, "Epidemiology of quadriceps strains in national collegiate athletic association athletes, 2009-2010 through 2014-2015," *Journal of Athletic Training*, vol. 52, no. 5, pp. 474–481, 2017.

[2] P. Edouard, P. Branco, and J. M. Alonso, "Muscle injury is the principal injury type and hamstring muscle injury is the first injury diagnosis during top-level international athletics championships between 2007 and 2015," *British Journal of Sports Medicine*, vol. 50, no. 10, pp. 619–630, 2016.

[3] J. Ekstrand, M. Hagglund, and M. Walden, "Epidemiology of muscle injuries in professional football (soccer)," *The American Journal of Sports Medicine*, vol. 39, no. 6, pp. 1226–1232, 2011.

[4] A. Kassarjian, R. M. Rodrigo, and J. M. Santisteban, "Current concepts in MRI of rectus femoris musculotendinous (myotendinous) and myofascial injuries in elite athletes," *European Journal of Radiology*, vol. 81, no. 12, pp. 3763–3771, 2012.

[5] D. D. Backous, K. E. Friedl, N. J. Smith, T. J. Parr, and Carpine WD Jr, "Soccer injuries and their relation to physical maturity," *American Journal of Diseases of Children*, vol. 142, no. 8, pp. 839–842, 1988.

[6] T. M. Cross, M. T. Houang, and M. Cameron, "Acute quadriceps muscle strains," *The American Journal of Sports Medicine*, vol. 32, no. 3, pp. 710–719, 2004.

[7] C. T. Hasselman, T. M. Best, C. Hughes, S. Martinez, and W. E. Garrett, "An explanation for various rectus femoris strain injuries using previously undescribed muscle architecture," *The American Journal of Sports Medicine*, vol. 23, no. 4, pp. 493–499, 1995.

[8] C. Hughes, C. T. Hasselman, T. M. Best, S. Martinez, and W. E. Garrett, "Incomplete, intrasubstance strain injuries of the rectus femoris muscle," *The American Journal of Sports Medicine*, vol. 23, no. 4, pp. 500–506, 1995.

[9] A. Kassarjian, R. M. Rodrigo, and J. M. Santisteban, "Intramuscular degloving injuries to the rectus femoris: findings at MRI," *American Journal of Roentgenology*, vol. 202, no. 5, pp. W475–W480, 2014.

[10] R. Balius, A. Maestro, C. Pedret et al., "Central aponeurosis tears of the rectus femoris: practical sonographic prognosis," *British Journal of Sports Medicine*, vol. 43, no. 11, pp. 818–824, 2009.

[9] A. Kassarjian, R. M. Rodrigo, and J. M. Santisteban, "Intramuscular degloving injuries to the rectus femoris: findings at MRI," *American Journal of Roentgenology*, vol. 202, no. 5, pp. W475–W480, 2014.

[10] R. Balius, A. Maestro, C. Pedret et al., "Central aponeurosis tears of the rectus femoris: practical sonographic prognosis," *British Journal of Sports Medicine*, vol. 43, no. 11, pp. 818–824, 2009.

20

Utilization of a Continuous Pericapsular Nerve Group (PENG) Block with an Opioid-Sparing Repair of a Femoral Neck Fracture in a Pediatric Patient

Karla Wyatt, Moustafa Zidane, and Chyong-jy Joyce Liu

Department of Anesthesiology, Perioperative and Pain Management, Baylor College of Medicine/Texas Children's Hospital, Houston, TX, USA

Correspondence should be addressed to Chyong-jy Joyce Liu; cjliu@texaschildrens.org

Academic Editor: Kaan Erler

In the pediatric population, femoral neck fractures are usually associated with high-impact trauma and often present with pain in the groin area. Regional anesthesia can offer adjunctive therapy for acute pain management. Various techniques have been employed to circumvent pain related to hip fractures and resultant hip surgery. Neuraxial, lumbar plexus, caudal, epidural, fascia iliaca, and femoral continuous nerve block techniques are advantageous in mitigating hip pain. However, these approaches require patient repositioning during placement and carry the potential for motor blockade with resultant weakness. A newly described method, the Pericapsular Nerve Group (PENG) block, allows for analgesia of the anterior hip capsule via the obturator, accessory obturator, and femoral nerves while sparing motor blockade. PENG blockade has demonstrated efficacy in both adult and pediatric patients. Herein, we describe the perioperative course of a 9-year-old girl with a transcervical femoral neck fracture who underwent an opioid-sparing open repair with the utilization of a continuous PENG block. PENG blockade via a continuous nerve block resulted in optimal analgesia and markedly reduced perioperative opioid consumption with preserved motor function. Our experience facilitated early discharge and rehabilitation mobility while reducing potential rebound hyperalgesia and enabling parental/patient satisfaction.

1. Introduction

Nonpathologic femoral neck fractures in the pediatric population are generally associated with high-impact trauma [1]. Optimal management involves prompt diagnosis, hip stabilization, and open versus closed fixation. Perioperative pain control is of paramount importance following pediatric hip surgery. Inadequate analgesia can contribute to patient and parental dissatisfaction, prolonged recovery, and increased hospital length of stay. While there is a paucity of pediatric data, adult literature has described an association between the utilization of regional anesthesia and decreased postoperative delirium, hospital length of stay, intensive care admission, and overall mortality among geriatric patients undergoing hip replacement surgery [2]. As such, regional anesthesia is advantageous in providing sufficient analgesia while reducing the adverse effects of opioids. Lumbar plexus blockade, neuraxial techniques (caudal or epidural), and combined femoral nerve and fascia iliaca blockade have been shown in a myriad of pediatric studies to exhibit opioid-sparing effects and lower postoperative pain scores in patients who are suffering from hip pain [3–6].

Despite the success of neuraxial techniques in decreasing postoperative pain scores in pediatric patients undergoing hip surgery [4–6], positioning requirements, bilateral sensory and motor blockade, and urinary retention limit their use. Our institutional practice includes administration of a general anesthetic combined with a lumbar plexus continuous nerve block for children undergoing unilateral hip surgery. This effectively blocks the femoral, lateral femoral cutaneous,

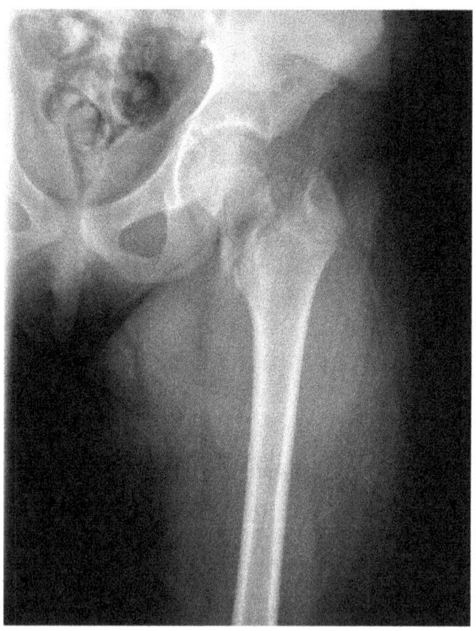

(a)

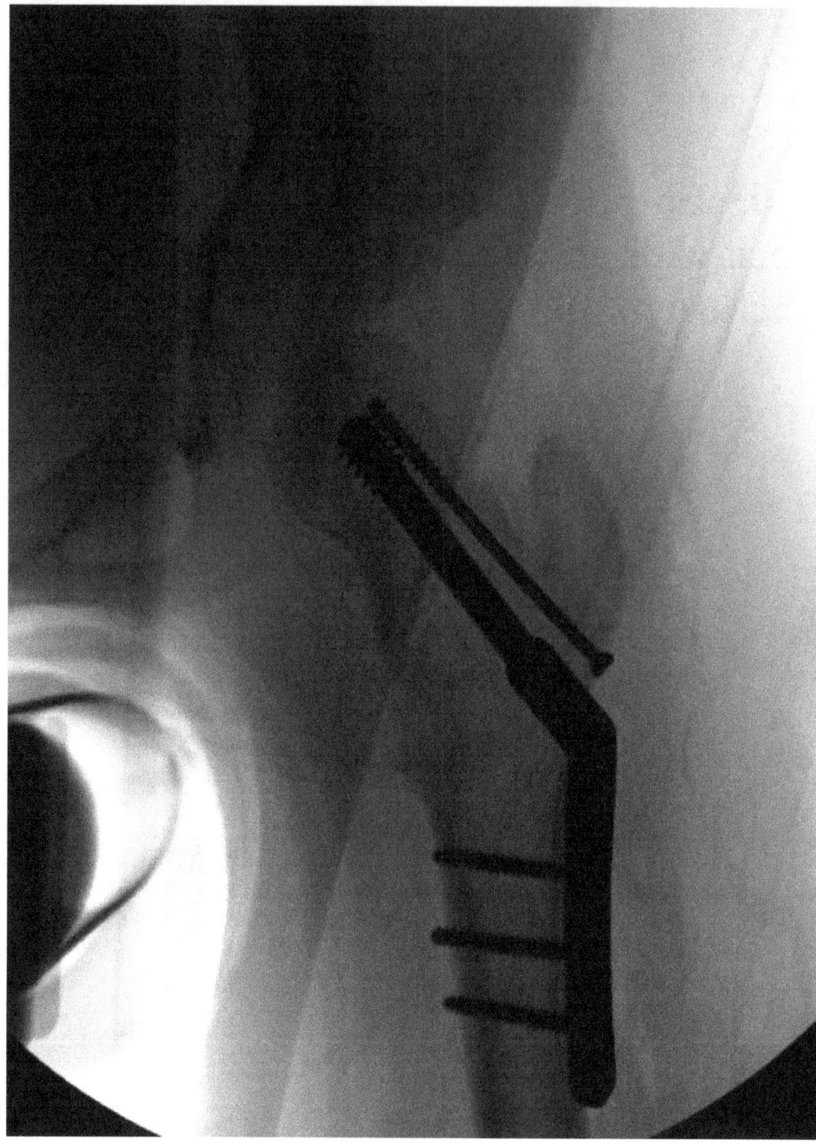

(b)

Figure 1: (a) X-ray image of patient's injury; (b) open reduction and internal fixation RIF of intertrochanteric left femur fracture with dynamic hip screw.

and obturator nerves which innervate the hip while maintaining functional status on the nonsurgical side, albeit the operative side is still susceptible to motor weakness.

Pericapsular Nerve Group (PENG) block was first described in 2018 by Girón-Arango et al. [7] for perioperative analgesia in hip fracture patients via blockade of the articulating branches of the hip: the accessory obturator nerve (AON), obturator nerve (ON), and the femoral nerve (FN) [7–11]. This technique was confirmed by a cadaveric dye study [12] showing a "true" pericapsular spread that only targeted the sensory branches of the anterior hip capsule with subsequent motor-sparing effects [7]. PENG block was also successfully demonstrated by Mistry et al. whereby five patients with hip fractures all reported pain relief within 15 minutes without resultant quadriceps weakness [13].

Herein, we present the utilization of a continuous PENG block for perioperative pain management in a pediatric patient undergoing hip surgery. To our knowledge, this is the first report describing a continuous PENG block analgesia for a pediatric patient.

Written informed consent was obtained from the parent for this scientific contribution.

2. Case Report

A 9-year-old, 45.7 kg, healthy girl presented following a fall from the top of a bounce house with inability to bear weight and hip pain. Imaging revealed a transcervical fracture of the left proximal femur with lateral displacement of the distal femoral segment (Figure 1(a)). There were no distal femoral fractures, intra-abdominal, or spine-related injuries. She was splinted and placed in traction in preparation for an open reduction with internal fixation. Upon discussion with the surgical team, the goals of care included a 2-day

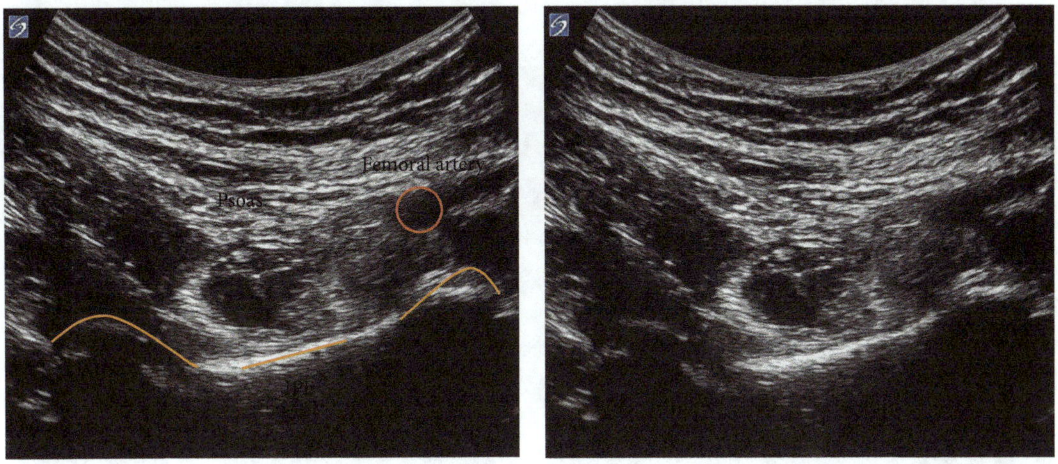

(a) (b)

Figure 2: (a) Visualization of the psoas muscle, femoral artery, and anterior inferior iliac spine (AIIS), iliopubic eminence (IPE), and the superior pubic (SP) ramus on sonoanatomy with identification. (b) Sonoanatomy.

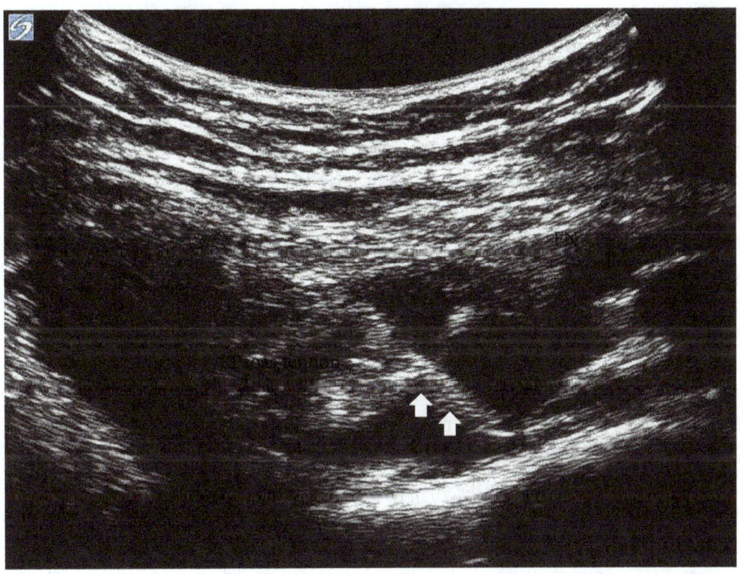

Figure 3: Echogenic needle isolation following contact with the iliopubic eminence. FA: femoral artery; FN: femoral nerve. Arrow represents the needle placement.

admission for postoperative pain control and physical therapy, with complete avoidance of motor blockade. Given the degree of traction, injury-related positioning restraints, and the postoperative motor assessment concern, we offered a PENG block catheter for postoperative pain in lieu of a lumbar plexus or combined femoral and fascia iliaca blockade.

Proceeding general anesthesia, the patient was maintained in the supine position with the left lower extremity in traction and satisfactory reduction, confirmed with X-ray imaging. A curvilinear, low-frequency transducer (2-5 MHz) was placed in the transverse plane along the left anterior inferior iliac spine (AIIS) to identify the iliopsoas muscle, femoral artery, and femoral nerve. The probe was then rotated counterclockwise, aligned with the pubic ramus to visualize the AIIS, iliopubic eminence (IPE), femoral artery, psoas muscle, and the superior pubic ramus (Figure 2). Under direct visualization, a 22-gauge (G), 80 mm echogenic needle was advanced in-plane, lateral to medial between the psoas tendon and pubic ramus until the needle made contact with the IPE (Figure 3). The needle was slightly withdrawn, and following negative aspiration, 14 ml of bupivacaine 0.25% (~0.75 mg/kg) was injected in incremental doses. The block performance took 7 minutes. This bolus dose single injection was sufficient for intraoperative surgical analgesia. Preparation and surgical positioning allowed for maximal time for block onset.

While an incision was made along the lateral proximal femur from the vastus ridge distally proceeding to the iliotibial band, there were no changes in heart rate or blood pressure. Following exposure of the lateral surface of the femur, a starting guide pin was placed in the femoral head just short of the physis. The guide pin was used for measurement and placement confirmation prior to the placement of hip screw and plate. The compression and shaft screws were then

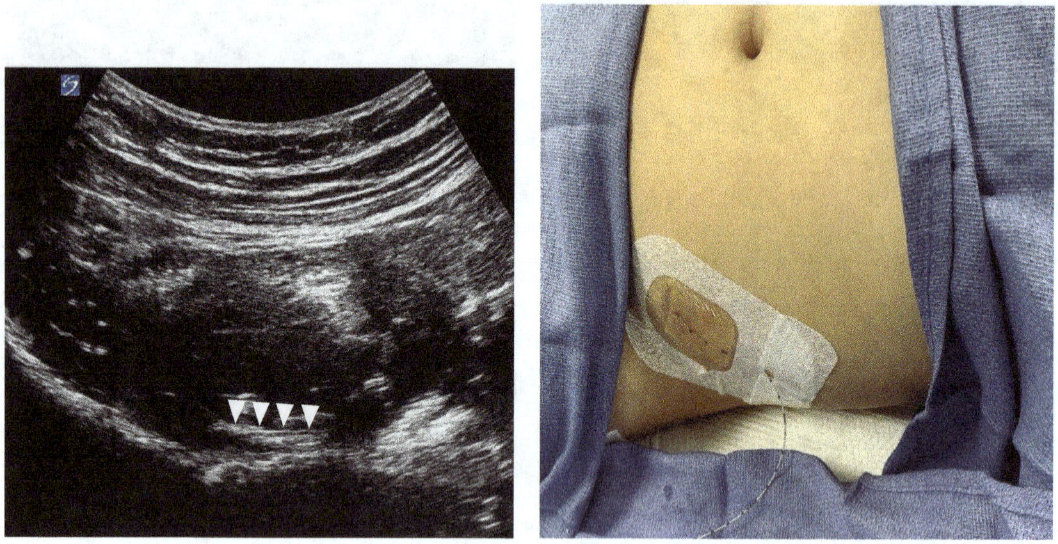

(a) (b)

Figure 4: (a) PENG catheterization and corresponding sonoanatomy with isolation of the proximal portion of the peripheral nerve catheter positioned above the iliopubic eminence. Arrow presents the catheter; (b) PENG catheter placement.

drilled, measured, and placed through the plate. An additional partially threaded cannulated screw was placed into the neck as an antirotation screw. The final location of implants was confirmed on anterior-posterior and lateral X-ray imaging before irrigation and closure (Figure 1(b)). The patient was maintained on 0.8 MAC of desflurane with no intraoperative opioid requirements. The total operating time was 102 minutes. The procedure was uneventful without any apparent complications. The estimated blood loss was 200 ml.

A nerve block catheter was placed following surgical repair to avoid location interference with operative access. At the conclusion of the case, image acquisition was again obtained as previously described. Similarly, a 22 G, 80 mm echogenic needle was advanced in-plane (Figure 4). Following lateral to medial advancement, contact with the IPE occurred at a sonographic depth of about 2.5 cm; however, given the lateral approach, the total needle length inserted was 5 cm. An end-hole peripheral nerve catheter was threaded to a depth of 7 cm (2 cm beyond the needle tip) with visualization of the femoral neurovascular structures. Catheter placement was performed in 12 minutes. The procedural anesthesia time was 45 minutes including the induction, emergence, and performance of both regional blocks.

Postoperatively, the patient appeared to be comfortable with numeric pain scores of 2-3/10. The anesthetic infusion via a PENG catheter was initiated with ropivacaine 0.1% at 6 ml/hr (0.13 mg/kg/hr rate). The patient was non-weight-bearing to the left lower extremity per surgical team, but no motor weakness was observed. Physical exam revealed no sensation to light touch on the anteromedial or lateral hip and intact flexion at the knee. Overnight, she did not require any breakthrough opioids or muscle relaxants. FLACC and subjective pain scores were 0/10 for the ensuing 12 hours, and the parents reported good pain control. On postoperative day (POD) 1, the patient was able to participate in physical therapy and gait training with ease. The anesthetic infusion was discontinued on POD 1 (>24 hours since placement of the catheter) after a trial of an oral acetaminophen-opioid preparation. The patient was discharged on the evening of POD1 with as needed diazepam for muscle spasms and an acetaminophen-opioid preparation for pain control. There was no evidence of block complication.

3. Discussion

Pediatric hip fractures can be divided into 4 subtypes with type II (transcervical fractures) being the most prevalent, extending through the middle of the femoral neck [1]. Cannulated screw fixation is usually required for older children in whom transcervical fracture is unstable, and the determination of open versus closed approach commonly depends on the success of surgical traction for reduction. Regional anesthetic techniques are safe in children [14–16] and can provide analgesia for pediatric patients undergoing hip surgery [3–6]. Adequate analgesia results in faster rehabilitation, decreased opioid consumption, and avoidance of the untoward side effects associated with opioids.

The single-shot PENG block has recently been described in adult and pediatric literature for perioperative analgesia for hip surgery by blocking the articulating branches of the femoral nerve, accessory obturator nerve (AON), and obturator nerve (ON) [7–11]. Short et al. demonstrated the consistent anatomical contribution of the FN and AON to the anterior hip capsule [11]. The motor-sparing effect and technical ease of image acquisition in the traction-immobilized patient made this blockade ideal for our patient. We also observed similar pain relief in our patient without quadriceps weakness as reported in other studies [12, 13].

A major drawback of the single-shot peripheral nerve blockade is the limited timeframe for analgesic relief. In addition, the potential for rebound hyperalgesia after a single-shot nerve block was described at 12-24 hours [17, 18]. Rebound hyperalgesia is postulated to be due to subjective pain perception or an inadequate pain regimen when single-shot blockade ceases. We would expect the pain associated with major hip surgery to span about 24-72 hours [19]. While additives such as dexamethasone and alpha-2 adrenoreceptor agonists have been documented to prolong the analgesia of single-shot peripheral nerve blocks, their use is off-label and perineural toxicity is lacking in the pediatric literature [19]. Given the potential extent for pain beyond the expected provision of a single-shot nerve block, our decision was to proceed with a continuous infusion via a catheter for this patient.

The use of continuous peripheral nerve blockades in children is safe and efficacious [20–23]. Infusion with optimal concentrations and dosages of local anesthetic can provide sensory analgesia while preserving motor function. Pediatric studies reviewing inpatient and outpatient regimens have replicated decreased opioid consumption with continuous peripheral nerve block and a low incidence of complication [20, 22, 23]. The most common complications cited in children were paresthesias (which resolved with local anesthetic discontinuation), mechanical malfunction, and nausea or vomiting [21]. Given the safety profile of a continuous nerve block and the potential for ongoing postoperative pain, we performed a PENG block for this patient to balance surgical neurovascular and musculoskeletal considerations with optimized regional pain management.

Consistent with the adult literature, our experience demonstrated motor preservation and opioid-sparing analgesia with the utilization of the PENG block. We chose to use the safe and accepted pediatric range of 0.5-1.5 mg/kg bupivacaine for the initial lower extremity bolus dosing with a conservative infusion rate of ~0.13 mg/kg/hr via the catheter [20]. We recognize that the efficacy of the PENG block has not been established with prospective clinical studies. While our observations were promising, future investigation into the efficacy, bolus and infusion rates, and safety of the PENG in the pediatric population is needed.

References

[1] T. Palocaren, "Femoral neck fractures in children: a review," *Indian Journal of Orthopaedics*, vol. 52, no. 5, pp. 501–506, 2018.

[2] E. J. Ahn, H. J. Kim, K. W. Kim, H. R. Choi, H. Kang, and S. R. Bang, "Comparison of general anaesthesia and regional anaesthesia in terms of mortality and complications in elderly patients with hip fracture: a nationwide population-based study," *BMJ Open*, vol. 9, no. 9, article e029245, 2019.

[3] O. Ahmed, M. Mohamed, and A. Kamal, "Psoas compartment block for acute postoperative pain management after hip surgery in pediatrics: a comparative study with caudal analgesia," *Regional Anesthesia and Pain Medicine*, vol. 36, no. 2, pp. 121–124, 2011.

[4] M. A. Villablobos, G. Veneziano, R. Miller et al., "Evaluation of postoperative analgesia in pediatric patients after hip surgery: lumbar plexus versus caudal epidural analgesia," *Journal of Pain Research*, vol. 12, pp. 997–1001, 2019.

[5] B. R. Miller, "Ultrasound-guided fascia iliaca compartment block in pediatric patients using a long-axis, in-plane needle technique: a report of three cases," *Paediatric Anaesthesia*, vol. 21, no. 12, pp. 1261–1264, 2011.

[6] M. E. Steinhaus, J. Rosneck, C. S. Ahmed, and T. S. Lynch, "Outcomes after peripheral nerve block in hip arthroscopy," *The American Journal of Orthopedics*, vol. 47, no. 6, 2018.

[7] L. Girón-Arango, P. W. H. Peng, K. J. Chin, R. Brull, and A. Perlas, "Pericapsular Nerve Group (PENG) block for hip fracture," *Regional Anesthesia and Pain Medicine*, vol. 43, no. 8, pp. 859–863, 2018.

[8] S. Orozco, D. Munoz, S. Jaramillo, and A. M. Herrera, "Pediatric use of Pericapsular Nerve Group (PENG) block for hip surgical procedures," *Journal of Clinical Anesthesia*, vol. 57, pp. 143-144, 2019.

[9] C. Aksu, S. Cesur, and A. Kus, "Pericapsular nerve group (PENG) block for postoperative analgesia after open reduction of pediatric congenital dysplasia of the hip," *Journal of Clinical Anesthesia*, vol. 61, article 109675, 2020.

[10] H. Ueshima and H. Otake, "Pericapsular nerve group (PENG) block is effective for dislocation of the hip joint," *Journal of Clinical Anesthesia*, vol. 52, p. 83, 2019.

[11] A. J. Short, J. J. G. Barnett, and M. Gofeld, "Anatomic study of innervation of the anterior hip capsule: implication for image-guided intervention," *Regional Anesthesia and Pain Medicine*, vol. 43, no. 2, pp. 186–192, 2018.

[12] J. Tran, A. Agur, and P. Peng, "Is pericapsular nerve group (PENG) block a true pericapsular block?," *Regional Anesthesia & Pain Medicine*, vol. 44, no. 2, p. 257, 2019.

[13] T. Mistry, K. B. Sonawane, and E. Kuppusamy, "PENG block: points to ponder," *Regional Anesthesia and Pain Medicine*, vol. 44, pp. 423-424, 2019.

[14] B. J. Walker, J. B. Long, M. Sathyamoorthy et al., "Complications in pediatric regional anesthesia an analysis of more than 100, 000 blocks from the pediatric regional anesthesia network," *Anesthesiology*, vol. 129, no. 4, pp. 721–732, 2018.

[15] X. Capdevila, P. Pirat, S. Bringuier et al., "Continuous peripheral nerve blocks in hospital wards after orthopedic surgery: a multicenter prospective analysis of the quality of postoperative analgesia and complications in 1, 416 patients," *Anesthesiology*, vol. 103, no. 5, pp. 1035–1045, 2005.

[16] P. Lonnqvist, C. Ecoffey, A. Bosenberg, S. Suresh, and G. Ivani, "The European Society of Regional Anesthesia and Pain Therapy and the American Society of Regional Anesthesia and Pain Medicine Joint Committee practice advisory on controversial topics in pediatric regional anesthesia I and II," *Current Opinion in Anaesthesiology*, vol. 30, no. 5, pp. 613–620, 2017.

[17] F. W. Abdallah, S. H. Halpern, K. Aoyama, and R. Brull, "Will the real benefits of single-shot Interscalene block please stand up? A systematic review and meta-analysis," *Anesthesia and Analgesia*, vol. 120, no. 5, pp. 1114–1129, 2015.

[18] R. Y. Goldstein, N. Montero, S. K. Jain, K. A. Egol, and N. C. Tejwani, "Efficacy of popliteal block in postoperative pain control after ankle fracture fixation: a prospective randomized study," *Journal of Orthopaedic Trauma*, vol. 26, no. 10, pp. 557–561, 2012.

[19] S. Suresh, C. Ecoffey, A. Bosenberg et al., "The European Society of Regional Anaesthesia and Pain Therapy/American Society of Regional Anesthesia and Pain Medicine recom-

mendations on local anesthetics and Adjuvants dosage in pediatric regional anesthesia," *Regional Anesthesia and Pain Medicine*, vol. 43, no. 2, pp. 211–216, 2018.

[20] H. Gurnaney, W. Kraemer, L. Maxwell, W. T. Muhly, L. Schleelein, and A. Ganesh, "Ambulatory continuous peripheral nerve blocks in children and adolescents: a longitudinal 8-year single center study," *Anesthesia and Analgesia*, vol. 118, no. 3, pp. 621–627, 2014.

[21] A. Ganesh, J. B. Rose, L. Wells et al., "Continuous peripheral nerve blockade for inpatient and outpatient postoperative analgesia in children," *Anesthesia and Analgesia*, vol. 105, no. 5, pp. 1234–1242, 2007.

[22] C. Dadure, P. Pirat, O. Raux et al., "Perioperative continuous peripheral nerve blocks with disposable infusion pumps in children: a prospective descriptive study," *Anesthesia and Analgesia*, vol. 97, no. 3, pp. 687–690, 2003.

[23] C. Dadure, S. Bringuier, O. Raux et al., "Continuous peripheral nerve blocks for postoperative analgesia in children: feasibility and side effects in a cohort study of 339 catheters," *Canadian Journal of Anesthesia*, vol. 56, no. 11, pp. 843–850, 2009.

21

Shear Wave Elastography in the Diagnosis of Hand Tumours

Debora Schivo,[1] **Ergys Gjika**,[2] **Aurélien Traverso**,[3] **and Sébastien Durand**[1]

[1]*Department of Plastic, Reconstructive and Hand Surgery, University Hospital of Lausanne, CHUV, Lausanne, Switzerland*
[2]*Department of Hand Surgery, University Hospital of Geneva, HUG, Genève, Switzerland*
[3]*Department of Orthopaedics and Traumatology, University Hospital of Lausanne, CHUV, Lausanne, Switzerland*

Correspondence should be addressed to Debora Schivo; debora.schivo@gmail.com
and Sébastien Durand; sebastien.durand@chuv.ch

Academic Editor: Taketoshi Yasuda

Diagnosis of hand tumours by conventional imaging remains difficult. Shear wave elastography (SWE) is a noninvasive method used to quantitatively assess the mechanical properties of tissues. We provide the first report of "histoelastographic" data concerning a finger tumour. Our data support the notion of ultrasound assessment using multiple parameters including morphology, elasticity, viscosity, and microflow vascularization likely contributing towards a more precise diagnosis in the future.

1. Introduction

Tumours of the hand and wrist represent 12.8% of soft tissue lesions [1]. There remains no noninvasive solution to establish with certitude the diagnosis of musculoskeletal tumours and of the hand in specific [2]. Standard radiography reveals aspecific signs such as cortical condensation, erosion, or periosteal reaction. While B-mode ultrasound imaging can be used to classify soft tissue lesions as cystic or solid depending on their echogenicity [3], the use of ultrasound and/or MRI is insufficient. Histological examination of a targeted biopsy is considered to be the best method to provide a definitive diagnosis of a suspect lesion [2] but an error rate of 17.8% has been found [4], which significantly reduces their utility. The surveillance of certain recurrent tumours is currently poorly evaluated by simple morphological examination. Furthermore, progress towards less invasive procedures in the treatment of certain tumours imposes a precise diagnosis as prerequisite to any intervention [5–8].

All tissues, whether healthy or pathological, present specific biomechanical properties relating to their specific architecture and which can be expressed using stress/strain curves or Young's modulus. One could reasonably assume therefore that knowledge of the elastic properties of different tissues might be indicative of their nature.

Shear wave elastography (SWE) is a recent quantitative technique for assessing the elasticity of soft tissues. It uses an acoustic radiation force impulse (ARFI) generated by a focused ultrasound beam and quantifies the shear wave velocity (in meters per second) and stiffness (Young's modulus in kilopascal) of tissues [9]. Initially used in the early nineties in vitro [10], its use has since then progressively increased within clinical exploration as a diagnosis and sometimes prognostic tool examining breast, liver, thyroid, prostate, and musculoskeletal pathologies [7, 11–13]. SWE has been shown to provide quantitative and reproducible information on solid breast lesions and serve as an accurate diagnostic tool for discriminating malignant and benign lesions, thereby avoiding biopsy [14].

Elastography has been used to assess upper limb musculoskeletal tissue and seems to be interesting in the diagnosis of many pathologies: lateral epicondylitis [15], rotator cuff tendon pathology [16], trigger finger [17], carpal tunnel syndrome [18], upper limb tendon transfer [9], and finger pulp reconstruction [19]. The aim of this case is to demonstrate

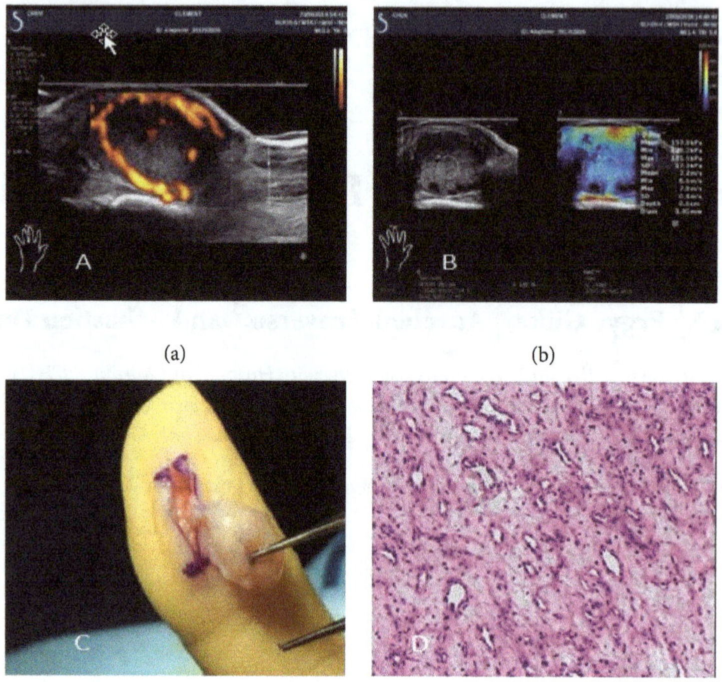

(a) (b) (c) (d)

Figure 1: (a) Doppler ultrasound angio PL.U.S mode. Peripheral ring-like vascularization of the mass. (b) SWE using a high-frequency probe (SHL 15-4, average frequency 12 kHz). (c) Surgical excision of the tumour. (d) Histology: lobular capillary haemangioma.

the technical feasibility of SWE for evaluating Young's modulus of infracentimetric tumours of the hand, which commonly occurs in hand surgery.

2. Case Report

A 45-year-old woman without any history of trauma presented with a painful and hard mass located within her right thumb pulp. The tumour showed adherence to deep tissues but not signs of local inflammation. Standard radiographs were unremarkable. The ultrasound examination of the tumour reported an encapsulated mass with regular and well-defined margins.

Doppler ultrasound using angio PL.U.S mode showed a homogenous ovoid mass with peripheral ring-like vascularization (Figure 1(a)).

SWE performed (Aixplorer®, Aix-en-Provence, France) using a high-frequency probe (SHL 15-4, average frequency 12 MHz) centred with a quantitative Q-box, with a circular region of interest of 3 mm diameter, on the mass revealed shear wave speed and modulus of elasticity of, respectively, 7.2 (6.6-7.8) m/s and 157.8 (129-181.5) kPa in the transverse plane and 5 (4.6-5.7) m/s and 75.8 (63.1-96.4) kPa in the sagittal plane (Figure 1(b)). The Q-box circle has a maximal precision of 1 mm; therefore, very small tumours can be detected and analysed.

Surgical excision of the tumour (Figure 1(c)) was carried out and the histopathological examination revealed a deep lobular capillary haemangioma (Figure 1(d)). The postoperative follow-up was without complications.

3. Discussion

Elastography is an imaging modality which maps the elastic properties and stiffness of soft tissue by different techniques. Strain elastography allows qualitative analysis, based on the deformation of the tissues (strain) for a given stress, and results in a qualitative map of the elastic modulus distribution, defined as an elastogram. While true quantitative measurements cannot be taken from this elastogram, a semiquantitative evaluation can be determined with the strain ratio, which represents an index of the relative elasticity between a chosen region of interest (ROI) and the surrounding tissues [20]. SWE does however provide quantitative information relating to tissue elasticity and is more reproducible than strain elastography owing to the standardised applied stress [21].

Studies into the use of SWE to investigate musculoskeletal tumours or masses are relatively few in number. Most previous studies on the use of sonoelastography for differentiating benign from malignant lesions adopted qualitative scales [22–26] (Table 1).

Different process models have been used to develop the SWE technique. The reproducibility, based on the results obtained using the different models, is unclear. The literature demonstrates certain discrepancies among the elastographic data obtained with different software [27]. We also found heterogeneity among the studies we analysed in terms of the probes used, with frequencies between 5 and 40 MHz (Table 1).

The data in the literature suggest that shear wave velocity measurements are reproducible and that

Table 1: Elastographic data for musculoskeletal tumours in the literature.

Article	Year	ROI	System	Technique	No.	Mass	Quantitative	Qualitative
Pass et al. [29]	2017	Dim. 2 × 2 mm VR 0-10 m/s	Acuson S3000 (9-4 MHz)	SWE (ARFI)	105	S	Long. 2.94 m/s; Trans. 2.93 m/s	Red
						H	Long. 2.57 m/s; Trans. 2.56 m/s	Blue
Taljanovic et al. [20]	2017	SW-velocity VR 0.5-15 m/s	Acuson S3000 (9-4 MHz)	SWE	7	S	Lipoma: 1.74-5.52 m/s Tophus: 7.32 m/s Fibroma: 5.93 m/s Epidermoid cyst: 2.76 m/s Baker cyst: 2.8 m/s Enchondroma: 9.21-15 m/s	Blue
						H	Osteosarcoma: 4.12 m/s	Red
Pass et al. [28]	2016	Dim. 6 × 7 mm VR 0-6 m/s	Acuson S2000 (9-4 MHz)	SWE (ARFI)	50	S	Long. 1.36 m/s; Trans. 1.92 m/s	Red
						H	Long. 2.17 m/s; Trans. 2.15 m/s	Blue
Hahn et al. [22]	2017	ROI A/B (A: lesion; B: adjacent area)	Acuson S2000 (5.5-18 MHz)	Strain elastography Strain ratio Elasticity score	73	S	/	SR: 1.03 ± 0.93 ES: 3.08 ± 1.44 Red
						H	/	SR: 0.49 ± 0.45 ES: 3.76 ± 0.97 Blue
Park et al. [23]	2015	ROI lesion	LOGIQ E9 (6-15 MHz) IU22 (5-12 MHz)	Strain elastography score (1-4)	103	S	/	Score 1-2 Red
						H	/	Score 3-4 Blue
Magarelli et al. [24]	2014	ROI lesion	My Lab 70 XVG (5-12 MHz)	Strain elastography score (1-5)	32	S	/	Score 1-3 Red
						H	/	Score 4-5 Blue
Lee et al. [25]	2014	ROI B/A	Acuson S2000 (5.5-18 MHz)	Strain elastography	34	S	/	Lipoma (19): SR 0.83 ± 0.18 Ganglia (6): SR 2.78 ± 0.48 Epiderm. cyst (5): SR 0.17 ± 0.21 Pilomatricoma (4): SR 0.13 ± 0.02 Blue
						H	/	Red
Lalitha et al. [26]	2011	ROI lesion	GE E8 (8-12 MHz)	Real-time compression elastography	Few	S	/	Haemangioma Ganglion cyst Lipoma Red
						H	/	Blue

S: soft; H: hard; SR: strain ratio; ES: elasticity score; ROI: region of interest; Long.: longitudinal; Trans.: transversal.

malignant masses may have slower shear wave velocities than benign masses [28, 29].

To our knowledge, only three published studies concerned with the application of SWE in assessing musculoskeletal soft tissue masses presented quantitative elastographic results [20, 28, 29].

Using SWE to analyse soft tissue tumours, Pass et al. [28] reported an average 30% slower longitudinal shear wave velocity of malignant masses as compared to benign masses. The authors concluded upon this finding representing some evidence of an association between lower shear wave velocities and malignancy. Taljanovic et al. [20] described the applications of SWE in the evaluation of various pathologic conditions of the musculoskeletal system and its utility in the characterization of soft tissue masses.

Larger prospective studies will be needed to establish the diagnostic value of SWE in musculoskeletal tumours. While B-mode and Doppler imaging provide information on acoustic impedance and vascular flow allowing a more detailed interpretation of the microvasculature inside a tissue lesion, SWE provides information about the tissue stiffness and could be a useful complementary tool.

Ultrasound imaging has been evolving towards multiparameter assessment of soft tissue tumours and different techniques have now been developed to allow their more detailed analysis. SWE has been shown to have potential as a diagnostic and therapeutic tool not only for diseases of the breast, liver, thyroid, and prostate but also for musculoskeletal pathologies and in particular those of the hand [9, 17–19].

Ultrasound elastography appears to be a good complementary tool used in conjunction with B-mode ultrasound. This technique is reliable and reproducible and can be used and further developed to reinforce the assessment and enhance diagnostic confidence in malignant lesions of the musculoskeletal system [24, 25, 28, 29].

In the future, we foresee the completion of hand tumour assessment with a measurement of tissue viscosity, which has already proven to be useful in the assessment of liver lesions.

In our centre, we are developing a database of "histoelastographic" data on soft tissue tumours of the hand obtained using ultrasound.

References

[1] H. Guerini, G. Morvan, V. Vuillemin et al., "Ultrasound of wrist and hand masses," *Diagnostic and Interventional Imaging*, vol. 96, no. 12, pp. 1247–1260, 2015.

[2] F. Traina, C. Errani, A. Toscano et al., "Current concepts in the biopsy of musculoskeletal tumors," *The Journal of Bone and Joint Surgery American Volume*, vol. 97, no. 2, p. e7, 2015.

[3] A. Bermejo, T. D. De Bustamante, A. Martinez, R. Carrera, E. Zabía, and P. Manjón, "MR imaging in the evaluation of cystic-appearing soft-tissue masses of the extremities," *Radiographics*, vol. 33, no. 3, pp. 833–855, 2013.

[4] H. J. Mankin, C. J. Mankin, and M. A. Simon, "The hazards of the biopsy, revisited. Members of the Musculoskeletal Tumor Society," *The Journal of Bone and Joint Surgery American Volume*, vol. 78, no. 5, pp. 656–663, 1996.

[5] P. Thornley, A. Habib, A. Bozzo, N. Evaniew, and M. Ghert, "The role of denosumab in the modern treatment of giant cell tumor of bone," *JBJS Reviews*, vol. 5, no. 4, p. e4, 2017.

[6] L. Zhang, H. W. Wu, W. Yuan, and J. W. Zheng, "Propranolol therapy for infantile hemangioma: our experience," *Drug Design, Development and Therapy*, vol. 11, pp. 1401–1408, 2017.

[7] L. Debernard, L. Robert, F. Charleux, and S. F. Bensamoun, "Characterization of muscle architecture in children and adults using magnetic resonance elastography and ultrasound techniques," *Journal of Biomechanics*, vol. 44, no. 3, pp. 397–401, 2011.

[8] S. Gaucher, D. Maladry, A. M. Silitra, D. Documet, and H. J. Philippe, "Removal of subcutaneous lipomas: interest of liposuction," *Journal of Cosmetic Dermatology*, vol. 16, no. 3, pp. 400-401, 2017.

[9] J. Lamouille, C. Müller, S. Aubry, S. Bensamoun, W. Raffoul, and S. Durand, "Extensor indicis proprius tendon transfer using shear wave elastography," *Hand Surgery and Rehabilitation*, vol. 36, no. 3, pp. 173–180, 2017.

[10] J. Ophir, I. Céspedes, H. Ponnekanti, Y. Yazdi, and X. Li, "Elastography: a quantitative method for imaging the elasticity of biological tissues," *Ultrasonic Imaging*, vol. 13, no. 2, pp. 111–134, 1991.

[11] E. E. Drakonaki, G. M. Allen, and D. J. Wilson, "Ultrasound elastography for musculoskeletal applications," *The British Journal of Radiology*, vol. 85, no. 1019, pp. 1435–1445, 2012.

[12] A. S. Klauser, H. Miyamoto, R. Bellmann-Weiler, G. M. Feuchtner, M. C. Wick, and W. R. Jaschke, "Sonoelastography: musculoskeletal applications," *Radiology*, vol. 272, no. 3, pp. 622–633, 2014.

[13] S. J. Kim, H. J. Park, and S. Y. Lee, "Usefulness of strain elastography of the musculoskeletal system," *Ultrasonography*, vol. 35, no. 2, pp. 104–109, 2016.

[14] W. A. Berg, D. O. Cosgrove, C. J. Doré et al., "Shear-wave elastography improves the specificity of breast US: the BE1 multinational study of 939 masses," *Radiology*, vol. 262, no. 2, pp. 435–449, 2012.

[15] T. De Zordo, C. Fink, G. M. Feuchtner, V. Smekal, M. Reindl, and A. S. Klauser, "Real-time sonoelastography findings in healthy Achilles tendons," *American Journal of Roentgenology*, vol. 193, no. 2, pp. W134–W138, 2009.

[16] S. W. Hou, A. N. Merkle, J. S. Babb, R. McCabe, S. Gyftopoulos, and R. S. Adler, "Shear wave ultrasound elastographic evaluation of the rotator cuff tendon," *Journal of Ultrasound in Medicine*, vol. 36, no. 1, pp. 95–106, 2017.

[17] H. Miyamoto, T. Miura, H. Isayama, R. Masuzaki, K. Koike, and T. Ohe, "Stiffness of the first annular pulley in normal and trigger fingers," *The Journal of Hand Surgery*, vol. 36, no. 9, pp. 1486–1491, 2011.

[18] H. Miyamoto, T. Miura, Y. Morizaki, K. Uehara, T. Ohe, and S. Tanaka, "Comparative study on the stiffness of transverse carpal ligament between normal subjects and carpal tunnel syndrome patients," *Hand Surgery*, vol. 18, no. 2, pp. 209–214, 2013.

[19] P. Jafari, C. Muller, A. Grognuz et al., "First insights into human fingertip regeneration by Echo-Doppler imaging and wound microenvironment assessment," *International Journal of Molecular Sciences*, vol. 18, no. 5, 2017.

[20] M. S. Taljanovic, L. H. Gimber, G. W. Becker et al., "Shear--wave elastography: basic physics and musculoskeletal applications," *Radiographics*, vol. 37, no. 3, pp. 855–870, 2017.

[21] N. Winn, R. Lalam, and V. Cassar-Pullicino, "Sonoelastography in the musculoskeletal system: current role and future directions," *World Journal of Radiology*, vol. 8, no. 11, pp. 868–879, 2016.

[22] S. Hahn, Y. H. Lee, S. H. Lee, and J. S. Suh, "Value of the strain ratio on ultrasonic elastography for differentiation of benign and malignant soft tissue tumors," *Journal of Ultrasound in Medicine*, vol. 36, no. 1, pp. 121–127, 2017.

[23] H. J. Park, S. Y. Lee, S. M. Lee, W. T. Kim, S. Lee, and K. S. Ahn, "Strain elastography features of epidermoid tumours in superficial soft tissue: differences from other benign soft-tissue tumours and malignant tumours," *The British Journal of Radiology*, vol. 88, no. 1050, article 20140797, 2015.

[24] N. Magarelli, C. Carducci, C. Bucalo et al., "Sonoelastography for qualitative and quantitative evaluation of superficial soft tissue lesions: a feasibility study," *European Radiology*, vol. 24, no. 3, pp. 566–573, 2014.

[25] Y. H. Lee, H. T. Song, and J. S. Suh, "Use of strain ratio in evaluating superficial soft tissue tumors on ultrasonic elastography," *Journal of Medical Ultrasonics*, vol. 41, no. 3, pp. 319–323, 2014.

[26] P. Lalitha, M. C. B. Reddy, and K. J. Reddy, "Musculoskeletal applications of elastography: a pictorial essay of our initial experience," *Korean Journal of Radiology*, vol. 12, no. 3, pp. 365–375, 2011.

[27] H. J. Shin, M. J. Kim, H. Y. Kim, Y. H. Roh, and M. J. Lee, "Comparison of shear wave velocities on ultrasound elastography between different machines, transducers, and acquisition depths: a phantom study," *European Radiology*, vol. 26, no. 10, pp. 3361–3367, 2016.

[28] B. Pass, M. Johnson, E. M. A. Hensor, H. Gupta, and P. Robinson, "Sonoelastography of musculoskeletal soft tissue masses: a pilot study of quantitative evaluation," *Journal of Ultrasound in Medicine*, vol. 35, no. 10, pp. 2209–2216, 2016.

[29] B. Pass, M. Jafari, E. Rowbotham, E. M. A. Hensor, H. Gupta, and P. Robinson, "Do quantitative and qualitative shear wave elastography have a role in evaluating musculoskeletal soft tissue masses?," *European Radiology*, vol. 27, no. 2, pp. 723–731, 2017.

22

Prepatellar Bursitis with Abscess due to *Corynebacterium ulcerans*

Sachin M. Patil,[1] Phillip Paul Beck,[2] Taylor B. Nelson,[2] Andres Bran Acevedo,[2] and William Roland[2]

[1]*Department of Medicine, Division of Pulmonary, Critical Care and Environmental Medicine, University of Missouri Hospital and Clinic, One Hospital Dr, Columbia, MO 65212, USA*
[2]*Department of Medicine, Division of Infectious Disease, University of Missouri Hospital and Clinic, One Hospital Dr, Columbia, MO 65212, USA*

Correspondence should be addressed to Sachin M. Patil; drssmp1@gmail.com

Academic Editor: Konstantinos Anagnostakos

Corynebacteria are ubiquitous and reside as skin and mucosa commensals in animals. They are considered contaminants in clinical specimens, but significant clinical data points to their virulence and pathogenic potential over the last two decades. *Corynebacteria* can cause both community-acquired and nosocomial infections. *Corynebacterium diphtheriae* (*C. diphtheriae*) responsible for diphtheria has declined over the previous two decades with an increase in a similar clinical syndrome by *Corynebacterium ulcerans* (*C. ulcerans*) in Europe. As per recent studies, *C. ulcerans* shares similar virulence factors with *C. diphtheriae*. *C. ulcerans* has been implicated in airway infections, skin and soft tissue infections, lymphadenitis, wound infections, and rarely necrotizing fasciitis. Pet or farm animals have been the source of these infections to humans, as per recent reports. Strains can be either toxigenic or nontoxigenic. Due to recent advances, methods to characterize strains have become easier with mass spectrometry. Antimicrobial susceptibility testing is a must for definite treatment as *C. ulcerans* can be resistant to first-line antibiotic therapy. If resources are available, it is prudent to find if there is any toxin production. Here, we describe a rural farmer in central Missouri presenting with acute-onset right knee pain diagnosed with right prepatellar bursitis with abscess due to *C. ulcerans* infection. He recovered with surgical debridement and antimicrobial therapy. This is the first case of *C. ulcerans* causing prepatellar bursitis with an abscess as per medical literature review.

1. Introduction

Corynebacterium is an aerobic nonsporulating gram-positive rod [1]. *Corynebacterium diphtheriae* (*C. diphtheriae*) is a well-known subspecies of this group, which causes diphtheria, a potentially lethal disease in the pediatric population and unvaccinated adults associated with significant morbidity and long-term sequelae. Diphtheria is a public health issue in countries with inadequate vaccination strategies. Incidence in the United States of America (USA) is <0.01 case per 100,000 persons [2]. Two other subspecies that produce a virulent factor toxin are *Corynebacterium pseudotuberculosis* (*C. pseudotuberculosis*) and *Corynebacterium ulcerans* (*C. ulcerans*) [3, 4]. Both produce disease in livestock such as cattle, goats, and sheep and pet animals (cats or dogs). Infected livestock and animal pets serve as reservoirs for this infection. Zoonotic transmission occurs via raw contaminated milk consumption or contact with wound discharge or animal secretions [3]. In some European countries, it is the leading cause of cutaneous diphtheria in adults [4, 5]. Respiratory diphtheria due to *C. ulcerans*, mostly from industrialized countries, has increased over the last few decades as well [3]. In the USA, from 1996 to 2018, *C. ulcerans* was responsible for causing airway disease in five patients (culture positive). All five individuals' vaccination status against diphtheria was inadequate [2]. A single conjunctivitis case by a toxigenic strain was reported from Missouri in 2018, possibly from a pet animal exposure [6]. Animal exposure is not the source for all human cases of *C. ulcerans*, although human-to-human transmission has not been proven yet [3, 4]. A

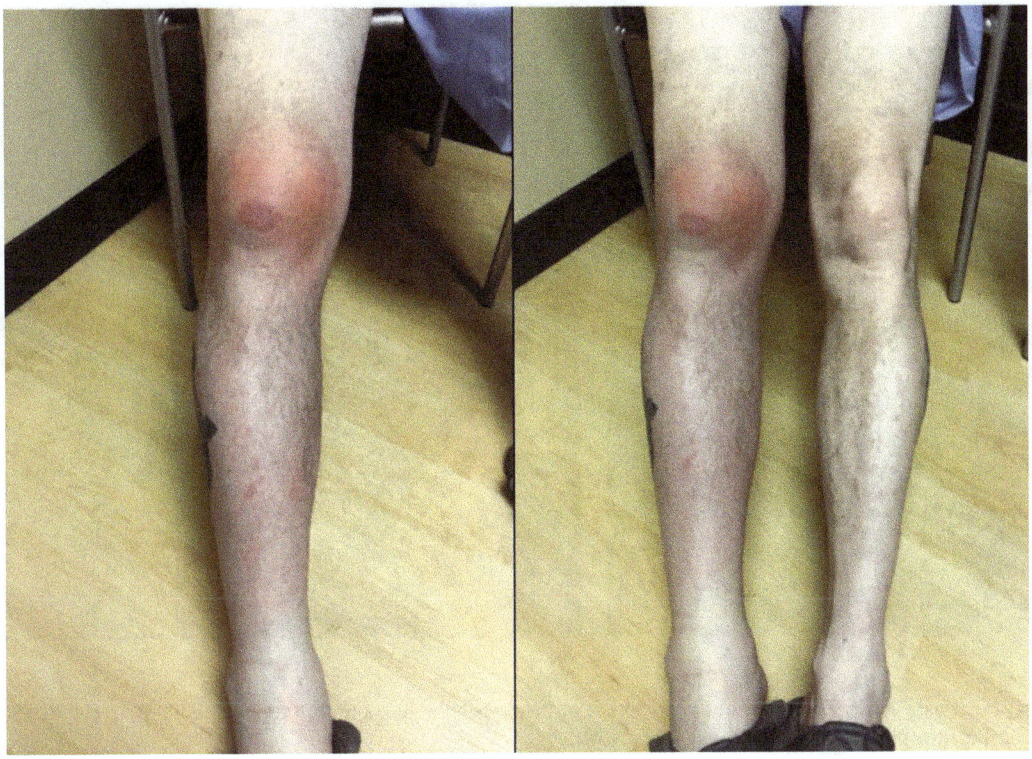

Figure 1: Right leg prepatellar bursitis with extension of inflammation to the upper medial thigh and lower leg.

PubMed literature search revealed no prior case reports of *C. ulcerans* as a cause of prepatellar bursitis with abscess. Here, we report the case of a rural hog farmer who presented with acute-onset right knee pain diagnosed with right prepatellar bursitis with abscess due to *C. ulcerans* infection.

2. Case Presentation

A 53-year-old male patient presented to the orthopedic clinic at our institution for new-onset right knee pain of two-day duration. His past medical history was significant for type two diabetes mellitus, acid reflux disorder, chronic obstructive pulmonary disease, and left shoulder osteoarthritis. His smoking history consisted of 1.5 packs per day with 40 pack-years with no alcohol or substance abuse. He is a self-employed hog farmer. One day before the presentation, he noticed progressive soft tissue swelling over the right knee with erythema extending from the midthigh down to below the knee. The right knee pain was described as intense and sharp with a grade of 10/10 with radiation to the right hip and difficulty in right lower extremity weight-bearing. There were no associated fevers, chills, night sweats, nausea, vomiting, or change in left shoulder pain. There was no history of right knee trauma, gout, or intra-articular steroid injection. His job demanded him to be on his knees during the day. A general observation revealed a middle-aged male in mild distress. Clinical examination showed stable vital signs and an antalgic gait. The direct clinical inspection was notable for right lower extremity diffuse swelling from the midthigh to the foot along with significant erythema (Figures 1 and 2). Palpation revealed tenderness over the superior portion of

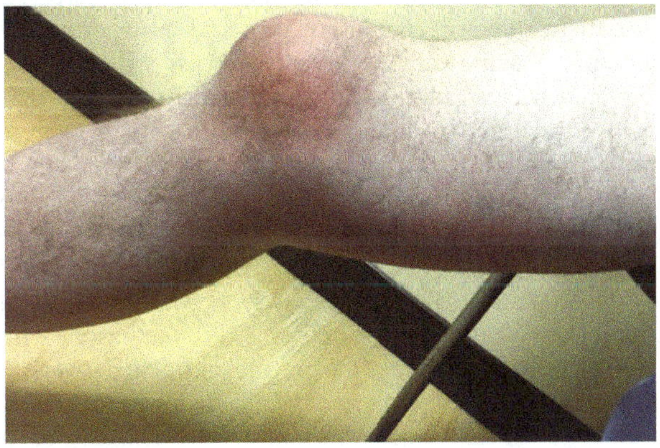

Figure 2: Lateral view of the right knee joint revealing right knee prepatellar bursitis with extension of inflammation.

the patella with no effusion. His knee flexion was limited to 100 degrees with no joint laxity. The right knee X-ray displayed prepatellar soft tissue swelling without osseous abnormality. A transfer to the emergency department (ED) for further care was initiated.

At the ED, the patient was tachycardic with stable blood pressure and oxygenation. Labs revealed a leukocytosis of 13,250/mL with an erythrocyte sedimentation rate of 76 mm/hr (0–40 mm/hr), C reactive protein of 6.74 mg/dL (<0.4 mg/dL), and a normal metabolic panel. Hemoglobin A1c was 7.4%, indicative of well-controlled diabetes mellitus. Right knee ultrasound showed generalized knee and calf subcutaneous edema. A $1.7 \times 1.6 \times 0.6$ cm fluid collection along the deep subcutaneous tissue at the knee joint level was

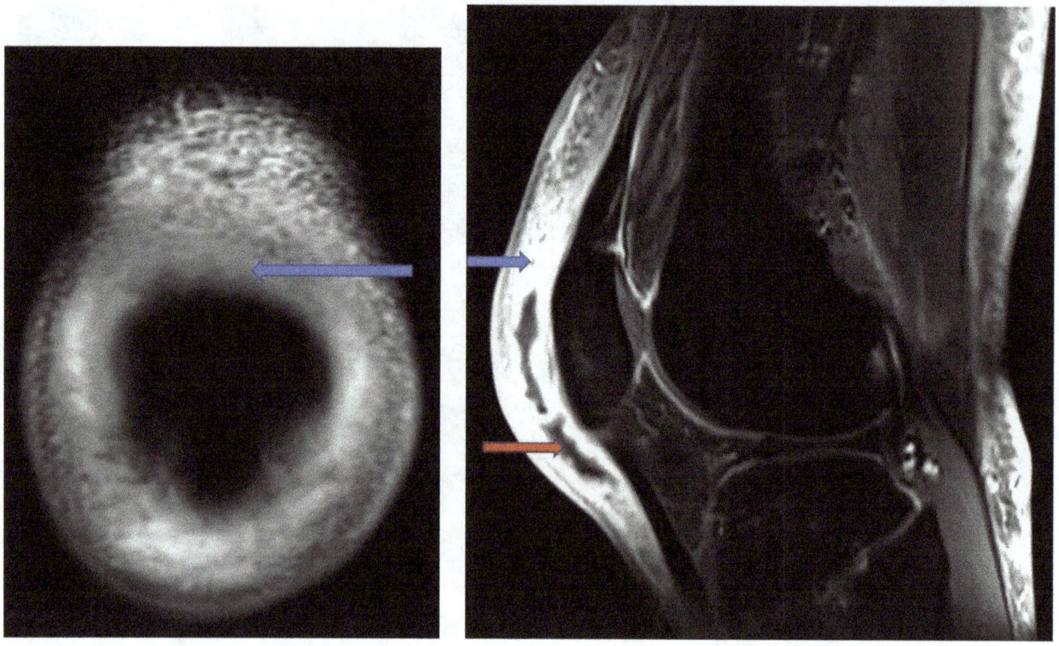

(a) (b)

Figure 3: (a) MRI coronal view reveals an area of hypodensity in the prepatellar bursa indicating bursitis (blue arrow). (b) Sagittal T1 view reveals prepatellar bursitis (blue arrow) and abscess (red arrow).

present along with the anterior medial knee with no knee joint involvement. Two sets of blood cultures were sent. The patient received Toradol for pain and intravenous (IV) clindamycin empirically. A bedside abscess aspiration was futile, and he was admitted to the internal medicine (IM). Orthopedic surgery recommended right knee magnetic resonance imaging (MRI). Due to suspected infection, IV clindamycin was stopped, and vancomycin was started. The next day, right knee MRI displayed a prepatellar bursa abscess (1 × 13.5 × 6 cm) with surrounding bursitis and myositis (Figures 3(a) and 3(b)). Preoperatively, he was given a single IV dose of cefazolin 2 gm (Gram) and dexamethasone 8 mg. An incision and drainage of the prepatellar bursitis revealed a small amount of murky fluid; it was sent for gram stain in addition to 14-day anaerobic, fungal, and acid-fast bacilli (AFB) cultures. Additionally, right prepatellar bursa tissue cultures were sent. Gram stain was positive for gram-positive rods. Postoperatively, he was continued on IV vancomycin. A positive abscess gram stain result necessitated an infectious disease (ID) consultation. The ID team recommended following final cultures and continuing empiric IV vancomycin. The patient did not oblige to staying inpatient as recommended by the ID team for culture-guided definite therapy but was willing to be followed up in the outpatient clinic. He discharged against medical advice (AMA); before discharge, he received a single IV dalbavancin 1.5 gm dose. An orthopedic, IM, and ID follow-up was arranged before discharge. Blood cultures, AFB cultures, and fungal cultures returned negative. The abscess fluid and the prepatellar tissue cultures both grew *C. ulcerans*. The susceptibility pattern indicated that it was intermediate to penicillin and sensitive to ceftriaxone, meropenem, and vancomycin (Table 1). At a two-week follow-up, the patient's pain had improved with decreased warmth and swelling. Clinical examination revealed superficial dehiscence and mild tenderness on palpation. He received another two weeks of oral cefdinir to complete therapy. At a six-week follow-up with the orthopedics, the incision site had healed with joint mobility and weight-bearing recovery.

Table 1: Antibiotic susceptibility.

Organism	*Corynebacterium ulcerans*	
Antibiotic	MIC (mcg/mL)	Interpretation
Penicillin	1	Intermediate
Ceftriaxone	1	Susceptible
Meropenem	≤0.25	Susceptible
Vancomycin	≤1	Susceptible

MIC = minimum inhibitory concentration.

3. Discussion

C. ulcerans is a nonlipophilic, fermentative *Corynebacterium* subspecies belonging to the *C. diphtheriae* group, which causes mastitis in cattle and airway disease in other livestock [1]. Its reservoir includes livestock, pet animals, squirrels, otters, camels, monkeys, and other wild animals [3]. It can produce the diphtheria toxin, which is 95% homologous to the toxin produced by *C. diphtheriae* [3]. Potential virulence factors are the diphtheria-like toxin (DT), phospholipase D, Shiga-like ribosome binding protein, endoglycosidase of the EndoE family, sialidase, adherence pili and complex cell wall containing peptidoglycan, and an outer mycolic acid layer [3]. Phospholipase D and DT can cause local tissue necrosis [4]. An experimental in vivo mouse model indicates that the high virulence of *C. ulcerans* is independent of DT production [3]. DT is a proteinaceous exotoxin with tropism for the myocardium, nervous system, kidneys, and suprarenal glands. Zoonotic transmission results in airway disease, skin and soft tissue infections, and tonsil, peritoneum, lymph node, and ear infections. Transmission occurs via raw milk consumption and contact with animal wounds or secretions. Transmission from wild animals to livestock has been suggested [3]. The incubation period is one to six days [4]. An increase in *C. ulcerans* zoonosis was observed in industrialized nations recently [4]. The prevalent risk factor has been animal contact in most cases. The zoonotic transmission has been verified in multiple cases, whereas human-to-human transmission has been proven in a single case [3].

Clinical manifestations are variable based on the infection site. Respiratory illness similar to diphtheria is the most common manifestation, and in some countries, it is more frequent than *C. diphtheria* [5]. Upper airway disease presents with a sore throat which can progress to a swollen bull neck with clinical examination revealing a firmly adherent pseudomembrane. If unattended, this can cause airway obstruction. Lower airway disease is rare in comparison. The next most common presentation is the cutaneous disease, which manifests as an erythematous tender rolled edge ulcer with adjacent edema. DT can also cause myocarditis, peripheral neuropathy, and bulbar dysfunction. It is seen commonly with respiratory illness and is rare in extensive cutaneous disease [5]. Rare clinical presentations include peritonitis, caseous lymphadenitis, and bronchopneumonia [3, 7, 8].

Diagnosis is arrived at by reviewing symptomatology, physical examination, and microbiologic evaluation. Clinical specimens include oropharyngeal and nasal mucosa, cutaneous lesions of both patients, and suspected animal contacts for the prior two weeks. Bacterial growth media selected are blood agar and tellurite-containing agar [3]. Species-level identification is favored if cultured from sterile sites (blood or cerebrospinal fluid) or is the prevalent organism on gram stain or urine culture [1]. Vitek or matrix-assisted laser desorption ionization-time of flight mass spectrometry is used to identify the bacteria precisely. A modified Elek test or a polymerase chain-based genotypic test can detect toxin production [3]. A matrix-assisted laser desorption ionization-time of flight mass spectrometry (MALDI-TOF MS) review reveals exceptional results in comparison to conventional methods and helps in identifying accurately up to genus and species level (>90%) [9]. A MALDI-TOF MS-based instrument database needs to be updated when used to detect the *Corynebacterium* microorganism. Based on Clinical and Laboratory Standards Institute breakpoints, 76% of *C. ulcerans* are intermediate to penicillin, 97% are susceptible to erythromycin, and 100% are susceptible to vancomycin. Only 3% of *Corynebacterium* species are resistant to erythromycin [10]. Dalbavancin is as efficacious as vancomycin against *Corynebacterium* species [11, 12]. Erythromycin is the drug of choice for *C. ulcerans* infections [10]. For severe disease, diphtheria antitoxin (DAT) at the earliest is recommended as it inhibits the systematic toxin effects [5]. Antimicrobial susceptibility can detect resistance patterns to modify, deescalate, or use an alternative agent for therapy. Antibodies against diphtheria toxoid decline by 10% annually, so decennial vaccination is needed [4]. Diphtheria toxoid possibly decreases disease severity with no effect on colonization and infection [2, 4]. Most patients with *C. ulcerans* infections have partial or complete diphtheria toxoid vaccination and are above 60 yrs [4]. Droplet and contact precautions should be followed as in diphtheria [13]. Disease elimination will require immediate antibiotic therapy, decreasing symptomatic carrier transmission risk, and decennial vaccination in adults.

Our patient had multiple sources of infection, including hogs and pet animals. He has recurrent minor abrasions over the knee during his farm work. He likely suffered less severe disease due to his full diphtheroid toxoid vaccination status. Our institution lacked laboratory capability to identify toxin production. Appropriate antimicrobial therapy and surgical intervention resulted in an excellent recovery. Physicians should use the guidance provided for diphtheria treatment for *C. ulcerans* infections. As *C. ulcerans* is not a notifiable disease, no surveillance measures were available to identify the transmission source. A PubMed literature review reveals no prior cases. The toxigenicity of isolated cultures should be assessed. *C. ulcerans* disease's infrequent occurrence and the lack of specimen culture sampling result in delayed diagnosis with grave implications.

4. Conclusion

This is the first case of prepatellar bursitis with abscess due to *C. ulcerans*. *C. ulcerans* needs to be considered in the correct epidemiological setting, particularly where zoonotic transmission is suspected. Physicians must be cognizant of disease acquisition from pet animals and its pathogenicity. Only a few cases have been described before in the USA. It is not a notifiable disease, as per the Centers for Disease Control and Prevention. For toxigenicity and species confirmation, it is ideal to send the isolate to a reference laboratory. Animal reservoirs can perpetuate infection in the community. In the future, the incidence may increase, leading to more diverse disease manifestations. Disease monitoring is essential to detect and prevent its spread. A recommendation for close contacts is vaccination. DAT therapy should be considered in patients with severe disease. Diphtheria vaccine decennial boosters in adults may provide some immunity against this infection, especially against toxin production, and decrease clinical severity. Current clinical laboratories in the USA cannot detect toxins due to a lack of expertise. The presence of *Corynebacteria* in clinical specimens should be processed judiciously.

Consent

The patient provided consent for this case report.

References

[1] R. Kim and A. C. Reboli, *Mandell, Douglas, and Bennett's Prin-*

ciples and Practice of Infectious Diseases, Elsevier, Philadelphia, 9th edition, 2020.

[2] J. O. Otshudiema, A. M. Acosta, P. K. Cassiday, S. C. Hadler, S. Hariri, and T. S. P. Tiwari, "Respiratory illness caused by Corynebacterium diphtheriae and C. ulcerans, and use of diphtheria anti-toxin in the United States, 1996-2018," *Clinical Infectious Diseases*, no. article ciaa1218, 2020.

[3] E. Hacker, C. A. Antunes, A. L. Mattos-Guaraldi, A. Burkovski, and A. Tauch, "Corynebacterium ulcerans, an emerging human pathogen," *Future Microbiology*, vol. 11, no. 9, pp. 1191–1208, 2016.

[4] A. A. Dias, L. S. Santos, P. S. Sabbadini et al., "Difteria pelo Corynebacterium ulcerans: uma zoonose emergente no Brasil e no mundo," *Revista de Saúde Pública*, vol. 45, no. 6, pp. 1176–1191, 2011.

[5] L. S. P. Moore, A. Leslie, M. Meltzer, A. Sandison, A. Efstratiou, and S. Sriskandan, "*Corynebacterium ulcerans* cutaneous diphtheria," *The Lancet Infectious Diseases*, vol. 15, no. 9, pp. 1100–1107, 2015.

[6] L. M. Weil, C. Butler, K. R. Howell et al., "Notes from the field: conjunctivitis caused by toxigenic Corynebacterium ulcerans - Missouri, 2018," *MMWR. Morbidity and Mortality Weekly Report*, vol. 68, no. 27, pp. 615-616, 2019.

[7] Y. Kimura, Y. Watanabe, N. Suga et al., "Acute peritonitis due to Corynebacterium ulcerans in a patient receiving continuous ambulatory peritoneal dialysis: a case report and literature review," *Clinical and Experimental Nephrology*, vol. 15, no. 1, pp. 171–174, 2011.

[8] I. Yasuda, H. Matsuyama, T. Ishifuji et al., "Severe pneumonia caused by toxigenic Corynebacterium ulcerans infection, Japan," *Emerging Infectious Diseases*, vol. 24, no. 3, pp. 588–591, 2018.

[9] A. A. Zasada and E. Mosiej, "Contemporary microbiology and identification of Corynebacteria spp. causing infections in human," *Letters in Applied Microbiology*, vol. 66, no. 6, pp. 472–483, 2018.

[10] D. V. Marosevic, A. Berger, G. Kahlmeter, S. K. Payer, S. Hörmansdorfer, and A. Sing, "Antimicrobial susceptibility of Corynebacterium diphtheriae and Corynebacterium ulcerans in Germany 2011-17," *The Journal of Antimicrobial Chemotherapy*, vol. 75, no. 10, pp. 2885–2893, 2020.

[11] E. J. Goldstein, D. M. Citron, C. V. Merriam, Y. Warren, K. Tyrrell, and H. T. Fernandez, "In vitro activities of dalbavancin and nine comparator agents against anaerobic gram-positive species and corynebacteria," *Antimicrobial Agents and Chemotherapy*, vol. 47, no. 6, pp. 1968–1971, 2003.

[12] A. C. Gales, H. S. Sader, and R. N. Jones, "Antimicrobial activity of dalbavancin tested against Gram-positive clinical isolates from Latin American medical centres," *Clinical Microbiology and Infection*, vol. 11, no. 2, pp. 95–100, 2005.

[13] M. F. Lartigue, X. Monnet, A. le Flèche et al., "Corynebacterium ulcerans in an immunocompromised patient with diphtheria and her dog," *Journal of Clinical Microbiology*, vol. 43, no. 2, pp. 999–1001, 2005.

23

Isolated Posterior Medial Ankle Dislocation with Associated Os Trigonum Dislocation after Low-Energy Mechanism

Devan Irving, Brent Geers, and Bruce Lawrence

Ascension Genesys Hospital, 1 Genesys Parkway, Grand Blanc, MI. 48439, USA

Correspondence should be addressed to Devan Irving; devanirving7@gmail.com

Academic Editor: Athanassios Papanikolaou

We describe a case of an isolated posteromedial ankle dislocation, without malleolar fracture, with associated dislocation of an os trigonal process after a low-energy tennis injury. We demonstrate that nonoperative treatment results in excellent functional outcome scores with minimal arthritic progression at 2 years of follow-up. We discuss pathoanatomic risk factors of pure dislocations and propose that an os trigonum is a risk factor for isolated dislocations of the ankle.

1. Introduction

Ankle dislocation without an associated fracture (pure ankle dislocation) is a rare injury accounting for only 0.065% of all ankle injuries [1]. Due to its rarity, pure ankle dislocations are not well understood with only case reports and small case series being described in the literature [2–10]. Even more unusual is a pure ankle dislocation with associated dislocation of an os trigonal process. This phenomenon has been described only once by Segal et al., in conjuncture with an anterior dislocation of the ankle [11]. Currently, risk factors for pure ankle dislocation are thought to be ligamentous hyperlaxity, medial malleolar hypoplasia, talar undercoverage, and history of prior ankle sprains [4, 6–9]. We present a case of posterior ankle dislocation with associated os trigonal dislocation following low-energy trauma and discussion of an os trigonal process as a possible risk factor for pure ankle dislocation.

2. Case Report

A 17-year-old female, LL, presented to our level 2 emergency room with pain and gross deformity of her left ankle. She sustained a plantarflexion and inversion injury while playing tennis. She reported pain in the ankle but denied paresthesia or loss of strength distal to the injury. She did not have any prior medical or surgical history and denied allergies to medications. She had met all developmental milestones at appropriate times. She and her parents denied any family history of hypermobility syndromes. She had no history of pain, instability, recurrent sprains, or prior functional issues in the affected ankle.

Physical examination demonstrated an inversion and internal rotation deformity of the ankle (Figure 1). The lateral malleolus was prominent with a 1 cm by 0.5 cm overlying superficial abrasion, which did not extend deeper than the epidermis. Distally, her foot was neurovascularly intact with +2/4 pulses in the dorsalis pedis and posterior tibial arteries with brisk capillary refill and sensation present in all nerve distributions. Radiographs of the left ankle were obtained and demonstrated a posteromedial ankle dislocation without malleolar fracture (Figure 2). On the lateral view, a double density over the posterior process of the talus was noticed and suspected to be an anteriorly displaced os trigonum. The patient was sedated with IV ketamine, and closed reduction of the ankle was performed. Reduction maneuver consisted of flexion of the knee to 90 degrees, anterior translation, and external rotation of the foot with posteriorly directed counter pressure on the tibia. The ankle was not stressed after reduction. A well-padded, short-leg posterior splint with stirrups was placed with the ankle in a neutral dorsiflexed position. Post reduction radiographs demonstrated a congruent tibiotalar joint reduction and reduced position of the os trigonum. However, persistent lucency of

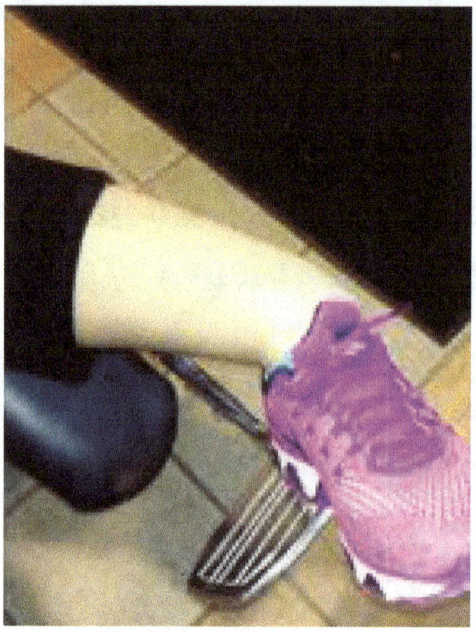

Figure 1: Gross internal rotation and inversion injury of the left ankle.

2 mm between the os trigonum and the talar body remained. Post reduction computed topography was obtained and demonstrated no fracture, but well corticated and unfused posterior lateral process of the talus, consistent with an os trigonum (Figure 3).

The patient was treated nonoperatively with nonweight-bearing management initially in a short leg splint for two weeks and then cast for 4 weeks. At 6 weeks, she began to weight bear as tolerated in a walking boot. She resumed all normal activities by 3 months.

The final follow-up was 2 years from initial injury at which time the patient was very happy with her outcome. She admitted to mild, painless swelling in the injured ankle after activity and the occasional sensation of painless instability approximately once every 2 months. She was able to return to playing tennis the season after her injury. The patient was assessed with The American Orthopedic Foot and Ankle Society (AOFAS) Ankle-Hindfoot Score, visual analog scale (VAS), and Beighton score for hypermobility [12–14]. She scored perfectly in all categories of the AOFAS (pain, function, and alignment) for a final score of 100/100 points, indicating normal ankle function. She reported a 0/10 VAS score. Finally, the patient scored a 3 on the Beighton scale indicating no hypermobility. She had no pain over her os trigonum and no pain with forced plantar flexion. There was no laxity with drawer or talar tilt testing. Radiographs of bilateral ankles were obtained, and the injury side demonstrated medial talar and tibial osteophyte formation with mild anterior joint space narrowing. This is consistent with Kellgren-Lawrence Grade 1 changes of post traumatic osteoarthritis [15]. Medial malar hypoplasia was not present using the method described by Elise et al. [16]. Talar coverage was also found to be within normal limits according to the method described by Shaik et al. [7]. Notably, radiographs of the contralateral ankle also showed an os trigonum. When comparing os trigonums, the injured left side demonstrated more diastasis between the talus and os trigonum than the uninjured right side (Figure 4).

3. Discussion

Pure ankle dislocations and bilateral os trigonums are uncommon entities. Pure ankle dislocations represent only 13 per 20,000 ankle injuries, with the two most common causes being sporting injuries and motor vehicle accidents [1]. The rarity of this injury is attributed to the mechanical stability of the ankle mortise, with the ligamentous structures being relatively stronger than the boney malleoli. This results in the fracture of the malleoli prior to disruption of the ligaments and consequently a fracture dislocation rather than a pure dislocation [2]. Pure dislocations are classified by the direction of talar displacement: anterior, posterior, medial, or lateral. Posteromedial displacement is the most common, accounting for 46% [1]. In posteromedial dislocations, the deltoid ligament generally remains intact leading to the more medial orientation of the talus. Generally, this allows for avoidance of talar avascular necrosis because of the maintained talar blood flow through the deltoid ligament [1]. In our patient, we suspect the deltoid ligament remained intact given the posteromedial displacement and the lack of talar collapse at 2 years of follow-up. The exact mechanistic sequence of a posterior pure dislocation is debated in the literature. There is consensus that the position of the foot during injury is inversion and extreme plantarflexion. However, there is disagreement on how the talus comes to reside posteriorly. Fernandez, in his cadaveric study, was able to demonstrate pure dislocation only through anterior extrusion. Because of this, he reasoned that after anterior dislocation, the Achilles pulled the talus posteriorly [17]. Conversely, other authors feel that in the unstable equinus position, an appropriately directed force could result in direct posterior extrusion [7, 18–20].

An os trigonum is an accessory ossicle which overlies the posterior-lateral process of the talus. In normal development, the secondary talar ossification center (os trigonum) appears at 7-14 years and fuses to the talar body within 1 year of ossification [21, 22]. If fusion does not occur, an os trigonum results and is attached to the talus by a fibrous synchondrosis. Like pure ankle dislocations, bilateral os trigonum is uncommon. Zwiers et al. found the incidence of bilateral os trigonums to be only 14.3% in their retrospective CT evaluation of 628 patients [20]. Injury of the os trigonum can occur by two different mechanisms. Extreme equinus results in compression of the os between the calcaneus and posterior tibia, which may result in a "nutcracker" type of fracture. Conversely, an inversion injury can lead to avulsion of the os by tensioning through the posterior talofibular ligament (PTFL) [23].

We present a case of a pure posteromedial ankle dislocation with a dislocated os trigonum in the setting of low-energy trauma. To the author's knowledge, this is the first case of this specific injury to be presented in the literature. Segal and colleges described a nearly opposite case of a pure anterior ankle dislocation with os trigonum dislocation following a motor vehicle accident. Segal hypothesized that in his case, violent plantarflexion with the calcaneus resting

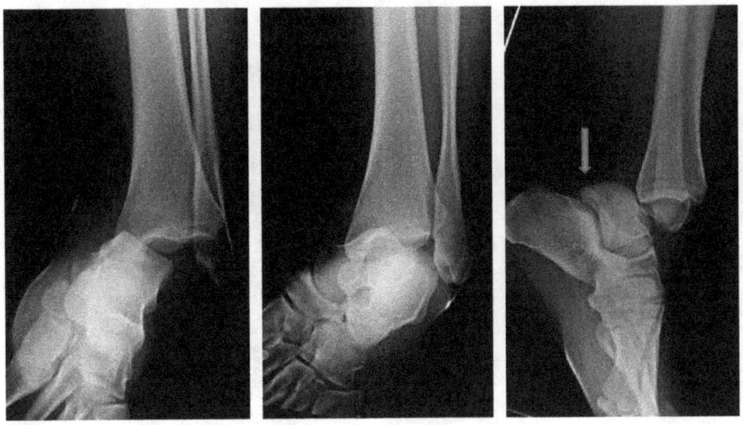

Figure 2: AP, lateral, and mortise radiograph demonstrating posteromedial ankle dislocation. The arrow on lateral view points towards double density over posterior talus representing displaced os trigonum.

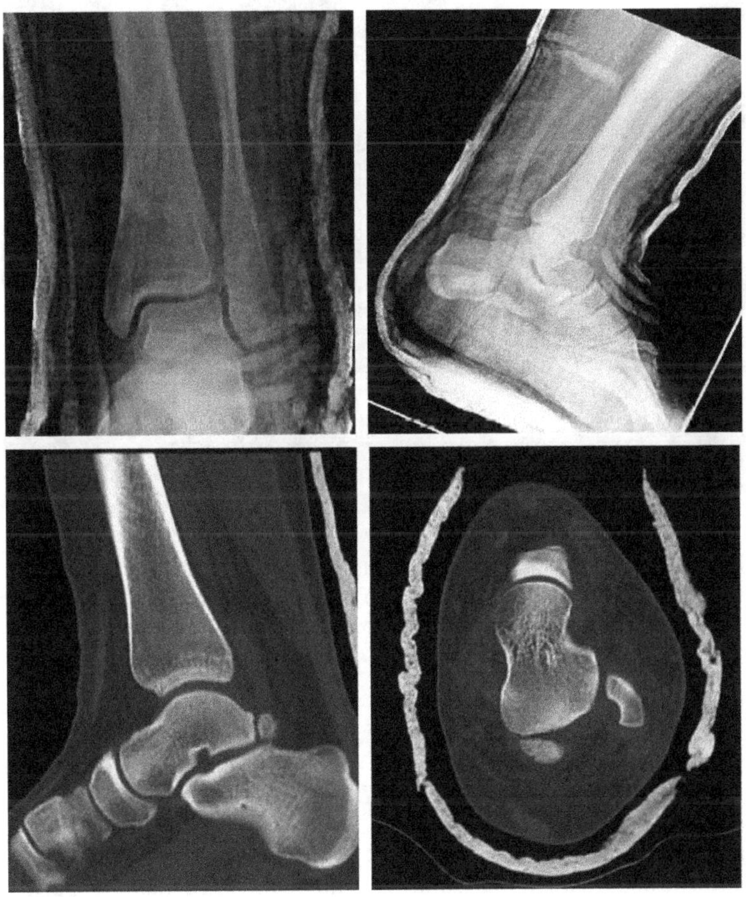

Figure 3: Mortise and lateral radiographs demonstrating reduced tibiotalar joint. Axial and lateral CT scans demonstrate displaced os trigonum without the fracture.

on the motorcycles' foot peg resulted in anterior dislocation and a compression-type fracture of the os trigonum [11]. In lower energy trauma, anatomic variations and prior injuries are thought to predispose individuals to sustaining this rare injury. Current risk factors include medial malleolar hypoplasia, talar undercoverage, hypermobility, and history of recurrent ankle sprains [6–9, 21].

Our patient demonstrated no known risk factors, and we believe the presence of an os trigonum may be a new risk factor. Normally, the PTFL short fibers run from the fibula to the lateral talus whereas the long fibers run from the fibula to the posterior-lateral process of the talus [24]. If an os trigonum is present, then the long fibers attach directly onto the os, which is only attached to the talus by a synchondrosis

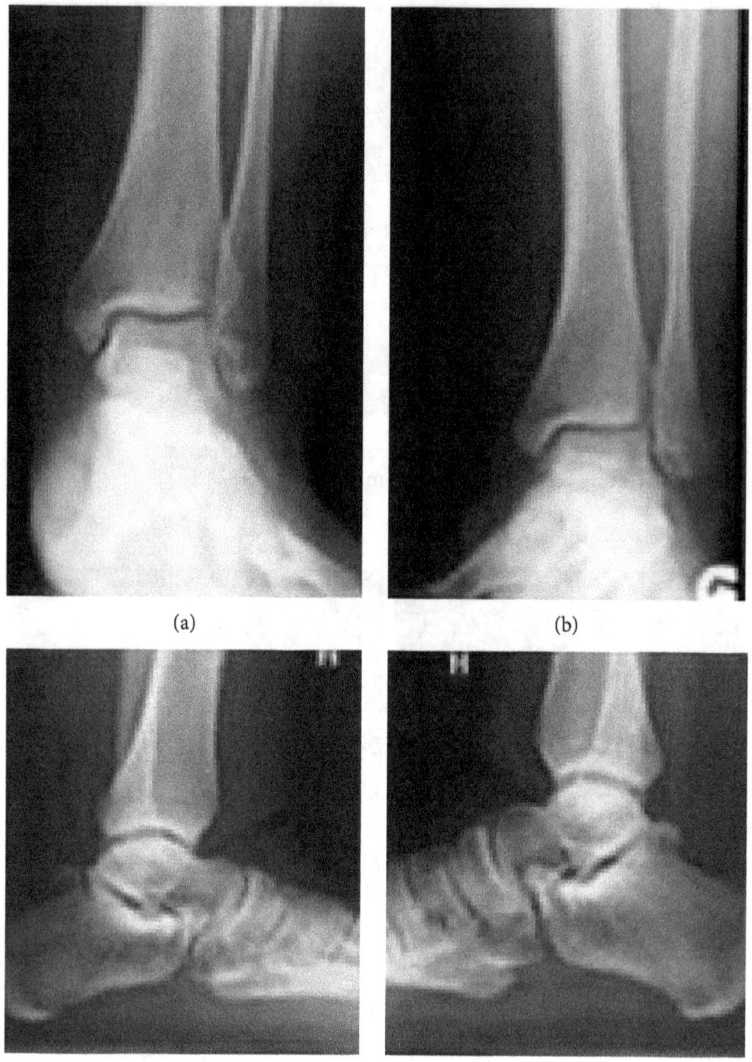

(a) (b) (c) (d)

FIGURE 4: (a) AP view of the left ankle demonstrating mild medial tibial and talar osteophyte formation. (b) Mortise view of the left ankle again demonstrating medial osteophyte formation. (c) Lateral view of the left ankle demonstrating anterior tibial osteophyte formation and mild narrowing with mildly displaced os trigonum. (d) Lateral view of right ankle demonstrating nondisplaced os trigonum.

[25]. We hypothesize that this results in an anatomic "weak link" in the ankle due to the synchondrosis being less robust than the bony malleolus and the normal PTFL attachment. The position of equinus and inversion is known to cause both injuries to the relatively weak ATFL, as well as, avulsion of the os trigonum through its synchondrosis [23, 26]. In this scenario, the lateral ligamentous complex would be significantly weakened, possibly pre-disposing to posterior dislocation [27]. This theory is supported by Gursoy et al.'s findings in their 2015 retrospective MRI study. In this study, they found an association between the presence of an os trigonum and an increase in signal intensity throughout the lateral ankle ligaments, which pointed towards chronic instability [25]. Despite this, pure ankle dislocation has not been reported as a complication following excision of symptomatic os trigonum without repair of the PTFL insertion. However, the literature on the subject is primarily small level IV studies [28–34]. Given that pure ankle dislocation is such a rare entity, it is possible these small studies were underpowered to detect its increased rate postoperatively.

Furthermore, our study corroborates the findings of multiple other authors in that ankle dislocations, without malleolar fracture, can be treated nonoperatively with good results [2–10]. This is likely due to the intact deltoid ligament and maintained blood supply. At two years, our patient reported a perfect score on the AOFAS and 0/10 pain on VAS. Radiographically, her ankle demonstrated only very mild arthritic changes which were likely a result of the initial injury. She occasionally experienced sensations of instability but this could not be reproduced on physical exam and was not symptomatic enough to prevent her from returning to sport. The injured ankle did continue to demonstrate slight widening of the os trigonum synchondrosis compared to the contralateral side, but this was asymptomatic.

In conclusion, pure ankle dislocation with associated os trigonum dislocation is a rare entity. The pathologic mechanism of pure ankle dislocations is not well understood. Known risk factors for pure dislocation include hyperlaxity, medial malleolar hypoplasia, talar undercoverage, and history of recurrent ankle sprains. We propose that the presence of an os trigonum may be a risk factor for pure ankle dislocation due to alternations in the attachment of PTFL.

References

[1] L. Wight, D. Owen, D. Goldbloom, and M. Knupp, "Pure ankle dislocation: a systematic review of the literature and estimation of incidence," *Injury*, vol. 48, no. 10, pp. 2027–2034, 2017.

[2] A. D'Anca, "Lateral rotatory dislocation of the ankle without fracture," *The Journal of Bone & Joint Surgery*, vol. 52, pp. A1643–AA164, 1970, https://www-ncbi-nlm-nih-gov.proxy1.cl.msu.edu/pubmed/4991681.

[3] T. Lui and K. Chan, "Posteromedial ankle dislocation without malleolar fracture: a report of six cases," *Injury*, vol. 43, no. 11, pp. 1953–1957, 2012.

[4] H. D. Moehring, R. T. Tan, R. A. Marder, and G. Lian, "Ankle dislocation," *Journal of Orthopaedic Trauma*, vol. 8, no. 2, pp. 167–172, 1994.

[5] I. Mubark, S. Anwar, and K. Hayward, "Closed posterior ankle dislocation without associated fractures: a case report," *Journal of Surgical Case Reports*, vol. 2017, no. 8, 2017.

[6] F. Rivera, C. Bertone, M. D. Martino, D. Pietrobono, and F. Ghisellini, "Pure dislocation of the ankle," *Clinical Orthopaedics and Related Research*, vol. 382, pp. 179–184, 2001.

[7] M. M. Shaik, T. Tandon, Y. Agrawal, A. Jadhav, and L. J. Taylor, "Medial and lateral rotatory dislocations of the ankle after trivial trauma-pathomechanics and management of two cases," *The Journal of Foot and Ankle Surgery*, vol. 45, no. 5, pp. 346–350, 2006.

[8] T. Thangarajah, N. Giotakis, and E. Matovu, "Bilateral ankle dislocation without malleolar fracture," *The Journal of Foot and Ankle Surgery*, vol. 47, no. 5, pp. 441–446, 2008.

[9] J. S. Toohey and R. A. Worsing, "A long-term follow-up study of tibiotalar dislocations without associated fractures," *Clinical Orthopaedics and Related Research*, vol. 239, pp. 207–210, 1989, https://www.ncbi.nlm.nih.gov/pubmed/2912624.

[10] Y. T. Wang, X. T. Wu, and H. Chen, "Pure closed posteromedial dislocation of the tibiotalar joint without fracture," *Orthopaedic Surgery*, vol. 5, no. 3, pp. 214–218, 2013.

[11] L. Segal, L. CLiffortd, and S. Stauffer, "Anterior Ankle Dislocation With Associated Trigonal Process Fracture," *Clinical Orthopaedics and Related Research*, vol. 278, pp. 171–176, 1992.

[12] A. M. Boomstra, H. R. Schiphorst Preuper, M. F. Reneman, J. B. Posthumus, and R. E. Stwert, "Reliability and validity of the visual analogue scale for disability in patients with chronic musculoskeletal pain," *International Journal of Rehabilitation Research*, vol. 31, no. 2, pp. 165–169, 2008.

[13] J. J. Cook, E. Cook, B. Rosenblum, A. Landsman, and T. S. Roukis, "Validation of the American College of Foot and Ankle Surgeons Scoring Scales," *The Journal of Foot and Ankle Surgery*, vol. 50, no. 4, pp. 420–429, 2001.

[14] L. Remvig, D. V. Jensen, and R. C. Ward, "Are diagnostic criteria for general joint hypermobility and benign joint hypermobility syndrome based on reproducible and valid tests? A review of the literature," *The Journal of Rheumatology*, vol. 34, no. 4, pp. 798–803, 2007.

[15] N. Holzer, D. Salvo, A. C. Mariinissen et al., "Radiographic evaluation of posttraumatic osteoarthritis of the ankle: the Kellgren–Lawrence scale is reliable and correlates with clinical symptoms," *Osteoarthritis and Cartilage*, vol. 23, no. 3, pp. 363–369, 2015.

[16] S. Elise, C. Maynou, H. Mestdagh, P. Forgeois, and P. Labourdette, "Simple tibiotalar luxation. Apropos of 16 cases," *Acta Orthopaedica Belgica*, vol. 64, no. 1, pp. 25–34, 1998.

[17] T. Fernandes, "The mechanism of talo-tibial dislocation without fracture," *Journal of Bone and Joint Surgery (British)*, vol. 56, pp. 364-365, 1976.

[18] W. D. Coltart, "Aviator's astragalus," *The Journal of Bone and Joint Surgery. British volume*, vol. 34-B, no. 4, pp. 545–566, 1952.

[19] R. R. Wroble, J. V. Nepola, and T. A. Malvitz, "Ankle Dislocation without Fracture," *Foot & Ankle*, vol. 9, no. 2, pp. 64–74, 1988.

[20] R. Zwiers, T. A. Baltes, K. M. Opdam, J. I. Wiegerinck, and C. V. Dijk, "Prevalence of os trigonum on CT imaging," *Foot & Ankle International*, vol. 39, no. 3, pp. 338–342, 2018.

[21] D. P. Grogan, A. K. Walling, and J. A. Ogden, "Anatomy of the os trigonum," *Journal of Pediatric Orthopaedics*, vol. 10, no. 5, pp. 618–622, 1990.

[22] A. Mcdougall, "The os trigonum," *The Journal of bone and joint surgery. British volume*, vol. 37-B, no. 2, pp. 257–265, 1955, https://www.ncbi.nlm.nih.gov/pubmed/14381471.

[23] B. Kleiger and M. Ahmed, "Injuries of the talus and its joints," *Clinical orthopaedics and related research*, vol. 121, pp. 243–262, 1976, https://www.ncbi.nlm.nih.gov/pubmed/991510.

[24] A. Courvoisier, R. Vialle, C. Thevenin-Lemoine, P. Mary, and J. P. Damsin, "The posterior talofibular ligament: an anatomical study with clinical implication in clubfoot surgery," *Surgical and Radiologic Anatomy*, vol. 30, no. 8, pp. 633–637, 2008.

[25] M. Gursoy, F. Dag, B. D. Mete, T. Bulut, and M. E. Uluc, "The anatomic variations of the posterior talofibular ligament associated with os trigonum and pathologies of related structures," *Surgical and Radiologic Anatomy*, vol. 37, no. 8, pp. 955–962, 2015.

[26] D. T. Fong, Y. Y. Chan, K. M. Mok, P. S. Yung, and K. M. Chan, "Understanding acute ankle ligamentous sprain injury in sports," *Sports Medicine, Arthroscopy, Rehabilitation, Therapy & Technology: SMARTT*, vol. 1, p. 14, 2009.

[27] O. Rasmussen, I. T. Jensen, and J. Hedeboe, "An analysis of the function of the posterior talofibular ligament," *International Orthopaedics*, vol. 7, no. 1, pp. 41–48, 1983.

[28] Y. Abramowitz, R. Wollstein, Y. Barzilay et al., "Outcome of resection of a symptomatic os trigonum," *The Journal of Bone and Joint Surgery. American Volume*, vol. 85, no. 6, pp. 1051–1057, 2003.

[29] J. H. Ahn, Y. C. Kim, and H. Y. Kim, "Arthroscopic Versus Posterior Endoscopic Excision of a Symptomatic Os Trigonum: A Retrospective Cohort Study," *The American Journal of Sports Medicine*, vol. 41, no. 5, pp. 1082–1089, 2013.

[30] J. D. Calder, S. A. Sexton, and C. J. Pearce, "Return to training and playing after posterior ankle arthroscopy for posterior impingement in elite professional soccer," *The American Journal of Sports Medicine*, vol. 38, no. 1, pp. 120–124, 2010.

[31] M. Galla and P. Lobenhoffer, "Technique and results of arthroscopic treatment of posterior ankle impingement," *Foot and Ankle Surgery*, vol. 17, no. 2, pp. 79–84, 2011.

[32] Q. W. Guo, Y. L. Hu, C. Jiao, Y. F. Ao, and X. Tian, "Open versus endoscopic excision of a symptomatic os trigonum: a comparative study of 41 cases," *Arthroscopy: The Journal of Arthroscopic & Related Surgery*, vol. 26, no. 3, pp. 384–390, 2010.

[33] T. Ogut, E. Ayhan, K. Irgit, and A. I. Sarikaya, "Endoscopic treatment of posterior ankle pain," *Knee Surgery, Sports Traumatology, Arthroscopy*, vol. 19, no. 8, pp. 1355–1361, 2011.

[34] C. H. Park, S. Y. Kim, J. R. Kim, and W. C. Lee, "Arthroscopic excision of a symptomatic os trigonum in a lateral decubitus position," *Foot & Ankle International*, vol. 34, no. 7, pp. 990–994, 2013.

24

Carpometacarpal Dislocation of the Third to Fifth Fingers and an Associated Fracture of the Hamate in a Military Paratrooper

Georgios Kalinterakis,[1] Emmanouil Antonogiannakis,[1] Arezoo Abdi,[1] Georgios Demetriades,[1] Alexandros Koulouktsis,[1] Athanasios Syllaios,[2] Antonios Koutras,[2] Sotiria Vrouva,[1] Anastasios Papagiavis,[1] and Miltiadis Ziogas[1]

[1]*First Department of Orthopedics, 401 General Military Hospital of Athens, Athens 11525, Greece*
[2]*First Department of Surgery, Laiko General Hospital, National and Kapodistrian University of Athens, Athens 11527, Greece*

Correspondence should be addressed to Georgios Kalinterakis; gkalinterakis@gmail.com

Academic Editor: Mark K. Lyons

Multiple carpometacarpal dislocations with a simultaneous fracture of the hamate represent less than 1% of all injuries to the hand and wrist regions, with a scarcity of published cases. These injuries usually require a great force, and diagnosis can be missed or delayed because of the high likelihood of other severe concomitant injuries. We report a case of acute closed dislocation of the third through fifth carpometacarpal joints and an associated fracture of the hamate in a military paratrooper. The injury was caused by a wrong landing technique during parachuting. The patient was managed with primary surgical repair, and after a six-month follow-up, he has excellent functional results. The fact that both this clinical entity and the mechanism of injury are very unusual a high index of suspicion is needed, especially for orthopedic surgeons working in military hospitals. Additionally, given that there is a paucity of published cases and optional treatment is controversial, this study corroborates the superiority of surgical repair in a long-term basis.

1. Introduction

Carpometacarpal (CMC) dislocations of the hand with a simultaneous fracture of the hamate have been infrequently cited in the medical bibliography occurring in less than 1% of osseous hand injuries. The most common mechanism of the injury is the hyperflexion of the metacarpal heads. These injuries usually require a great force, and diagnosis can be missed or delayed because of the high likelihood of other severe concomitant injuries. Applying a high index of suspicion and performing a good clinical examination play a prominent role in recognizing this rare condition. Treatment is controversial and can be either conservative or operative [1–3]. We report a case of acute closed dislocation of the third through fifth carpometacarpal joints and an associated fracture of the hamate in a military paratrooper.

2. Case Presentation

A 22-year-old right-handed paratrooper was presented to the orthopedic emergency department because he fell on his outstretched right hand after having attempted a wrong landing technique. The accident took place in the island of Rodos where he received first aids and was then transported to our hospital for further treatment.

On physical examination, there was swelling and pain over the dorsum of the hand. Despite the swelling, it was feasible to notice deformity and to palpate the characteristic step-off created by the bases of the metacarpals. Active movement of the wrist and the fingers was limited while the patient was unwilling to cooperate due to pain. Neurovascular assessment revealed both a strong palpable radial pulse and a lively capillary refill while sensation of the hand was normal.

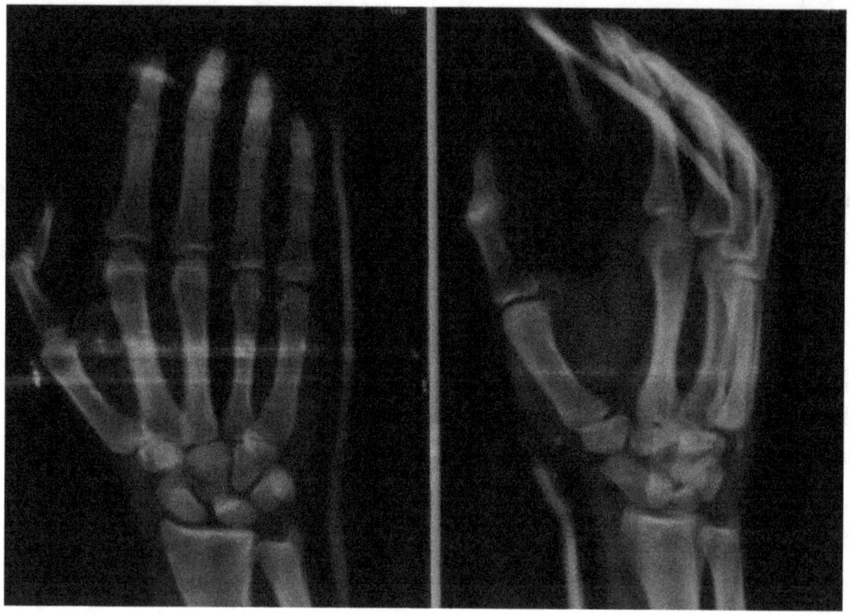

FIGURE 1: Anteroposterior and oblique radiographs of the right hand demonstrating complete dorsal dislocation of the three ulnar CMC joints.

Plain radiographs (a dorsopalmar and an oblique view) of the right hand showed complete dorsal dislocation of the three ulnar CMC joints (Figure 1). In order to achieve a better assessment of the injured joint surfaces, an additional CT scan of the right hand was conducted. The latter not only confirmed the diagnosis but also revealed a bony fragment at the base of the fifth metacarpal that originated from the hamate (Figures 2(a) and 2(b)).

At the emergency department, closed reduction was attempted by applying longitudinal traction to the involved digits with pressure over the bases of the dislocated metacarpals. After that, the wrist was immobilized with a plaster. Three days later, the patient was operated under general anaesthesia in supine position. The surgical treatment chosen was open reduction and internal fixation (ORIF). Two longitudinal incisions were made over the second and fourth web spaces addressing adjacent respective joints. At this point, it is of note that when the subcutaneous hematoma was evacuated and the extensor tendons were retraced with the surrounding loose connective tissues, we noticed that our initial closed reduction which took place in the emergency room has been lost. Therefore, a new one was achieved under image intensifier guidance, and then, internal fixation was accomplished with K-wires 1.6. In detail, the third and fourth metacarpals were transfixed on the trapezoid and on the capitate, respectively. The fifth metacarpal was pinned similarly on the hamate (Figure 3). Regarding the fracture of the hamate, it was extra-articular and its reduction was secured by an interosseous suture vicryl 2-0. After the fracture alignment and joint reduction were evaluated under image intensifier, all wounds were meticulously irrigated and then closed in layers. Lastly, a sterile dressing and volar splint were applied for six weeks.

Both the splint and the K-wires were removed in six weeks' time (Figures 4(a)–4(c)). At this point, active ROM exercises were started. The DASH score one week after the splint removal was 62.5. At 8 weeks, physiotherapy was begun emphasizing on both strengthening exercises and earning full range of motion. In total, 10 sessions were done and the patient was reevaluated after one month. The DASH score was then 12.5. The patient was able to fully return to former activities in six months' time. The DASH score was 0.0. The last follow-up that took place 6 months after the injury revealed great functional results with full return of strength as well as satisfactory cosmetics results. The patient did not mention any difficulties in his labor and everyday life activities.

3. Discussion

Multiple carpometacarpal dislocations with a simultaneous fracture of the hamate are uncommon incidents, with a scarcity of published cases. They represent less than 1% of all injuries to the hand and wrist regions [3–6]. Additionally, owing to extensive swelling and overlapping of bones on the radiograph, up to 70% of them are missed or misdiagnosed [2, 7–9]. These injuries more commonly occur as a result of high-energy trauma as in our case (parachuting accident) while the predominant mechanism is direct force in the axial direction which causes secondary flexion or extension forces. The direction of CMC joint dislocation may be volar or dorsal depending on the direction of the force, with dorsal dislocations being the most common [5, 9, 10]. The CMC joint is the only joint not having a gliding configuration but instead is a modified saddle-shaped joint. Stability at the finger CMC joints is provided by static and dynamic constraints. The former refers to multiple articular facets while the latter to a system of four ligaments (dorsal, palmar, and 2 sets of interosseous) with surrounding muscles and tendons. What is more, it is essential to note that the third

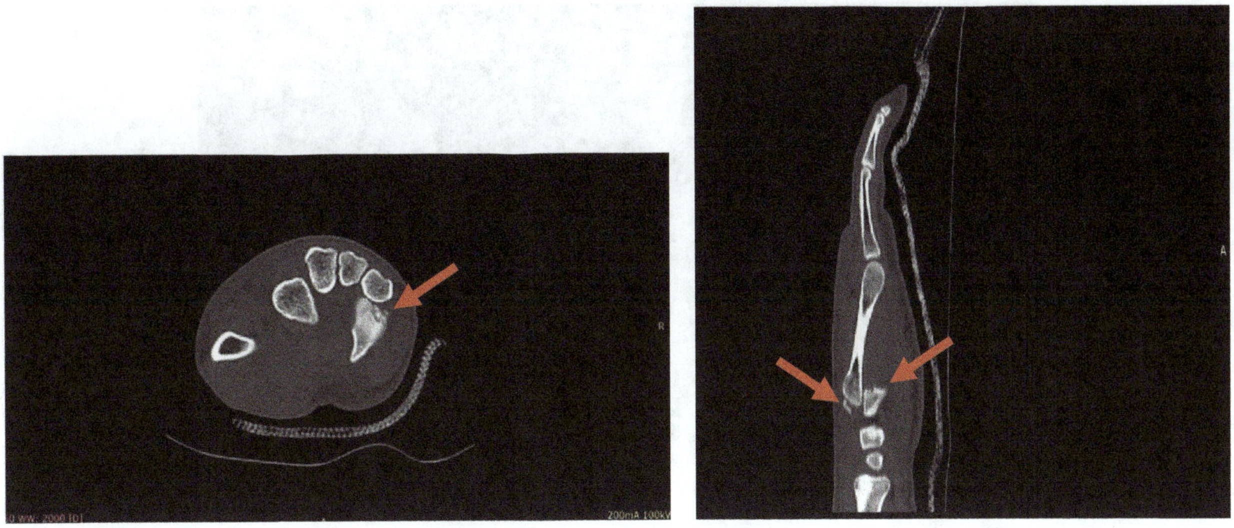

(a) (b)

Figure 2: (a, b) CT images showing the dorsal dislocation of the fifth CMC joint and a bony fragment at the base of the fifth metacarpal that originated from the hamate (red arrows).

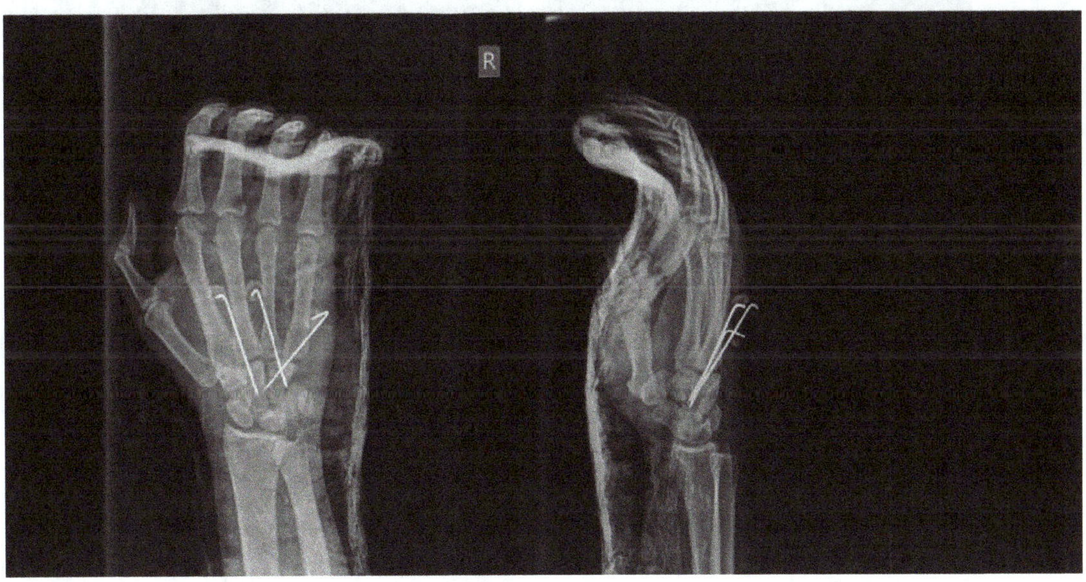

Figure 3: Radiographs after open reduction and fixation with Kirschner wires.

metacarpocapitate articulation is located more proximal than that of the other CMC joints, creating a so-called keystone relationship. As a result, reduction and stabilization of the third metacarpal CMC joint is fundamental for reduction of the remaining CMC joints. The same approach was also followed in our case. Furthermore, because of the tough attachments of the CMC ligaments, these injuries are often combined with avulsion fractures of the base of the metacarpal or the carpal bones, a finding noticeable in our case [3, 5, 6].

Dislocations of the CMC joint can be easily missed in the acute setting. Thus, it is recommended that three radiographs should be taken: a dorsopalmar, a true lateral, and an oblique view of the hand. However, a computed tomography (CT scan) is sometimes necessary in order to confirm the diagnosis and show missed carpal bone fractures, assisting in this way to preoperative planning [3, 11].

Because of the paucity of the published cases, treatment of carpometacarpal injuries is debatable. Two case reports by Horneff et al. and Agarwal A. and Agarwal R. demonstrated satisfactory results with closed reduction and splinting regarding the maintenance of reduction and the recovery of hand function [12, 13]. Operative treatment includes closed reduction and K-wire fixation or open reduction and internal fixation. The former is mostly chosen when either the joint surfaces are intact or in the absence of carpal

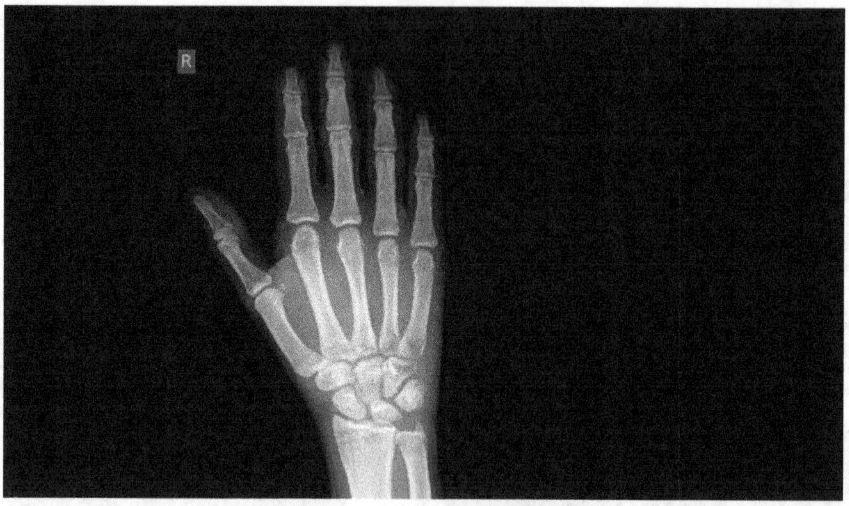

(a)

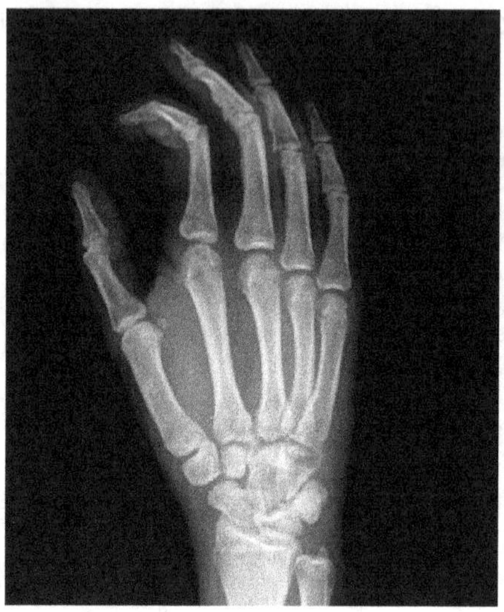

(b)

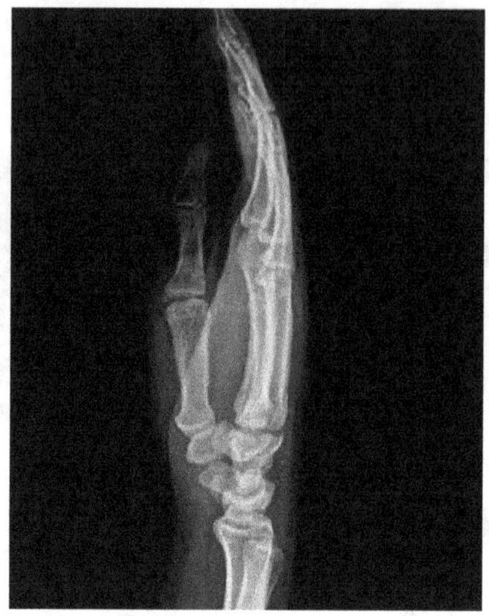

(c)

FIGURE 4: (a–c) Radiographs 6 weeks postoperatively after the K-wires' removal.

fractures; otherwise, there is a high risk of redislocation. Fracture-dislocations often require open reduction and fixation (ORIF). This approach has been noted to have some distinct advantages as opposed to a closed reduction, including a more anatomical joint restoration, the drainage of local hematoma, and the prevention of tendon transfixation. The fixation can be achieved with K-wires or miniplates depending on the characteristics of the injury. In our case, due to the morphology of the injury, we used K-wires with excellent intra- and postoperative results [3, 5, 10, 11]. Finally, regardless of the treatment chosen, follow-up protocols suggest a period of immobilization, on average 4 to 6 weeks, at which point the splint and the pins (in case of surgical treatment) are removed, followed by hand and wrist physiotherapy so as to prevent postoperative stiffness and to improve the functional outcome.

Carpometacarpal (CMC) dislocations of the hand with a simultaneous fracture of the hamate comprise a rare injury. Despite the fact that the landing phase of a parachute jump mostly causes injuries in the lower extremities [14], upper extremities run also the risk of being injured. Thus, orthopedic surgeons must be aware of this clinical feature especially if they work in military hospitals. Given that there is a scarcity of published cases and optional treatment is controversial, this study corroborates the superiority of surgical repair in a long-term basis and acts as a contributory factor in medical literature in terms of guiding treatment.

Data Availability

The data used to support the findings of this study are available from the corresponding author upon request.

Consent

Informed consent was obtained from the patient.

References

[1] L. J. Prokuski and W. A. Eglseder, "Concurrent dorsal dislocations and fracture-dislocations of the index, long, ring, and small (second to fifth) carpometacarpal joints," *Journal of Orthopaedic Trauma*, vol. 15, no. 8, pp. 549–554, 2001.

[2] R. S. Gaheer and R. D. Ferdinand, "Fracture dislocation of carpometacarpal joints: a missed injury," *Orthopedics*, vol. 34, no. 5, p. 399, 2011.

[3] J. N. Brinkman, K. A. Hartholt, and M. R. de Vries, "Multiple carpometacarpal dislocations and an associated fracture of the hamate: an uncommon injury," *BMJ Case Reports*, vol. 2016, 2016.

[4] W. J. Peace and R. A. Abrams, "Simultaneous dorsal dislocations of the carpometacarpal joints of all four fingers," *Orthopedics*, vol. 33, no. 2, pp. 121–123, 2010.

[5] G. T. Pundkare and A. M. Patil, "Carpometacarpal joint fracture dislocation of second to fifth finger," *Clinics in Orthopedic Surgery*, vol. 7, no. 4, pp. 430–435, 2015.

[6] J. J. Mueller, "Carpometacarpal dislocations: report of five cases and review of the literature," *The Journal Hand Surgery*, vol. 11, no. 2, pp. 184–188, 1986.

[7] M. Gurland, "Carpometacarpal joint injuries of the fingers," *Hand Clinics*, vol. 8, no. 4, pp. 733–744, 1992.

[8] J. J. Henderson and M. A. Arafa, "Carpometacarpal dislocation. An easily missed diagnosis," *Journal of Bone and Joint Surgery. British Volume*, vol. 69-B, no. 2, pp. 212–214, 1987.

[9] M. Davis, E. Erel, and J. Webb, "Simultaneous bilateral third to fifth carpometacarpal joint dislocations; a boxing first?," *European Journal of Plastic Surgery*, vol. 34, no. 1, pp. 57–59, 2011.

[10] C. Y. L. Woon, K. C. Chong, and C. O. Low, "Carpometacarpal joint dislocations of the index to small finger: three cases and a review of the literature," *Injury Extra*, vol. 37, no. 12, pp. 466–472, 2006.

[11] C. Büren, S. Gehrmann, R. Kaufmann, J. Windolf, and T. Lögters, "Management algorithm for index through small finger carpometacarpal fracture dislocations," *European Journal of Trauma and Emergency Surgery*, vol. 42, no. 1, pp. 37–42, 2016.

[12] A. AGARWAL and R. AGARWAL, "An unusual farm injury: divergent carpometacarpal joint dislocations," *Journal of Hand Surgery*, vol. 30, no. 6, pp. 633-634, 2016.

[13] J. G. Horneff, M. J. Park, and D. R. Steinberg, "Acute closed dislocation of the second through fourth carpometacarpal joints: satisfactory treatment with closed reduction and immobilization," *Hand*, vol. 8, no. 2, pp. 227–231, 2013.

[14] M. C. M. Bricknell and S. C. Craig, "Military parachuting injuries: a literature review," *Occupational Medicine*, vol. 49, no. 1, pp. 17–26, 1999.

25

Management of Instability following Pyogenic Sacroiliitis: Technical Case Report

C. Passaplan, A. Simonin, G. Maestretti, and E. Gautier

Orthopaedic Surgery, Cantonal Hospital of Fribourg (HFR), Chemin des Pensionnats 2, 1700 Fribourg, Switzerland

Correspondence should be addressed to A. Simonin; alexandresimonin21@gmail.com

Academic Editor: Christian W. Müller

Background. Septic arthritis of the sacroiliac joint (SI-joint) is a rare and often delayed diagnosis. Management usually consists of intravenous antibiotics and debridement of infected tissue. However, very few reports consider the management of the secondary instability of the sacroiliac joint. *Case Presentation.* We report a case of a 16-year-old girl diagnosed with *S. aureus* pyogenic sacroiliitis who benefited from aggressive surgical debridement and primary arthrodesis for infection-related SI-joint instability in the acute infection phase. *Conclusion.* Diagnosis of pyogenic sacroiliitis is often delayed. Destruction of the joint can lead to chronic pain and instability. In cases of obvious intraoperative instability, primary arthrodesis could be considered in young patients.

1. Introduction

Infectious sacroiliitis represents less than 2% of septic arthritis [1–3]. Diagnosis is often delayed because of nonspecific clinical findings. *S. aureus* is the most common causative pathogen. Management usually consists of intravenous antibiotics. SI-joint aspiration may be challenging. However, it is recommended, if blood cultures remain sterile. Surgical debridement of infected tissue is mandatory in cases of unfavorable evolution despite parenteral antibiotics. Only few authors have addressed the definitive management of the SI-joint instability secondary to infection in the chronic phase (more than one month after onset of clinical symptoms). There is no clear consensus in the literature regarding the technique of SI-joint arthrodesis in patients with chronic infection. Different techniques using transarticular screws, anterior plate fixation, bone graft, or cage interposition are reported to perform SI-joint arthrodesis [4, 5].

2. Case Report

A 16-year-old girl with no medical history presented to the primary care physician with fever and low back pain radiating to the left buttock. There was no history of trauma. A viral coxitis was diagnosed, and the patient was sent home with NSAIDs and bed rest. Because of progressing pain and inability to walk, the patient presented in the emergency room 5 days later. Upon examination, she was febrile, and palpation of the SI-joint and coccyx was painful. Neurological examination was normal. Laboratory findings showed increased C-reactive protein (318 mg/l) and leucocytosis (14.2 G/l).

MRI of the pelvis and SI-joints showed a bulge in the intra-articular capsule of the left SI-joint and bone remodelling (Figure 1). Blood cultures were sampled, and ultrasound-guided aspiration was performed. Direct examination revealed gram-positive cocci. Intravenous antibiotics (daptomycin 350 mg/day) were started following the aspiration. Cultures became positive for *S. aureus*, and antibiotic treatment was switched to gentamicin. Because of aortic murmur, transthoracic echocardiogram was performed to rule out endocarditis. Antibiotherapy was subsequently switched to flucloxacillin. Five days after initial treatment, because of increasing fever and inflammation markers, a new MRI was performed, showing abscesses anterior to the left SI-joint. Surgical debridement was performed, using the Olerud approach to the SI-joint. After aggressive debridement and evacuation of pus, there was obvious instability of

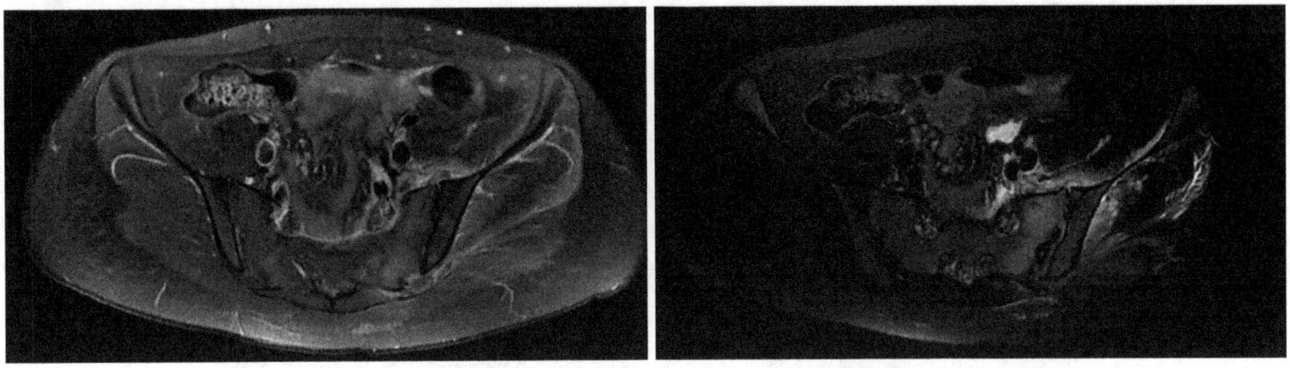

FIGURE 1: MRI of the pelvis: T1-enhanced and T2 axial views showing signal abnormality of the left sacroiliac joint, predominant in the sacral wing, characterized by hyperintensity on T2. There are significant signal abnormalities and gadolinium uptake of the musculature adjacent to the left sacroiliac joint. Anterior effusion of the left sacroiliac joint is visible with additional bulging of the posterior articular capsule.

the SI-joint in the lateral-medial and craniocaudal directions. Therefore, even in the absence of significant joint destruction in the preoperative MRI, an arthrodesis was performed using two titanium reconstruction plates angulated with each other. In addition, Vancomycin-loaded calcium sulphate (Osteoset™ resorbable beat) pellets were added inside and around the articulation to provide a high local concentration of Vancomycin as described before [6] (Figure 2(a)).

Four days later, because of recurring pain, a new MRI was performed, showing a surgical site hematoma, which was evacuated. Subsequent clinical course was favorable; the patient was discharged at day 26 with some residual pain, normalized inflammation markers of infection, and 15 kg partial weight-bearing on the operated leg. After 6 weeks, she did not have any episode of fever and only little pain on palpation of her left SI-joint. Intravenous antibiotics were given for 9 weeks in our outpatient department, and 30 kg partial weight-bearing on the operated leg was allowed for 6 more weeks. Biological inflammatory markers were normal, and an anteroposterior pelvic radiograph was satisfactory after 3 months (Figure 2(b)). After 4 months, the patient was pain-free and could perform her usual activities without any restriction. Before allowing heavier sports activities, a CT scan was performed at 4 months revealing the first signs of joint fusion without osteolysis or secondary displacement (Figure 3). One year after surgery (Figure 2(c)), the SI-joint was no more visible on the pelvic radiograph as a sign of complete SI-joint fusion.

3. Discussion

Pelvic ring stability relies on osseoligamentous structures. Instability is mainly caused by traumatic injuries. However, chronic conditions like infectious or inflammatory diseases may also affect the integrity of the sacroiliac joint [2]. Pyogenic sacroiliitis is rare and diagnosis is often delayed. However, it is usually not associated with instability when appropriate treatment is conducted before destruction of the SI-joint. Management usually consists of surgical debridement and several weeks of intravenous antibiotherapy. However, very few reports consider the infection-related SI-joint instability. Many authors recommend 2-3 months of non-weight-bearing [2]. Long-term outcome is lacking in most of the series and case reports [7–21]. Chronic SI-joint pain is reported in a high proportion of cases (33% to 43.5%) [3, 22, 23]. The cause of the pain has not been investigated in retrospective studies. But chronic SI-joint instability could be a causative phenomenon.

Arthrodesis is normally reserved as a salvage procedure in case of ineffective conservative therapy or by severity criteria as septicaemia or neurological deficits in the acute phase or secondary instability due to joint destruction in the chronic phase of the infection. The most appropriate surgical regime is still discussed controversially in the literature: open procedure for extensive debridement and fusion of the joint are described in some series as a current approach [1, 2, 22]. The surgical approach can be posterior, anterior, or mixed, depending on the location of the abscess on the MRI. Schubert et al. [24] described the first series of primary arthrodesis with autologous bone graft with a posterior approach of the sacroiliac joint in case of neurological deficits, abscess formation, or septicaemia, with good clinical results. Ahmed et al. [4] described a series of eleven cases of debridement combined to arthrodesis performed with a variety of surgical techniques (posterior or combined approaches, bone graft with/without cage and/or screws) and recommended a joint fusion in chronic cases or in patients in bad general condition even with moderate destruction of the sacroiliac joint. Recently, some cases of minimal invasive sacroiliac joint fusion were recently described in the literature showing good results in case of chronic sacroiliac dysfunction. Anton et al. [25] described a pyogenic sacroiliitis treated with minimally invasive joint fusion (SI Fusion System Medtronic) with a good long-term outcome. Wandermann et al. [26] reported a case of chronic infectious sacroiliitis treated with a combination of joint debridement, biologic fusion with bone graft, and nonbiologic functional fusion using titanium ingrowth rods, all performed in a minimally invasive fashion with good results at 2 years of follow-up. Wise and Dall [27] described a series of patients presenting after failed conservative therapy of pyogenic sacroiliitis. Fusion was achieved by percutaneous insertion of cages on the posterior side of the SI-joint.

In cases presenting a destruction of the SI-joint or obvious intraoperative instability, like in our case, primary arthrodesis could be considered, in order to prevent chronic

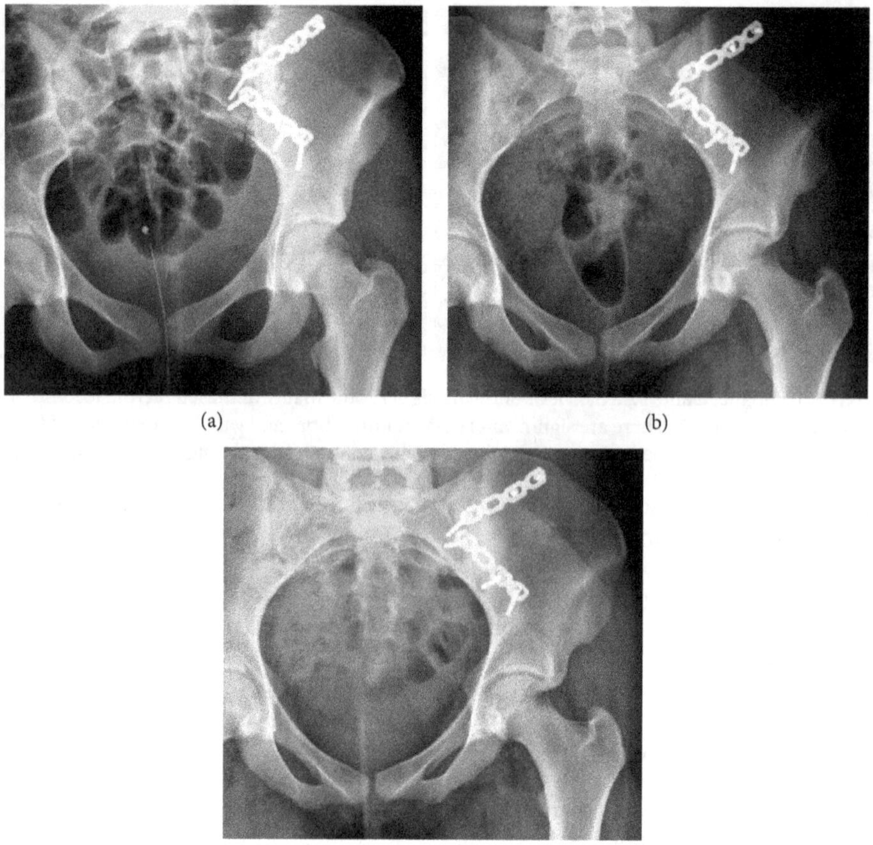

(a) (b)

(c)

Figure 2: Postoperative anteroposterior pelvic radiograph showing the SI-joint arthrodesis using two plates with radiographically visible Vancomycin-loaded calcium sulphate pellets (a). Three months after surgery (b), the calcium sulphate pellets are totally resorbed. There are no signs of secondary displacement of the SI-joint, implant loosening, or failure. One year after surgery (c), the SI-joint is completely fused.

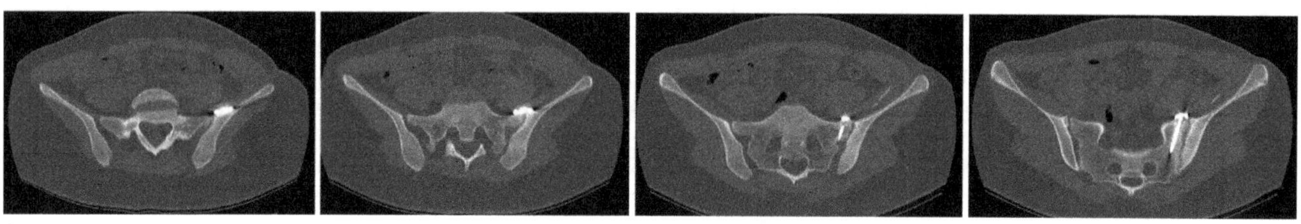

Figure 3: Series of axial CT scan showing early signs of fusion of the SI-joint without osteolysis of the adjacent bone.

pain and instability. Minimally invasive techniques are described for the treatment of sacroiliac joint infection showing good results, low complication rates, and short recovery. Nevertheless, in case of pyogenic SI-joint infection, an open procedure is a successful alternative. The anterior approach to the SI-joint allows debridement of all infected tissue, complete removal of the infected cartilage by distraction of the SI-joint, local administration of antibiotics using Vancomycin-loaded calcium sulphate pellets, and stable fixation by means of two reconstruction plates.

4. Conclusion

Diagnosis of pyogenic sacroiliitis is often delayed. The infectious process can lead to the destruction of the SI-joint with chronic pain due to persistent infection and instability. In cases with destruction of the SI-joint and obvious intraoperative instability, primary arthrodesis could be considered even in the acute phase of the infection in order to prevent chronic pain and instability. Our case is to our knowledge the first report of a one-stage debridement and primary plate fixation of an acute pyogenic SI-joint infection.

References

[1] U. B. Schaad, McCracken GH Jr, and J. D. Nelson, "Pyogenic arthritis of the sacroiliac joint in pediatric patients," *Pediatrics*, vol. 66, no. 3, pp. 375–379, 1980.

[2] N. K. Kanakaris, S. Psarakis, B. Chalidis, G. Kontakis, and P. V. Giannoudis, "Management of pelvic instability secondary to

chronic pyogenic sacroiliitis: case report," *Surgical Infections*, vol. 10, no. 4, pp. 353–358, 2009.

[3] Y. Horai, K. Izumikawa, S. Oka et al., "Methicillin-resistant Staphylococcus aureus-related septic pulmonary embolism and sacroiliitis treated with long-term linezolid in a patient with adult-onset Still's disease," *Internal Medicine*, vol. 53, no. 9, pp. 1023–1027, 2014.

[4] H. Ahmed, A. E. Siam, G. M. Gouda-Mohamed, and H. Boehm, "Surgical treatment of sacroiliac joint infection," *Journal of Orthopaedics and Traumatology*, vol. 14, no. 2, pp. 121–129, 2013.

[5] W. R. Spiker, B. D. Lawrence, A. L. Raich, A. C. Skelly, and D. S. Brodke, "Surgical versus injection treatment for injection-confirmed chronic sacroiliac joint pain," *Evidence-Based Spine-Care Journal*, vol. 3, no. 4, pp. 41–53, 2012.

[6] P. Wahl, M. Guidi, E. Benninger et al., "The levels of vancomycin in the blood and the wound after the local treatment of bone and soft-tissue infection with antibiotic-loaded calcium sulphate as carrier material," *Bone & Joint Journal*, vol. 99-B, no. 11, pp. 1537–1544, 2017.

[7] A. Donzelli, E. Samara, V. Spyropoulou, C. Juchler, and D. Ceroni, "Pediatric sacroiliitis: clinical and microbiologic differences between infants and children-adolescents," *The Pediatric Infectious Disease Journal*, vol. 36, no. 7, pp. 631–634, 2017.

[8] L. Ghedira Besbes, S. Haddad, A. Abid, C. Ben Meriem, and M. N. Gueddiche, "Pyogenic sacroiliitis in children: two case reports," *Case Reports in Medicine*, vol. 2012, 4 pages, 2012.

[9] S. Kim, K. L. Lee, H. L. Baek, S. J. Jang, S. M. Moon, and Y. K. Cho, "A case of acute pyogenic sacroiliitis and bacteremia caused by community-acquired methicillin-resistant Staphylococcus aureus," *Infect Chemother*, vol. 45, no. 4, pp. 441–445, 2013.

[10] A. Shemer, I. Eshed, and M. Levinkopf, "Septic sacroiliitis: a diagnostic challenge for the clinician," *The Israel Medical Association Journal*, vol. 20, no. 1, pp. 58-59, 2018.

[11] M. Hermet, E. Minichiello, R. M. Flipo et al., "Infectious sacroiliitis: a retrospective, multicentre study of 39 adults," *BMC Infectious Diseases*, vol. 12, no. 1, 2012.

[12] W. D. Jayamali, H. M. M. T. B. Herath, and A. Kulatunga, "A young female presenting with unilateral sacroiliitis following dengue virus infection: a case report," *Journal of Medical Case Reports*, vol. 11, no. 1, p. 307, 2017.

[13] M. J. Antonelli and M. Magrey, "Sacroiliitis mimics: a case report and review of the literature," *BMC Musculoskeletal Disorders*, vol. 18, no. 1, p. 170, 2017.

[14] M. Doita, S. Yoshiya, Y. Nabeshima et al., "Acute pyogenic sacroiliitis without predisposing conditions," *Spine*, vol. 28, no. 18, pp. e384–e389, 2003.

[15] A. Zejden and A. G. Jurik, "Anatomy of the sacroiliac joints in children and adolescents by computed tomography," *Pediatric Rheumatology Online Journal*, vol. 15, no. 1, p. 82, 2017.

[16] R. C. McHugh, J. M. Tiede, and T. N. Weingarten, "Clostridial sacroiliitis in a patient with fecal incontinence: a case report and review of the literature," *Pain Physician*, vol. 11, no. 2, pp. 249–252, 2008.

[17] F. Bellazreg, Z. Alaya, Z. Hattab et al., "Infectious sacroiliitis in tunisian centre: retrospective study of 25 cases," *The Pan African Medical Journal*, vol. 24, 2016.

[18] F. Aydin, Z. B. Özçakar, N. Çakar et al., "Sacroiliitis in children with familial mediterranean fever," *Journal of Clinical Rheumatology*, vol. 25, no. 2, pp. 69–73, 2019.

[19] M. O. Almoujahed, R. Khatib, and J. Baran, "Pregnancy-associated pyogenic sacroiliitis: case report and review," *Infectious Diseases in Obstetrics and Gynecology*, vol. 11, 5 pages, 2003.

[20] P. J. Woytala, A. Sebastian, K. Błach, J. Silicki, and P. Wiland, "Septic arthritis of the sacroiliac joint," *Reumatologia*, vol. 56, no. 1, pp. 55–58, 2018.

[21] M. Elsammak, H. Hanna, A. Ghazal, F. B. Edeen, and M. Kandil, "Diagnostic value of serum procalcitonin and C-reactive protein in Egyptian children with streptococcal tonsillopharyngitis," *The Pediatric Infectious Disease Journal*, vol. 25, no. 2, pp. 174–176, 2006.

[22] J. Leroux, I. Bernardini, L. Grynberg et al., "Pyogenic sacroiliitis in a 13-month-old child: a case report and literature review," *Medicine*, vol. 94, no. 42, article e1581, 2015.

[23] H. E. Ennis, M. N. Ialenti, J. Jose, and M. Baraga, "A rare case of isolated salmonella species group B sacroiliitis in a healthy collegiate-level swimmer: a case report," *JBJS Case Connector*, vol. 7, no. 3, article e55, 2017.

[24] T. Schubert, J. Bruns, and G. Dahmen, "Results of surgical therapy of bacterial sacroiliitis with primary arthrodesis," *Langenbecks Archiv für Chirurgie*, vol. 378, no. 6, pp. 335–338, 1993.

[25] G. Anton, D. Tong, T. Little, and T. M. Soo, "Minimally invasive sacroiliac joint fusion for the treatment of brucella pyogenic sacroiliitis: a case report," *Cureus*, vol. 11, article e6212, 2019.

[26] N. Wanderman, J. Thurn, M. Wyffels, and J. N. Sembrano, "Successful treatment of *Mycobacterium gordonae* sacroiliitis using a novel minimally invasive sacroiliac joint arthrodesis: A case report," *JBJS Case Connector*, vol. 6, no. 3, article e55, 2016.

[27] C. L. Wise and B. E. Dall, "Minimally invasive sacroiliac arthrodesis: outcomes of a new technique," *Journal of Spinal Disorders & Techniques*, vol. 21, no. 8, pp. 579–584, 2008.

26

Engaging Posterior Capitellum Fracture and Elbow Posterolateral Rotatory Instability: Is it Always Necessary to Treat the Bone Defect?

Juan M. Patiño and Juan M. Torres Moirano

Departamento de Ortopedia y Traumatologia, Servicio de Cirugía de Miembro Superior, Hospital Militar Central "Cosme Argerich", Buenos Aires., Argentina

Correspondence should be addressed to Juan M. Patiño; drpatinojm@gmail.com

Academic Editor: Paul E. Di Cesare

Case. We present a 23-year-old male with 7 episodes of left elbow dislocation during a two-year period. He had a positive pivot shift test with engaging. The original treatment plan included lateral ulnar collateral ligament reconstruction and eventually bone defect grafting and osteosynthesis. However, a bone graft was not performed. After 2 years of follow-up, the DASH score was 3.3. The Mayo Score was 90. *Conclusion.* Posterolateral instability associated with an engaging bone defect, in every elbow extension and pivot shift test, was not found in the literature. The capitellum defects are associated with PLRI and make it worse. Bone reconstruction may not be indicated.

1. Introduction

In 1966, Osborne and Cotterill described a posterior capitellum defect in recurrent elbow dislocation (Osborne-Cotterill lesion) [1–4]. Posterolateral rotatory instability (PLRI) was, more recently, described by O'Driscoll in 1991 [5].

Impression fractures of the distal portion of the capitellum could contribute to the loss of radiocapitellar stability and may be unrecognized, especially in a dislocation fracture of the elbow [6].

Information about the treatment guides and outcomes of the Osborne-Cotterill fractures is scarce [2].

It is given by case reports and short series that show a lack of consensus.

Cases of posterolateral instability associated with an engaging bone defect, in every elbow extension and pivot shift test, were not found in the literature.

In this particular case that we are presenting, a question emerges during surgical planning. Could the instability be treated without fixing the engaging bone defect?

Therefore, we report a case in which the instability was treated without fixing the bone defect.

Informed consent was obtained from the patient included in the study, and the institutional Ethical Committee approved the retrospective medical chart review.

2. Case

We report a case of a 23-year-old male with a history of 7 episodes of left elbow dislocation during a two-year period. The first dislocation was the result of a bicycle fall with the arm in extension and mild supination. Treatment in another center included closed reduction and immobilization with the elbow in 90 degrees for 10 days. The other elbow dislocation episodes occurred while the patient performed daily activities; these dislocations reduced spontaneously. Daily activities were significantly limited by subjective instability and apprehension.

Our first examination showed elbow extension apprehension, a positive pivot shift test with engaging, audible clank,

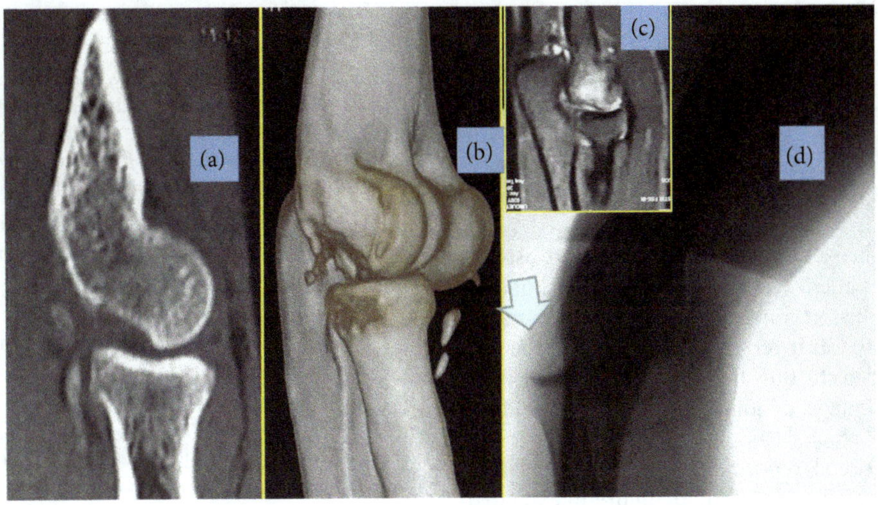

FIGURE 1: (a, b, and c) TC scan and MRI showing capitellum fracture. (d) Engaging pivot shift.

and pain in the lateral aspect of the elbow. Elbow medial ligaments remained stable during the stress (valgus and varus) tests. AP and lateral elbow x-rays did not show bone injuries. A pivot shift test was positive with engaging due to the bone defect, resulting in difficult reduction under fluoroscopy.

The preoperative Disabilities of the Arm, Shoulder, and Hand (DASH) score was 76.7 points, and the Mayo Elbow Performance Score was 5 points.

A left elbow CT scan showed a bone deficit at the posterior capitellum site. This finding appeared to be related with the erosion produced by the impact of the radial head in recurrent dislocations.

MRI revealed distal humerus bone edema (Figure 1).

The preoperative treatment plan included lateral ulnar collateral ligament reconstruction and eventually bone defect grafting and osteosynthesis. The examination under anesthesia and image intensifier confirmed posterolateral rotatory dislocation and engaging (Video 1).

A Kocher incision of 8 centimeters long was performed. A lateral capsular and ligamentous deficit was observed. An autologous graft was taken from the palmaris longus tendon. Two holes were performed in the proximal ulna: one in the supinator crest tubercle and the other at 2 centimeters proximal to the former, close to the annular ligament insertion, keeping the bone bridge between them. The humerus hole was placed 2 millimeters anteriorly and distally from the lateral condyle. Using a tendon hook, the palmaris longus graft was passed through the holes.

Stability was tested. Intraoperative observation revealed that the posterior capitellum deficit was not implicated in the elbow excursion after lateral ligament reconstruction. Therefore, a bone graft was not performed. Elbow immobilization in 90 degrees and full pronation for 4 weeks were performed.

3. Results

After 3 weeks, active and passive flexion exercises were indicated. Then, progressive elbow extension was allowed, initially in 90 degrees of flexion and increasing 10 degrees of extension each week until the full extension was achieved in 8 weeks.

The DASH (Disabilities of the Arm, Shoulder, and Hand) score was used to evaluate the function of the elbow and symptoms during a 3-month period; the obtained score was 24.4 points. After 2 years of follow-up, the DASH score increased to 3.3. The Mayo Elbow Performance Score was 70 after 3 months and 90 after 2 years.

4. Discussion

We report a patient with unstable elbow and engaging bone defect. The joint was stabilized with no need of bone defect repair, and a favorable outcome was achieved. In this particular case that we are presenting, a question emerges during surgical planning. Could the instability be treated without fixing the engaging bone defect?

PLRI and ligament reconstruction have been well described [7].

In cases of bone defect associated with instability, some authors treat the instability but not the bone defect; some others treat both. Lateral elbow reconstruction has shown predictable results, but scarce information was found in the literature (cases reports and short series) about this kind of chronic impression fractures, even more when this bone defect is associated with elbow engaging.

The bone stock deficit in the posterior capitellum could be a significant indicator of PLRI. In 2008, a study based on images of the elbow reported a high prevalence (82%) of PLRI in injuries of LCL in patients with capitellum defect [1, 4].

Faber and King published in 1998 an isolated case of a 27-year-old female with capitellum fracture and PLRI but with no engagement. This defect was described as an impression of the posterior capitellum, and the treatment was only ligament reconstruction [8].

Capitellum height reduction decreases the tension of the LCL complex, potentially leading to instability.

In addition, changes in the structure of the capitellum could comprise joint stability due to the radiocapitellar congruence alteration. Ligament reconstruction techniques in addition to bone defect correction using bone graft were successful in patients with bone defect greater than one-fourth of the joint surface. The biomechanical evaluation could be important to determine the exact relevant amount of bone loss secondary to PLRI in order to establish the optimal surgical treatment for this patient population [2, 9].

Clark et al. described a case of capitellum fracture associated with PLRI. The patient was treated with osteochondral autograft and LCL ulnar reconstruction. The author stated that the elbow stability was inversely proportional to the size of the capitellum defect. But he emphasized that it is unknown what percentage of joint surface loss should be treated using surgical repair [10].

Shukla and O'Driscoll reported 2 cases: a 38-year-old female patient with a history of traumatic injury in extended arm resulting in impression fracture at the anterolateral radius head border associated with capitellum impression fracture (superior posterolateral aspect) and displaced avulsion of the supinator crest tubercle at the LCL ulna insertion site. Intraoperative examination revealed engaging elbow and subluxation with greater than 25-degree extension with the forearm in supination. It was not reported if the engaging appeared with each maneuver.

The article described the capitellum impression fracture reposition using cancellous bone graft. In the 2nd case, ligament reconstruction was performed, in a 35-year-old female with instability and depressed comminuted fracture involving the inferior aspect of the capitellum [11].

Many questions arise as regards the surgical intervention and evaluation of patients with posterolateral rotatory instability associated with posterior engaging fracture. Information is scarce; the options for distal humerus bone reconstruction appear to have pitfalls and uncertain results.

No studies were found describing what type of injuries leads to engaging the proximal radius in each trial of elbow extension and which of these injuries should be fixed. We consider that the bone defect size added to capsular insufficiency and laxity could result in this condition.

5. Conclusions

The capitellum defects are associated with PLRI and could make it worse. However, once the ligaments have been reconstructed, probably the mentioned defect could be excluded from the joint excursion. Consequently, bone reconstruction may not be indicated, since the procedure could lead to complications and the results are uncertain.

More studies are needed to determine in which bone defect (size localization and depth) the surgical treatment is necessary.

References

[1] I. H. Jeon, I. D. Micic, N. Yamamoto, and B. F. Morrey, "Osborne-cotterill lesion: an osseous defect of the capitellum associated with instability of the elbow," *American Journal of Roentgenology*, vol. 191, no. 3, pp. 727–729, 2008.

[2] I. H. Jeon, W. K. Min, I. D. Micic, H. S. Cho, and P. T. Kim, "Surgical treatment and clinical implication for posterolateral rotatory instability of the elbow: Osborne-Cotterill lesion of the elbow," *The Journal of Trauma: Injury, Infection, and Critical Care*, vol. 71, pp. 45–49, 2011.

[3] G. Osborne and P. Cotterill, "Recurrent dislocation of the elbow," *Journal of Bone and Joint Surgery. British Volume*, vol. 48, pp. 340–346, 1966.

[4] Z. S. Rosenberg, S. I. Blutreich, M. E. Schweitzer, J. S. Zember, and K. Fillmore, "MRI features of posterior capitellar impaction injuries," *American Journal of Roentgenology*, vol. 190, no. 2, pp. 435–441, 2008.

[5] S. W. O'Driscoll, "Classification and evaluation of recurrent instability of the elbow," *Clinical Orthopaedics and Related Research*, vol. 370, pp. 34–43, 2000.

[6] D. R. Shukla, A. R. Thoreson, J. S. Fitzsimmons, K. N. An, and S. W. O'Driscoll, "The effect of capitellar impaction fractures on radiocapitellar stability," *The Journal of Hand Surgery*, vol. 40, no. 3, pp. 520–525, 2015.

[7] J. Sanchez-Sotelo, B. F. Morrey, and S. W. O'Driscoll, "Ligamentous repair and reconstruction for posterolateral rotatory instability of the elbow," *Journal of Bone and Joint Surgery British Volume*, vol. 87-B, no. 1, pp. 54–61, 2005.

[8] K. J. Faber and G. J. W. King, "Posterior capitellum impression fracture: a case report associated with posterolateral rotatory instability of the elbow," *Journal of Shoulder and Elbow Surgery*, vol. 7, no. 2, pp. 157–159, 1998.

[9] M. T. Sabo, K. Fay, C. P. McDonald, L. M. Ferreira, J. A. Johnson, and G. J. King, "Effect of coronal shear fractures of the distal humerus on elbow kinematics and stability," *Journal of Shoulder and Elbow Surgery*, vol. 19, no. 5, pp. 670–680, 2010.

[10] T. A. Clark, R. William, and J. Leiter, "Posterior capitellum impaction fracture associated with posterolateral instability of the Elbow," *Techniques in Shoulder in Elbow Surgery*, vol. 9, no. 3, pp. 164–167, 2008.

[11] D. R. Shukla and S. W. O'Driscoll, "Atypical etiology of lateral collateral ligament disruption and instability," *Journal of Orthopaedic Trauma*, vol. 27, no. 6, pp. e144–e146, 2013.

27

Posttraumatic Pseudoarthrosis of a Clavicle Fracture in an 11-Year-Old Girl: A Case Report and Analysis

Marco Odorizzi, Maurice FitzGerald, Jorge Gonzalez, Dario Giunchi, Flurim Hamitaga, and Vincenzo De Rosa

Paediatric and Orthopaedic Surgical Department, Istituto Pediatrico della Svizzera Italiana (IPSI), Bellinzona and Valli Regional Hospital, Ticino, Switzerland

Correspondence should be addressed to Marco Odorizzi; marco.odorizzi3@gmail.com

Academic Editor: Johannes Mayr

Clavicular fractures are some of the most common bone injuries in the paediatric population, yet the rates of nonunion are very low under 18 years. To the best of our knowledge, posttraumatic nonunion of the clavicle in a paediatric population is rarely reported. We report the case of an 11-year-old girl who presented with a nondislocated fracture of the midshaft to the proximal third of the right clavicle. Initial conservative treatment by sling immobilization demonstrated radiologically confirmed healing at 3 months. However, at 1-year follow-up, she presented with painful nonunion. Diagnostic MRI and CT exams confirmed a pseudoarthrosis, requiring elective open reduction and internal fixation with the aid of an ipsilateral iliac crest bone graft.

1. Introduction

The clavicle is the most commonly fractured bone in children, representing 6% to 15% of all paediatric fractures [1]. The vast majority of these fractures involve the middle third, and the majority are ubiquitously treated conservatively, using sling immobilization and serial radiological check-ups [2, 3]. The reported incidence of nonunion in the paediatric population is extremely rare, in contrast to that known of the adult population, where the rate is from 8% to 14% [4]. A systematic review undertaken by Hughes et al. reported 21 paediatric cases of nonunion, the majority of which occurred after a displaced right-sided fracture and with typical presentation occurring at a distance of one year [5].

2. Case Report

An 11-year-old girl presented to our A&E department after a fall on an outstretched arm with immediate pain experienced at the right shoulder. The X-ray demonstrated a nondisplaced fracture of the middle to proximal third of the right clavicle (Figure 1). There were no other injuries, and neurovascular examination of the upper extremity was normal. The fracture was managed conservatively with sling immobilization for 6 weeks, and on clinical follow-up, it appeared to be healing well. The patient had no pain nor functional limitation, with adequate progression of periosteal reossification and callus formation seen on radiological examination. The patient was an amateur junior javelin thrower and was restricted from all sporting activity for a total of 3 months and until there was radiographic confirmation of callus formation (Figure 2).

The patient remained completely asymptomatic for 12 months, after which time she presented with new swelling at the callus midline, associated pain, and shoulder function loss, in the absence of additional trauma. The X-ray at 12 months confirmed the clinical suspicion of a pseudoarthrosis (Figure 3).

Following a multidisciplinary discussion, we decided to investigate the suspected nonunion and need for surgical intervention using CT and MRI (as seen below). The initial topographic examination was important to validate the pseudoarthrosis, which clearly identified two areas of hypertrophy without signs of bridging. The MRI was useful in

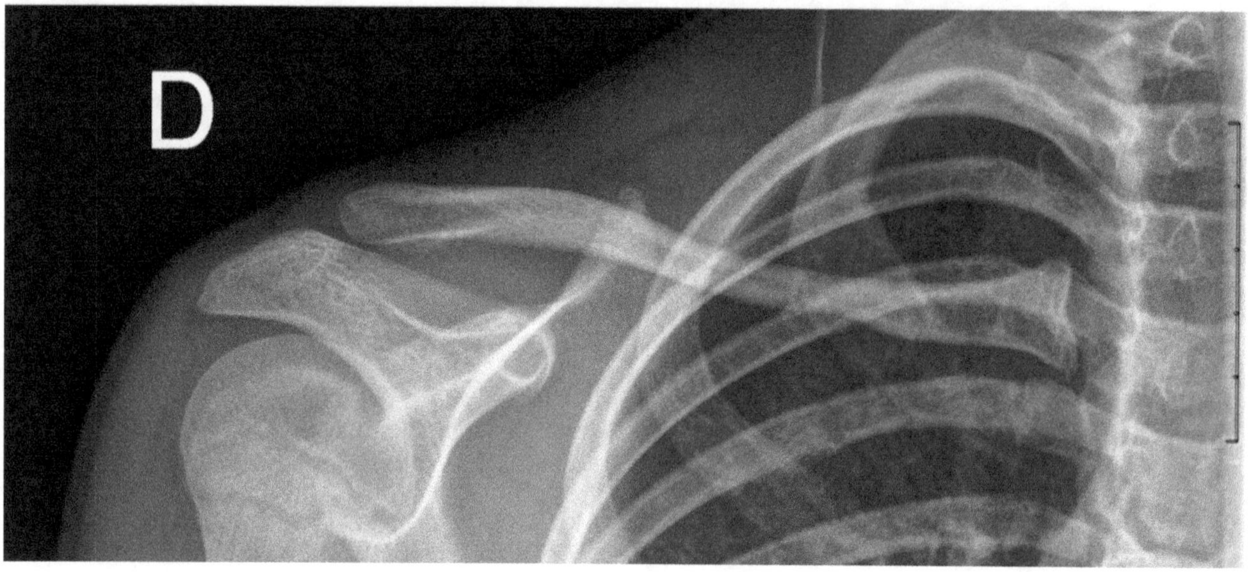

Figure 1: X-ray imaging showing the nondislocated fracture on the day of presentation to the paediatric A&E.

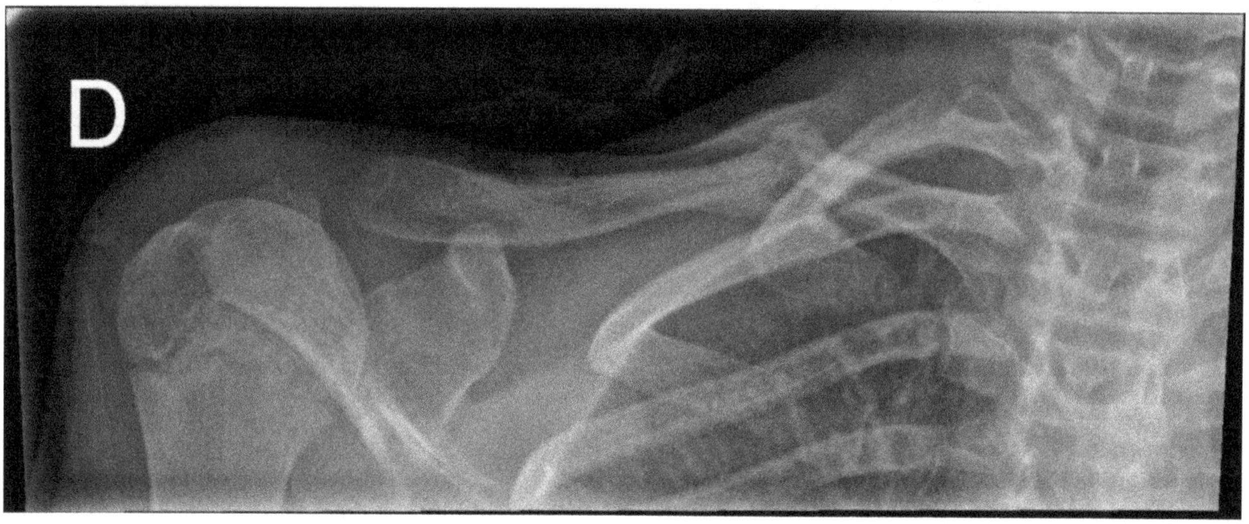

Figure 2: X-ray imaging showing callus formation after three months.

excluding an entrapment of surrounding articular structures and in evaluating the involvement of the neurovascular bundle with respect to the bone (Figure 4).

Following a discussion with the patient's parents, we opted for a surgical approach with open reduction and internal fixation and iliac crest bone graft from the ipsilateral hip $3 \times 3 \times 1$ cm. The nonunion was confirmed intraoperatively with debriding of the fracture site, with a loss of bone substance of 2 cm. The bone sample taken from the iliac crest was customised, molded, and inserted into the remaining gap. Following bone tissue transplant, the clavicle was reduced and internal fixation performed with a 3.5 mm seven-hole locking compression plate (LCP) (Synthes) in compression (Figure 5).

Following a normal postoperative course, clinical and radiological follow-up showed complete isometric anatomical healing at 1 year from the operation (Figure 5). The clinical examination showed no pain during shoulder movement, with a range of motion in antepulsion of 180°, abduction of 180°, internal rotation up to X thoracic vertebra, and external rotation of 80° (Figure 6).

3. Discussion

Clavicle fractures are common injuries in children and adults [1, 6], but generally the treatment is nonoperative with a sling immobilization and avoidance of high-risk activity such as contact sports for several weeks. The efficacy of this management is well described in the literature [2, 3, 7, 8]. Surgical treatment is very rarely performed with the most common indication being an exposed fracture, potential skin necrosis or perforation, and floating shoulder injuries [3]. Relative indications are a completely displaced fracture in high-performing adolescent athletes and/or for cosmetic purposes

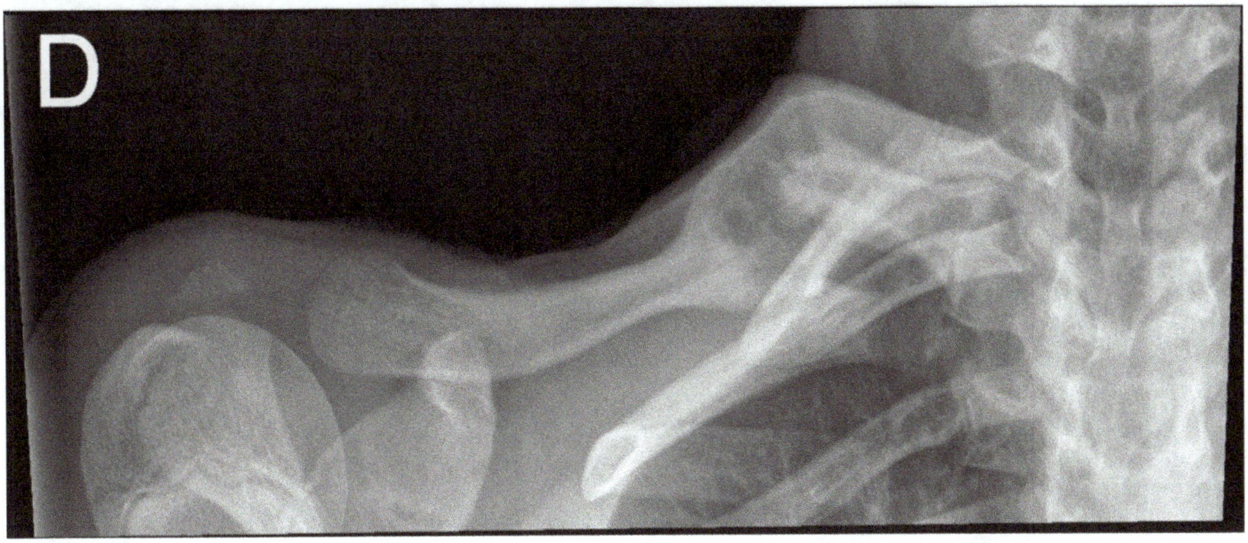

FIGURE 3: X-ray imaging showing partial callus formation, hypertrophic nonunion, and deformation at the boundary of the midshaft and proximal right clavicle.

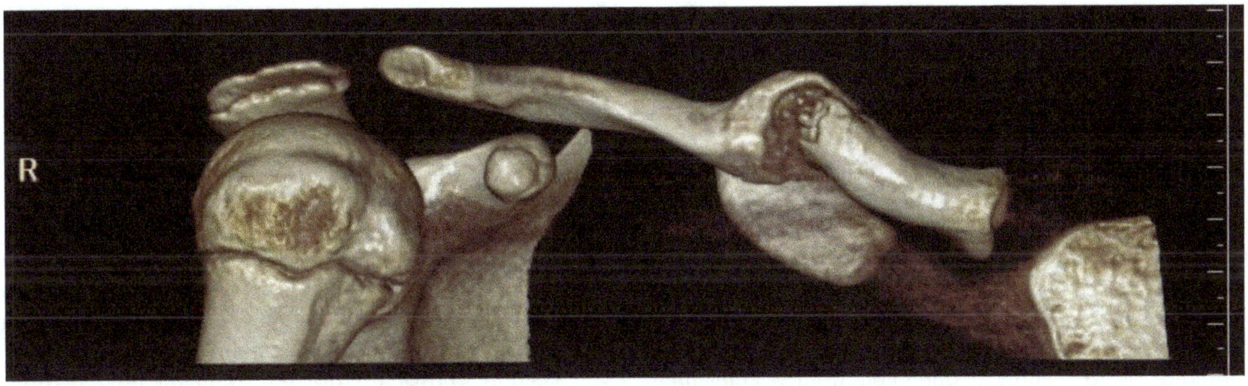

FIGURE 4: CT scan confirmed the diagnosis of the pseudoarthrosis.

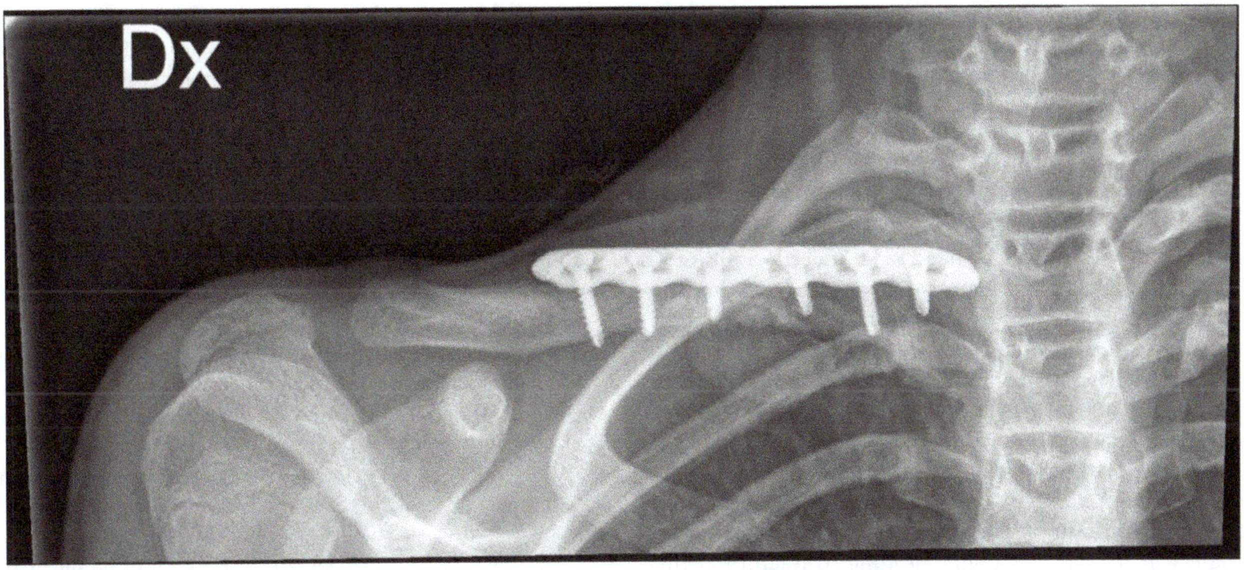

FIGURE 5: Postoperative X-rays.

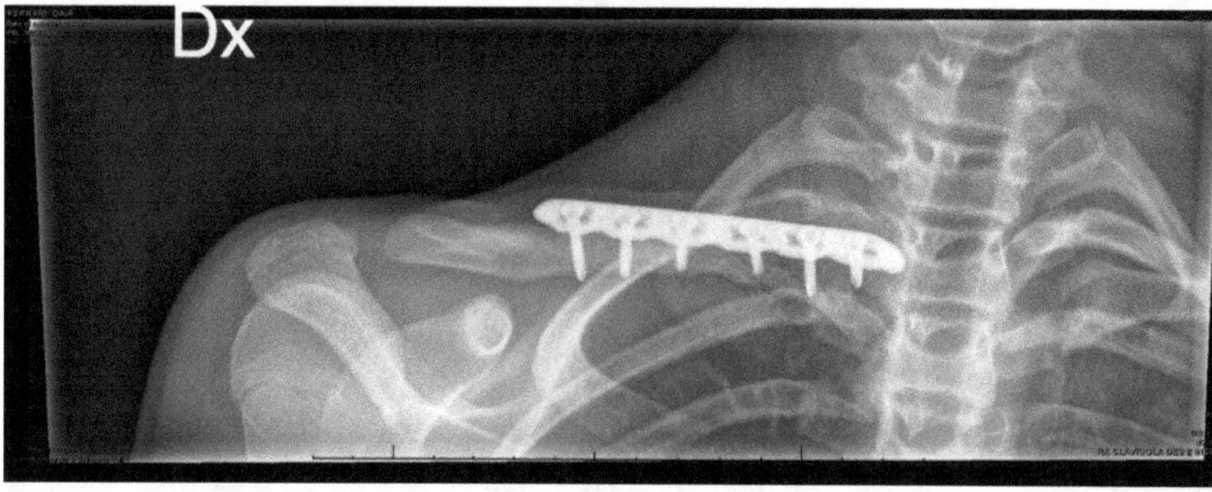

FIGURE 6: X-ray imaging at 1 year.

[2, 8–10]. In most cases, there is no difference in outcome between operative and nonoperative management [2, 11].

Paediatric clavicle fracture nonunion is a rare clinical occurrence [3, 7, 12, 13]. Even in large retrospective reviews of clavicle fracture in children, a precise nonunion rate is not yet known. For example, Kessler et al. [12] found no cases of nonunion, and Randsborg et al. [13] had only one case of nonunion out of 185 clavicle fractures. Completely displaced fractures and refractures of the ipsilateral clavicle may be predisposing factors for nonunion [3, 7] as described in the study by Strauss et al. [7]. Their findings demonstrated just one case of nonunion and three cases of delayed union out of 537 children. However, there is a limited number of reviews specifically evaluating paediatric nonunion.

A clinically relevant finding, that is of therapeutic importance, is to identify a nonunion from a congenital pseudoarthrosis of the clavicle from a posttraumatic nonunion [14]. These generally occur on the right side in females [15] and at birth present as a painless lump that may increase in size and become painful, without necessarily any history of trauma [14, 16]. Radiographic differences are well described by Owen and include that the medial half of the clavicle is large and protrudes forward and upwards, whereas the lateral half is situated below, pointing upwards and backwards and ending in a bulbous mass at the site of the pseudoarthrosis [16].

The prevalence of documented nonunion clavicle fractures result on the right-hand side. Indeed, Smith and William proposed a possible/probable connection of this predominance with the known predominance of congenitally acquired pseudoarthrosis, also occurring on the right-hand side [17]. The exact pathophysiological reason for such a connection is not further elaborated nor known, yet Smith and William identify the fact that many subclinical congenital pseudoarthrosis may not be identified or visible on X-ray nor by physical exam. This may lead to a lack of pathology recognition, thus predisposing such patients to a line of weakness in the case of trauma, leading to fracture at this pseudoarthritic site and subsequent misdiagnosis as a "posttraumatic nonunion" [5].

Another important aspect of case management is the necessity of performing serial imaging in asymptomatic children. Adamich et al. [18] demonstrated that the rate of detection does not change and therefore advocated against serial imaging. Instead, he advocated for an informative approach with patient or parent education of the possibility of nonunion and stressed the importance of "early presentation" as being critical as a clinical strategy, in order for early identification and prevention [18].

Paediatric posttraumatic clavicular nonunion is rare but remains a potential complication and therefore requires physician awareness and early identification. Though the case population is small and consensus is not unanimous as yet, it appears that clinical follow-up with serial X-ray imaging and radiation exposure, is a safe management option.

There is a possibility that posttraumatic pseudoarthrosis of the clavicle may have a congenital component, in that it is a population underdiagnosed until the time of presentation. However the discrimination between a "true" traumatic nonunion and a previously undiagnosed "congenital" nonunion may have little clinical impact on diagnosis, follow-up, and treatment strategies. Additionally, as in our case, when operative intervention is necessary, plate fixation and autologous graft usage proves an excellent therapeutic option.

References

[1] L. Rennie, C. M. Court-Brown, J. Y. Q. Mok, and T. F. Beattie, "The epidemiology of fractures in children," *Injury*, vol. 38, no. 8, pp. 913–922, 2007.

[2] J. A. Parry, M. van Straaten, T. D. Luo et al., "Is there a deficit after nonoperative versus operative treatment of shortened midshaft clavicular fractures in adolescents?," *Journal of Pediatric Orthopedics*, vol. 37, no. 4, pp. 227–233, 2017.

[3] B. J. O'Neill, A. P. Molloy, and W. Curtin, "Conservative management of paediatric clavicle fractures," *International Journal Of Pediatrics*, vol. 2011, Article ID 172571, 4 pages, 2011.

[4] W. Liu, J. Xiao, F. Ji, Y. Xie, and Y. Hao, "Intrinsic and extrinsic risk factors for nonunion after nonoperative treatment of

midshaft clavicle fractures," *Orthopaedics & Traumatology, Surgery & Research*, vol. 101, no. 2, pp. 197–200, 2015.

[5] K. Hughes, J. Kimpton, R. Wei et al., "Clavicle fracture non-union in the paediatric population: a systematic review of the literature," *Journal of Children's Orthopaedics*, vol. 12, no. 1, pp. 2–8, 2018.

[6] F. Postacchini, S. Gumina, P. De Santis, and F. Albo, "Epidemiology of clavicle fractures," *Journal of Shoulder and Elbow Surgery*, vol. 11, no. 5, pp. 452–456, 2002.

[7] B. J. Strauss, T. P. Carey, J. A. Seabrook, and R. Lim, "Pediatric clavicular fractures: assessment of fracture patterns and predictors of complicated outcome," *The Journal of Emergency Medicine*, vol. 43, no. 1, pp. 29–35, 2012.

[8] M. S. Caird, "Clavicle shaft fractures," *Journal of Pediatric Orthopedics*, vol. 32, pp. S1–S4, 2012.

[9] K. L. Vander Have, A. M. Perdue, M. S. Caird, and F. A. Farley, "Operative versus nonoperative treatment of midshaft clavicle fractures in adolescents," *Journal of Pediatric Orthopedics*, vol. 30, no. 4, pp. 307–312, 2010.

[10] N. J. Fanter, R. M. Kenny, C. L. Baker III, and C. L. Baker Jr., "Surgical treatment of clavicle fractures in the adolescent athlete," *Sports Health: A Multidisciplinary Approach*, vol. 7, no. 2, pp. 137–141, 2015.

[11] J. Schulz, M. Moor, J. Roocroft, T. P. Bastrom, and A. T. Pennock, "Functional and radiographic outcomes of nonoperative treatment of displaced adolescent clavicle fractures," *The Journal of Bone and Joint Surgery-American Volume*, vol. 95, no. 13, pp. 1159–1165, 2013.

[12] J. Kessler, I. Gardner, and J. Corral, "Pediatric clavicular shaft fractures treated nonoperatively: assessment of treatment results, fracture patterns, modes of injury, and patient demographics," *Annual Meeting of the Pediatric Orthopaedic Society of America*, vol. 30, 2009.

[13] P.-H. Randsborg, H. F. S. Fuglesang, J. H. Røtterud, O.-L. Hammer, and E. A. Sivertsen, "Long-term patient-reported outcome after fractures of the clavicle in patients aged 10 to 18 years," *Journal of Pediatric Orthopedics*, vol. 34, no. 4, pp. 393–399, 2014.

[14] D. L. Fitzwilliams, "Hereditary cranio-cleido-dysostosis: with a review of all the published cases of this disease: theories of the development of the clavicle suggested by this condition," *The Lancet*, vol. 176, no. 4551, pp. 1466–1475, 1910.

[15] D. A. Gibson and N. Carroll, "Congenital pseudarthrosis of the clavicle," *Journal of Bone and Joint Surgery*, vol. 52-B, no. 4, pp. 629–643, 1970.

[16] R. Owen, "Congenital pseudarthrosis of the clavicle," *The Journal of Bone and Joint Surgery. British volume*, vol. 52-B, no. 4, pp. 644–652, 1970.

[17] N. W. Smith and N. Williams, "Post-traumatic nonunion of a clavicle fracture in a 9-year-old child," *Journal of Pediatric Orthopaedics. Part B*, vol. 25, no. 1, pp. 74–77, 2016.

[18] J. S. Adamich, A. Howard, and M. Camp, "Do all clavicle fractures in children need to be managed by orthopedic surgeons?," *Pediatric Emergency Care*, vol. 34, pp. 706–710, 2018.

28

Intramedullary Nail Fixation with Autologous Bone Marrow Transplantation in an Incomplete Atypical Femoral Fracture Patient: Use of Bone Marrow Extracted from the Hollow Reamer

Ryutaro Iwasaki,[1] Masaaki Sakamoto,[2] Tomoyuki Rokkaku,[2] Hitoshi Watanabe,[2] Toshiyuki Yamada,[2] Takeshi Yamaguchi,[2] Yasushi Wako,[2] Hitoshi Kubosawa,[3] and Seiji Ohtori[1]

[1]*Department of Orthopaedic Surgery, Graduate School of Medicine, Chiba University, Japan*
[2]*Department of Orthopaedic Surgery, Chiba Municipal Aoba Hospital, Japan*
[3]*Department of Pathology, Chiba Municipal Aoba Hospital, Japan*

Correspondence should be addressed to Masaaki Sakamoto; ma-sakamo@nifty.com

Academic Editor: Athanassios Papanikolaou

The present report describes an incomplete atypical femoral fracture (AFF) patient who underwent simultaneous autogenous bone transplantation to the resected fracture region during intramedullary nail fixation. A 73-year-old female with a history of multiple myeloma had been undergoing treatment with intravenous drip injections of Zoledronic Acid. She was introduced to our department due to the left lateral thigh pain, with no trauma incidence. An anteroposterior radiograph showed a transverse thin fracture line with localized periosteal and endosteal thickening, which is compatible with subtrochanteric incomplete AFF. A biochemical investigation revealed the existence of severely suppressed bone turnover. She underwent intramedullary nail fixation for fear of a complete fracture. After the fixation, the cortical bone at the fracture region was excised as a wedge-shaped block, and bone marrow extracted from the hollow reamer was simultaneously transplanted to the resected fracture region. Histological examination showed few bone formation features at the fracture line in the excised lateral cortical bone. At 7 months after surgery, radiographs demonstrated complete bone repair, and no clinical problems were observed two years postoperatively. To the best of our knowledge, this is the first report in which autogenous bone marrow transplantation, noninvasive to the iliac crest, was performed in an incomplete AFF patient. We believe that this low invasive procedure can be a useful technique for AFF treatment.

1. Introduction

In 2005, Odvina et al. [1] reported that long-term alendronate therapy could cause severely suppressed bone turnover (SSBT), resulting in delayed healing of nonspinal fractures. Since then, SSBT after prolonged use of bisphosphonates (BPs) has been considered to be one of the causes of low-energy femoral fractures, called "atypical femoral fracture" (AFF). Delayed healing has long been a clinical problem in AFF cases under SSBT [2, 3]. Moreover, recent histological studies clarified few bone formation features at the thin fracture lines of incomplete AFF cases [4]. The present report shows a minimally invasive procedure, which could facilitate bone union in incomplete AFF. The clinical course and pathological results of the patient are presented with a review of the related literature.

2. Case Presentation

A 73-year-old female with a history of multiple myeloma had been undergoing treatment with intravenous drip injections of Zoledronic Acid over three years in our hospital. She was introduced to our department due to an increase of weight-bearing pain in her left lateral thigh, with no trauma incidence. Anteroposterior radiographs and magnetic resonance images were compatible with subtrochanteric incomplete

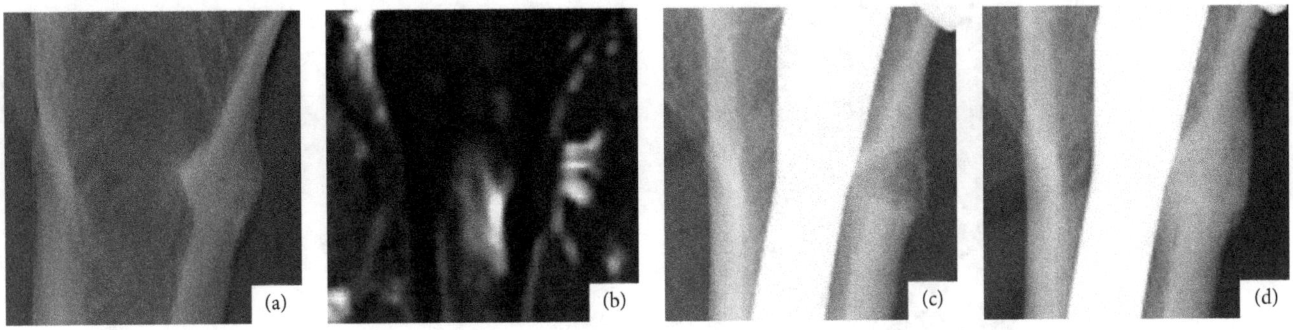

(a) (b) (c) (d)

FIGURE 1: Anteroposterior radiograph showing a transverse thin fracture line with localized periosteal and endosteal thickening at the left subtrochanteric lateral cortex (a). Coronal STIR image showing focal cortical thickening with minimal edema of the adjacent bone marrow (b). Anteroposterior radiographs showing fracture region just after surgery (c) and complete bone repair at 7 months after surgery (d).

AFF (Figures 1(a) and 1(b)) [2, 5, 6]. A biochemical investigation revealed a serum calcium of 9.2 mg/dl, phosphorus of 4.1 mg/dl, and 25-hydroxyvitamin D of 62 ng/ml, indicating vitamin D sufficiency. Tartrate-resistant acid phosphatase 5b was 245 mU/dl and bone-specific alkaline phosphatase level was 6.1 μg/l, clarifying the existence of SSBT [7]. Dual-energy X-ray absorptiometry at lumbar spine and hip revealed T scores of −1.0, −1.3, and Z scores of 1.1, 1.0. Although teriparatide was not used due to a medical contraindication, Zoledronic Acid treatment was discontinued based on the judgment of an internist. Since severe loading pain continued for approximately 3 months, surgical procedures were considered to be necessary for fear of a complete fracture.

After intramedullary nail fixation, the skin incision was extended 2 cm distally from the blade insertion. The cortical bone at the fracture region was excised as a wedge-shaped block to reach the medullary cavity with a chisel. Bone marrow remains inside the hollow reamer were extracted for use as an autologous bone graft (Figure 2(a)), which was transplanted to the resected fracture region.

Histological examination showed few bone formation features at the fracture line in the excised cortical bone (Figure 2(b)). No atypical cells were pathologically identified in the bone marrow pieces inside the hollow reamer. Anteroposterior radiograph just after surgery demonstrated bone marrow transplanted to the resected fracture region (Figure 1(c)). The postoperative course was uneventful, and pain decreased promptly. At 4 months after surgery, radiographs demonstrated apparent cortical bone remodeling, and complete bone repair was observed at 7 months after surgery (Figure 1(d)). No clinical problems were observed two years postoperatively.

3. Discussion

Since Odvina et al. [1] reported patients sustaining low-energy fractures after prolonged BPs use, there have been many reports regarding AFF including etiology, pathophysiology, and the treatment outcome [8, 9]. Delayed healing is one of the minor features in the American Society of Bone and Mineral Research task force, and as a matter of fact, we also experienced 2 AFF cases with unusual bone healing. The first reference case is a 74-year-old female who underwent intramedullary nailing for complete AFF. Although complete healing was observed throughout most of the whole cortex bone circumference at 2 years after surgery, the fracture surface in the lateral cortex, despite contact, showed little bone remodeling radiographically (Figures 3(a) and 3(b)). The second reference case is a 76-year-old female who underwent intramedullary nailing for incomplete AFF. Approximately 3 years later, a fall accident led to a complete fracture, which originated from the same prior fracture line in despite thick nailing (Figures 3(c) and 3(d)). Based on these clinical experiences, we focused on the thin fracture lines in the lateral cortex.

Koh et al. [10] named the thin fracture line "dreaded black line", which was considered as an indicator for the progression of complete fractures and as a state of chronic nonunion for microcrack accumulation under SSBT with continued BPs. In a histological study, Schilcher et al. [4] showed that the thin fracture line contained amorphous, nonmineralized materials. Histological findings in the present case also showed few bone formation features at the thin fracture line in the lateral cortex, which was compatible with previous reports.

Cortical bone repair is considered to be necessary for a complete bone union [11]. Several recent reports have described additional surgical techniques for the fracture region in AFF patients. Bögl et al. [12] reported incomplete AFF patients who underwent reamed intramedullary nail fixation with excision of the fracture region. This technique brought continuity over the defect with dense bone at a median of 17 months, which indicates remodeling activity in the bone adjacent to the thin fracture line. Lovy et al. [13] reported that the use of bone marrow aspirate concentrate from the iliac crest reduced time to bone union in AFF. Several basic studies have reported the significant role of myeloid cells in fracture healing; therefore, it can be assumed that bone marrow transplantation is certainly effective for bone union [14, 15]. The iliac crest is currently the most common donor site for obtaining the autogenous bone graft, which can be an invasive procedure. Consequently, bone marrow extracted from the hollow reamer was used to prevent invasive autogenous bone collection, resulting in smooth bone remodeling. We believe that the good result was brought by both excisions of the incomplete fracture

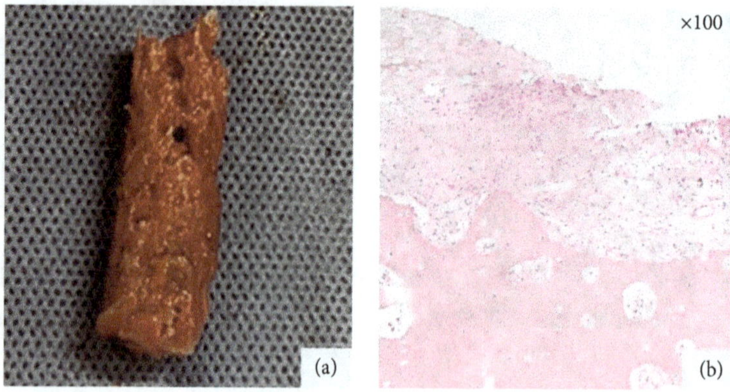

(a) (b)

Figure 2: Intraoperative photograph showing the cylindrical bone marrow extracted from the hollow reamer (a). Histologic image at the fracture line in the excised lateral cortical bone. Photomicrograph showing few osteoblasts and little woven bone (hematoxylin-eosin, original magnification x 100) (b).

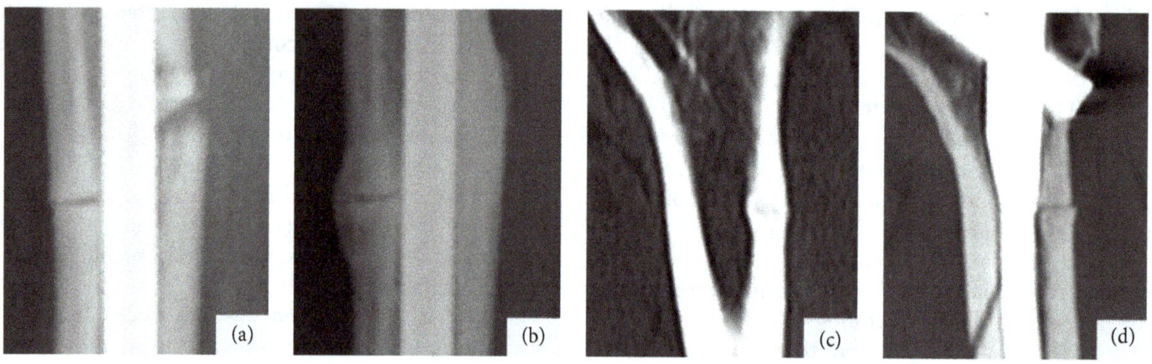

(a) (b) (c) (d)

Figure 3: Images of the first reference case (a, b) and the second reference case (c, d). Anteroposterior radiographs showing fracture region just after surgery (a) and incomplete bone remodeling in the lateral cortex at 2 years after surgery (b). Reconstructed coronal computed tomography (CT) scans showing a thin fracture line in the lateral cortex before surgery (c) and a complete fracture at approximately 3 years after surgery (d).

region with poor remodeling activity and bone marrow transplantation to the resected region.

To the best of our knowledge, this is the first report in which autogenous bone marrow transplantation, noninvasive to the iliac crest, was simultaneously performed during intramedullary nail fixation in incomplete AFF patients. Furthermore, the procedure brought about good clinical results. Although further research is necessary to verify the effectiveness and limitation of additional surgical techniques in the fracture region, our procedure can be considered to be a simple method in the acceleration of fracture healing in AFF.

4. Conclusion

A subtrochanteric incomplete AFF patient, who underwent autogenous bone marrow transplantation to the resected fracture region simultaneously with intramedullary nail fixation, is presented. Bone marrow extracted from the hollow reamer was used as an autogenous bone graft, resulting in a satisfactory bone union. We believe that this low invasive procedure can be a useful technique for AFF treatment.

Consent

The patient has been given informed consent for print and electronic publication of her case report. Institutional review board approval was not required for the publication of her report.

References

[1] C. V. Odvina, J. E. Zerwekh, D. S. Rao, N. Maalouf, F. A. Gottschalk, and C. Y. C. Pak, "Severely suppressed bone turnover: a potential complication of alendronate therapy," *The Journal of Clinical Endocrinology & Metabolism*, vol. 90, no. 3, pp. 1294–1301, 2005.

[2] E. Shane, D. Burr, B. Abrahamsen et al., "Atypical subtrochanteric and diaphyseal femoral fractures: second report of a task force of the American Society for Bone and Mineral Research," *Journal of Bone and Mineral Research*, vol. 29, no. 1, pp. 1–23, 2014.

[3] B. J. X. Teo, J. S. B. Koh, S. K. Goh, M. A. Png, D. T. C. Chua, and T. S. Howe, "Post-operative outcomes of atypical femoral subtrochanteric fracture in patients on bisphosphonate ther-

apy," *The Bone & Joint Journal*, vol. 96-B, no. 5, pp. 658–664, 2014.

[4] J. Schilcher, O. Sandberg, H. Isaksson, and P. Aspenberg, "Histology of 8 atypical femoral fractures," *Acta Orthopaedica*, vol. 85, no. 3, pp. 280–286, 2014.

[5] M. A. Png, J. S. B. Koh, S. K. Goh, S. Fook-Chong, and T. S. Howe, "Bisphosphonate-related femoral periosteal stress reactions: scoring system based on radiographic and MRI findings," *American Journal of Roentgenology*, vol. 198, no. 4, pp. 869–877, 2012.

[6] R. L. R. Vieira, Z. S. Rosenberg, M. B. Allison, S. A. Im, J. Babb, and V. Peck, "Frequency of incomplete atypical femoral fractures in asymptomatic patients on long-term bisphosphonate therapy," *American Journal of Roentgenology*, vol. 198, no. 5, pp. 1144–1151, 2012.

[7] S. Ikegami, S. Uchiyama, Y. Nakamura et al., "Factors that characterize bone health with aging in healthy postmenopausal women," *Journal of Bone and Mineral Metabolism*, vol. 33, no. 4, pp. 440–447, 2015.

[8] S. K. Goh, K. Y. Yang, J. S. B. Koh et al., "Subtrochanteric insufficiency fractures in patients on alendronate therapy: a caution," *The Journal of Bone and Joint Surgery. British volume*, vol. 89-B, no. 3, pp. 349–353, 2007.

[9] A. S. Neviaser, J. M. Lane, B. A. Lenart, F. Edobor-Osula, and D. G. Lorich, "Low-energy femoral shaft fractures associated with alendronate use," *Journal of Orthopaedic Trauma*, vol. 22, no. 5, pp. 346–350, 2008.

[10] J. S. B. Koh, S. K. Goh, M. A. Png, E. B. K. Kwek, and T. S. Howe, "Femoral cortical stress lesions in long-term bisphosphonate therapy: a herald of impending fracture?," *Journal of Orthopaedic Trauma*, vol. 24, no. 2, pp. 75–81, 2010.

[11] L. Bonifacio and P. Syson, "Construct failure in an atypical femoral fracture treated with intramedullary nailing: a case report," *Malaysian Orthopaedic Journal*, vol. 8, no. 1, pp. 82–84, 2014.

[12] H. P. Bögl, P. Aspenberg, and J. Schilcher, "Undisturbed local bone formation capacity in patients with atypical femoral fractures: a case series," *Osteoporosis International*, vol. 28, no. 8, pp. 2439–2444, 2017.

[13] A. J. Lovy, J. S. Kim, J. di Capua et al., "Intramedullary nail fixation of atypical femur fractures with bone marrow aspirate concentrate leads to faster Union," *Journal of Orthopaedic Trauma*, vol. 31, no. 7, pp. 358–362, 2017.

[14] S. Levy, J. M. Feduska, A. Sawant, S. R. Gilbert, J. A. Hensel, and S. Ponnazhagan, "Immature myeloid cells are critical for enhancing bone fracture healing through angiogenic cascade," *Bone*, vol. 93, pp. 113–124, 2016.

[15] L. Watson, S. J. Elliman, and C. M. Coleman, "From isolation to implantation: a concise review of mesenchymal stem cell therapy in bone fracture repair," *Stem Cell Research & Therapy*, vol. 5, no. 2, p. 51, 2014.

29

Myonecrosis in a Sickle Cell-Diseased Patient: A Case Report and Literature Review

Ali Wasel Almomen,[1] **Yaser Mansour Tawfeeq**,[2] **Ahmed Khalid Almuhaisin**,[2] **and Abdulraheem Ayman Altalib**[2]

[1]*King Fahad Specialist Hospital Dammam, Orthopedic Surgery, Saudi Arabia*
[2]*Imam Abdulrahman Bin Faisal University King Fahd Hospital of the University, Orthopedic Surgery, Saudi Arabia*

Correspondence should be addressed to Ali Wasel Almomen; aliwaselalmomen@gmail.com

Academic Editor: George Mouzopoulos

Myonecrosis is a condition that results in muscle tissue necrosis, and it is rarely seen in sickle cell patients and often missed because more common manifestations of sickle cell can overlap like vaso-occlusive crises (VOC), which results in pain in the extremities or spine; also osteomyelitis is commonly seen in sickle cell patients. In this article, we present a case of myonecrosis in a sickle cell-diseased patient who presented with left acute atraumatic left foot pain and MRI with contrast showing characteristic image of muscle infarction supportive therapy initiated, and 2-year follow-up did not reveal any physical disabilities; further study and follow-up are needed to know the nature of the disease and avoid improper management of those patients.

1. Introduction

Sickle cell disease (SCD) is the most common hematological inheritable condition worldwide [1]. The prevalence of SCD in the eastern province of Saudi Arabia is 145 cases/10,000 persons, which is the highest in the kingdom [2]. It is characterized by a single missense mutation in the beta-globin gene and can present as homozygous hemoglobin S (HbSS) or compound heterozygous hemoglobin S. When tension is lowered, hemoglobin becomes distorted and rigid and binds to postcapillary venules, which leads to vascular trapping and reduced blood flow, precipitating vaso-occlusive crisis (VOC), which can result in myonecrosis [3]. Myonecrosis in sickle cell patients is rare and is, therefore, frequently missed, partly because of its rarity in sickle cell patients, and in part to the scarcity of literature on this specific topic (to date, only 15 cases have been reported) [3]. Another reason that myonecrosis may be missed is that its signs and symptoms could be mistaken for VOC or osteomyelitis, both of which are common in SCD.

2. Case Presentation

Herein, we present a case of a 30-year-old Saudi Arabian gentleman known to have SCD (HBSS) and complaining of sudden onset right-foot pain for 3 days. The pain was continuous and nonradiating. There was no history of fever, trauma, or a similar prior episode. With respect to the patient's SCD history, he had had no major complications of SCD, with an average number of hospital admissions of one or two per year for VOC pain management. He had no history of previous intensive care unit (ICU) admissions, surgical interventions, or blood transfusions, and he had no current drug use.

On physical examination, the patient's vital signs were within the normal range. The patient had an antalgic gait and full active and passive range of movement with minimal pain. The right foot showed a swelling $4 \times 6\ cm^2$, 3 cm below the lateral malleolus, extending to the planter aspect of the foot. The swelling was firm, warm, and mildly tender with no signs of erythema, discharge, or fluctuation. Blood vessels were palpable (Figure 1).

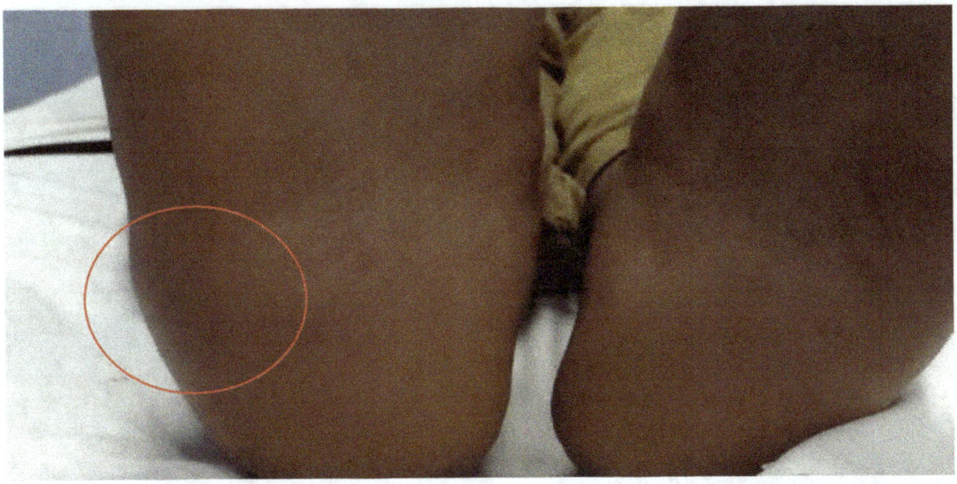

FIGURE 1: Clinical photograph with red circle showing swelling in the right foot.

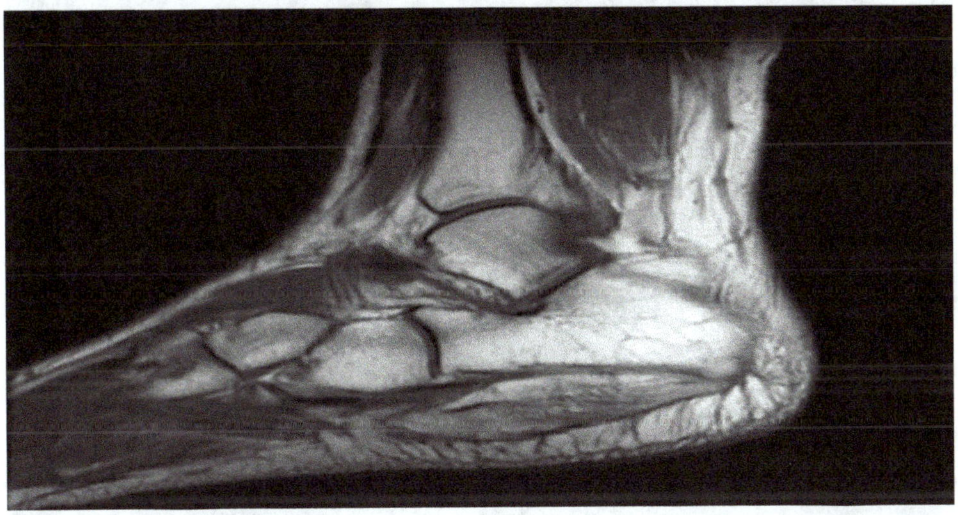

FIGURE 2: Magnetic resonance image of the right foot, Sag T1 showing diffuse enlargement of the muscle, with increased signal intensity. The muscle fibers are intact.

Laboratory investigations revealed the following findings: complete blood count (CBC): WBC: 11.5\L, hemoglobin (Hgb): 12.0 g\dl, and platelet (PLT): 149,000\L. Renal panel: normal. liver panel: normal. Lactic acid dehydrogenase (LDH), creatine kinase (CK), and CK-MB: normal. Erythrocyte sedimentation rate (ESR) = 20. C-reactive protein (CRP): negative. Alkaline phosphatase: normal.

Magnetic resonance imaging (MRI) with contrast showed increased signal intensity in T1 and T2 of the abductor digiti minimi and flexor digitorum brevis, diffuse muscular edema in short T1 inverse recovery (STIR), and heterogeneous enhancement of post gadolinium with no wall enhancement. There were no bony changes. This MRI reading together with the clinical picture was indicative of acute muscle infarction, indicative of myonecrosis (Figures 2–5).

The patient was managed with intravenous (IV) fluid hydration and NSAIDS and was advised not to bear weight on his right lower limb. In addition, he underwent extensive physiotherapy in the form of a range of motion and strengthening exercises of the left foot and ankle.

The patient was followed up after 2 weeks at 6 months, 1 year, and 2 years. The pain and swelling had resolved completely after two weeks. The 6-month outpatient follow-up also showed that he was pain-free with no complaints and no gross abnormality or deformity of the right foot and ankle.

3. Discussion

While the exact pathophysiology of myonecrosis in SCD is unknown, it is most likely due to the rigidity of the red blood cells, which, in turn, causes a decrease in blood supply to the muscle, causing ischemia. This tissue ischemia and hypoxia cause an inflammatory process that leads to muscular edema that can cause muscular infarction, which in turn leads to myofibrosis [12].

Myonecrosis in SCD patients is commonly missed probably because of the following two reasons: first, the lack of experience of the primary care providers with such cases; and second, the common association of SCD with

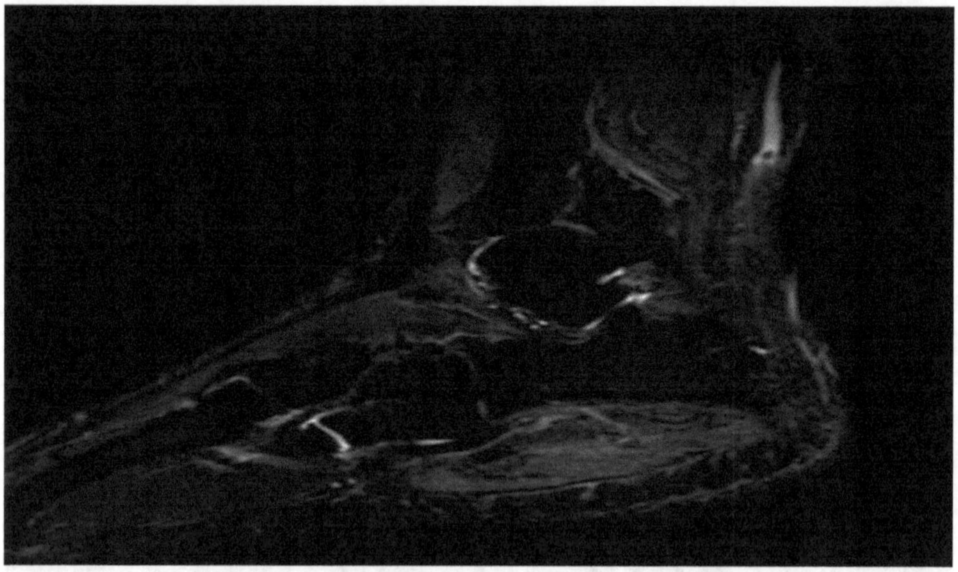

Figure 3: Short T1 inverse recovery (STIR) showing enlargement of the muscle with diffuse heterogeneous increase in signal intensity, with no drop of signal on fat-saturated image and normal signal intensity of the bone.

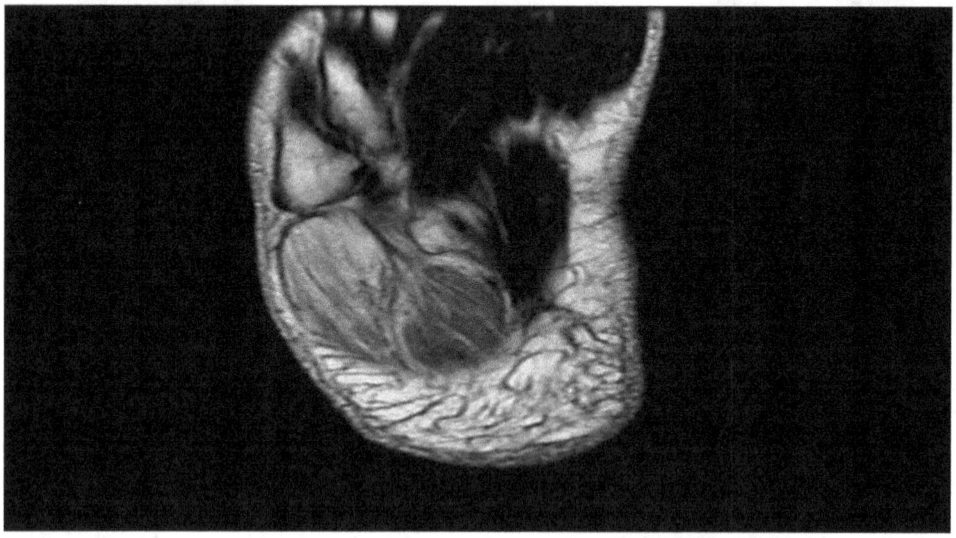

Figure 4: Axial T2 showing abnormally high T2 signal intensity along the muscle fibers with involvement of the adjacent muscle (flexor digitorum brevis).

VOC and infections. It is important to note that the latter reason will require the patient to undergo unnecessary treatment [13].

Up until January 2017, there have been 15 cases of sickle cell myonecrosis (including ours) reported (Table 1). Most patients were young adults, with a mean age of 28 years (with the exception of one patient, who was a child). The male to female ratio was 2 : 1. All the patients had HbSS disease with a history of previously treated pain crises [3].

Painful swelling is the most common presentation of myonecrosis. There have been no reports of fever. Ten of the reported patients had bilateral muscle involvement with the proximal large muscle group, usually involving the lower limbs, which are most commonly involved in a ratio of 2 : 1. The involvement of the joints is usually in the form of decreases in range of motion due to pain.

Misdiagnosis of myonecrosis will lead to a delay in treatment or leave the disease untreated, which will cause progressive necrosis of myocytes, leading to muscle atrophy, fibrosis, and contractures. Finally, liquefactive necrosis can occur, resulting in the formation of a sterile abscess. This abscess is typically nonpurulent on drainage [4, 5]. Other atypical features include the development of compartment syndrome (which necessitated fasciotomies in 2 of the reported patients) [6, 7].

Laboratory investigation, while not useful for determining a specific diagnosis of myonecrosis, may be useful to rule out a differential diagnosis such as infection. CPK and LDH

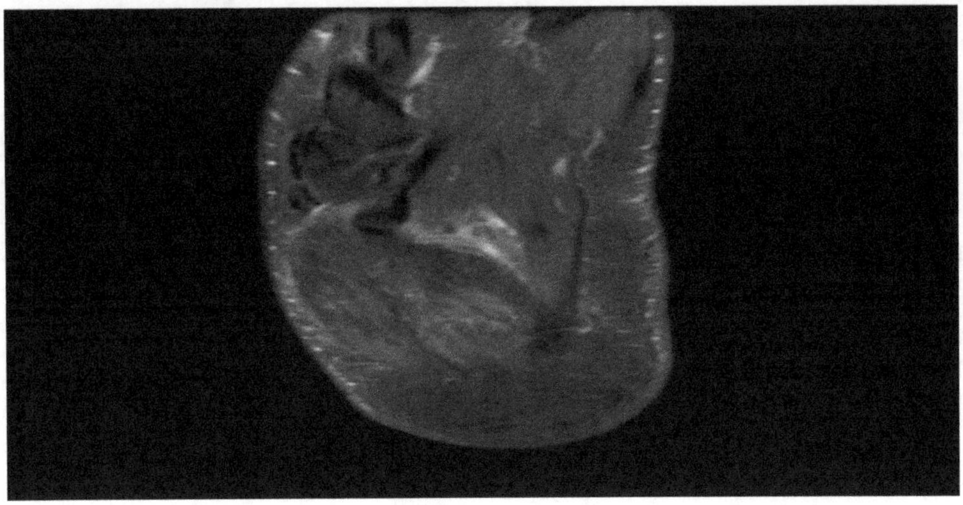

FIGURE 5: Axial T1 images post contrast demonstrating ill-defined heterogeneous enhancement of the abductor digiti minimi muscle, with no wall (ring) enhancement.

TABLE 1: Reported cases of myonecrosis in sickle cell patients.

Age (years)	Sex	Findings	CPK* (IU/L)	LDH/\ (IU/L)	Muscles involved	Reference
30	M	Pain, swelling, warmth, tenderness	300	—	B/L deltoids, B/L quadriceps	2
22	M	Pain, swelling, warmth, tenderness	—	—	B/L deltoids, B/L thighs	2
26	F	Pain, swelling, warmth, tenderness	300	—	B/L thigh and knee	3
4	M	Pain, swelling, tenderness	—	—	Right thigh and knee	3
44	F	Pain, swelling, indurated contracture	—	—	B/L deltoids	4
36	M	Pain, swelling, indurated contracture	—	—	B/L quadriceps	4
26	M	Pain, swelling induration	—	—	B/L quadriceps	4
30	M	Pain, swelling indurated contracture	—	—	B/L thighs	5
42	F	Induration	Normal	—	Left elbow	6
24	M	Pain, swelling, warmth, erythema	2140	592	Left leg	7
21	F	Pain, swelling, warmth, erythema	644	—	B/L thighs	8
28	M	Pain, swelling, warmth	185	1164	Left thigh	9
28	F	Pain, swelling, induration	624	431	B/L deltoids, B/L triceps	10
27	M	Pain, swelling, erythema	—	689	Plantar muscles	11
30	M	Pain, swelling, warmth	—	—	Plantar muscles	(our case)

Abbreviations: CPK: Creatine Phospho-Kinase; /\ LDH: Lactate Dehydrogenase, B/L: bilateral.

were reported to be high in 4 and 5 patients, respectively; however, all remaining patients showed normal levels of CPK and LDH, making these unreliable parameters for the diagnosis of myonecrosis [3].

Muscle biopsy is the gold standard for diagnosing myonecrosis; however, if the MRI and clinical findings are conclusive of a diagnosis of myonecrosis, biopsy is not indicated [5]. The necrosis of myocytes causes alteration in muscle size and shape, which increases signal intensity on T2-weighed images and gadolinium enhancement, as shown by MRI [8].

Intravenous nonsteroidal anti-inflammatory drugs (NSAIDS) have been reported as being sufficient for pain control. Aggressive physiotherapy in the form of nonweight bearing, pain-relieving modalities, and range of motion exercises to prevent fibrosis, which may cause contracture and stiffness of an involved joint, may be suggested as treatment options [3]. Swelling usually subsides within weeks, and the patient should be followed up for functional assessment of the affected limb.

Clear guidelines for treating myonecrosis have not yet been established; however, an early and accurate diagnosis and treatment, in addition to physical therapy, are essential for preventing complications such as contractures, fibrosis, and muscle atrophy [3].

4. Conclusion

Although myonecrosis is a well-known complication of SCD, treating physicians may not be aware of this as a possible diagnosis; therefore, it may frequently be missed, delaying necessary treatment. Moreover, further follow and study may be needed in order to help physicians to identify myonecrosis more easily.

References

[1] J. S. Hankins and W. C. Wang, "Sickle cell anemia and other sickling syndromes," in *Wintrobe's Clinical Hematology*, J. P. Greer, J. Foerster, G. M. Rodgers, F. Paraskevas, B. Glader, D. A. Arber, and R. T. Means Jr., Eds., pp. 1038–1082, Lippincott Williams & Wilkins, Philadelphia, 12th edition, 2008.

[2] M. M. Alotaibi, "Sickle cell disease in Saudi Arabia: a challenge or not," *Journal of Epidemiology and Global Health*, vol. 7, no. 2, pp. 99–101, 2017.

[3] N. Tageja, M. Racovan, J. Valent, and J. Zonder, "Myonecrosis in Sickle Cell Anemia—Overlooked and Underdiagnosed," *Case Reports in Medicine*, vol. 2010, 3 pages, 2010.

[4] B. Malekgoudarzi and S. Feffer, "Myonecrosis in sickle cell anemia," *The New England Journal of Medicine*, vol. 340, no. 6, p. 483, 1999.

[5] J. Groves and R. G. Stiles, "Sickle cell myonecrosis involving the plantar musculature," *Journal of the American Podiatric Medical Association*, vol. 87, no. 8, pp. 384–388, 1997.

[6] H. R. Schumacher Jr., W. M. Murray, and M. K. Dalinka, "Acute muscle injury complicating sickle cell crisis," *Seminars in Arthritis and Rheumatism*, vol. 19, no. 4, pp. 243–247, 1990.

[7] D. A. May, D. G. Disler, E. A. Jones, A. A. Balkissoon, and B. J. Manaster, "Abnormal signal intensity in skeletal muscle at MR imaging: patterns, pearls, and pitfalls," *Radiographics*, vol. 20, suppl_1, pp. S295–S315, 2000.

[8] L. P. Turaga, P. Boddu, S. Kipferl, A. Basu, and M. Yorath, "Myonecrosis in sickle cell anemia: case study," *American Journal of Case Reports*, vol. 18, pp. 100–103, 2017.

[9] V. C. Ejindu, A. L. Hine, M. Mashayekhi, P. J. Shorvon, and R. R. Misra, "Musculoskeletal manifestations of sickle cell disease," *Radiographics*, vol. 27, no. 4, pp. 1005–1021, 2007.

[10] B. B. Dorwart and T. G. Gabuzda, "Symmetric myositis and fasciitis: a complication of sickle cell anemia during vasoocclusion," *The Journal of Rheumatology*, vol. 12, no. 3, pp. 590–595, 1985.

[11] J. Valeriano-Marcet and L. D. Kerr, "Myonecrosis and myofibrosis as complications of sickle cell anemia," *Annals of Internal Medicine*, vol. 115, no. 2, pp. 99–101, 1991.

[12] G. J. Dennis and R. M. Keating, "Muscle infarction in sickle cell anemia," *Annals of Internal Medicine*, vol. 115, no. 10, pp. 831-832, 1991.

[13] S. Mani and T. P. Duffy, "Sickle myonecrosis revisited," *The American Journal of Medicine*, vol. 95, no. 5, pp. 525–530, 1993.

[14] P. Vicari, R. Achkar, K. R. B. Oliveira et al., "Myonecrosis in sickle cell anemia: case report and review of the literature," *Southern Medical Journal*, vol. 97, no. 9, pp. 894–896, 2004.

[15] M. Á. Rubio, L. Díez, N. Álvarez, and E. Munteis, "Afectacion muscular en la anemia drepanocitica," *Medicina Clínica (English Edition)*, vol. 145, no. 9, pp. 413-414, 2015.

30

Modified Arthroscopic Suture Fixation of Posterior Cruciate Ligament Tibial Avulsion Fracture in the Setting of Multiligament Knee Injury in Teenager

Miguel Quesado, Ana Sofia Esteves, Nuno Vieira da Silva, Tiago Costa, Nuno Ferreira, and Hélder Nogueira

Serviço de Ortopedia e Traumatologia, Centro Hospitalar do Tâmega e Sousa, Penafiel, Portugal

Correspondence should be addressed to Miguel Quesado; m_quesado@hotmail.com

Academic Editor: Hiroshi Takahashi

The posterior cruciate ligament (PCL) avulsion fracture is a rare injury and occurs mainly in young patients. The development of arthroscopic techniques and fixation methods has improved the treatment of this entity. This report describes a modified arthroscopic suture fixation of a small tibial avulsion fracture of the PCL. A 17-year-old male, injured in a motorcycle crash, was admitted to the Emergency Department and diagnosed with left knee PCL tibial avulsion fracture, lateral collateral ligament (LCL) femoral avulsion fracture, and patella fracture. The PCL was fixed arthroscopically using a Knee Scorpion and two SutureTapes (Arthrex, Munich-Germany) through of an interlaced configuration at the base of the fragment using a transseptal approach and fixed distally over a cortical button on the anterior cortex. The LCL was repaired with two cannulated screws by a percutaneous approach. At 1 year of follow-up, the fragment was healed with tibiofemoral congruence, and the knee was stable with complete range of motion. The Tegner Lysholm Knee Scoring Scale (TLKSS) was 92.

1. Introduction

PCL has a central role in knee biomechanics and stability. It represents the center of rotation of the knee, and it is the main structure to resist to posterior tibial translation [1]. Its damage impairs knee biomechanics with increased contact pressures in medial tibiofemoral and patellofemoral compartments and consequently progressive degenerative changes [2]. Avulsion fractures of PCL are more frequent in the younger age group and associated to high energy trauma [1, 3]. Reduction and fixation of the fragment assisted by arthroscopy favor minimal scarring, less tissue trauma, and early rehabilitation than open approaches, and it is actually indicated for PCL injuries with displacement and posterior instability [2, 4, 5]. Some procedures for suture fixation using different materials were described by several authors in the last 20 years. This report describes a new suture placement configuration for a small fragment and comminuted tibial PCL avulsion fracture that allows anatomical reduction and great compression at PCL footprint in one case of multiligament knee injury.

2. Case Presentation

A 17-year-old male was injured in a fall while riding a motorcycle. He presented left knee pain, swelling and partial active mobilities. The extensor mechanism was intact, and he had no neurovascular deficits. At clinical examination, he presented a positive posterior drawer test and positive varus stress test with a soft endpoint. The radiograph (X-ray) and computed tomography scan (CT scan) showed a displaced avulsion fracture of the PCL tibial attachment, a displaced avulsion fracture of the LCL femoral attachment and a comminuted fracture of the inferior pole of the patella (Figures 1 and 2). The PCL tibial avulsion fracture was better characterized by magnetic resonance imaging (MRI) (Figure 3). The limb

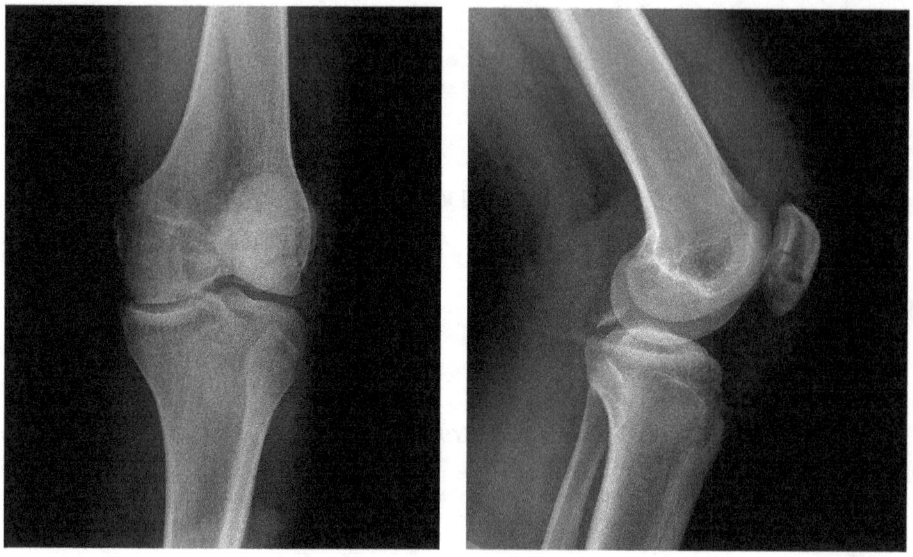

(a) (b)

Figure 1: Coronal (a) and sagittal (b) X-ray on admission to the Emergency Department.

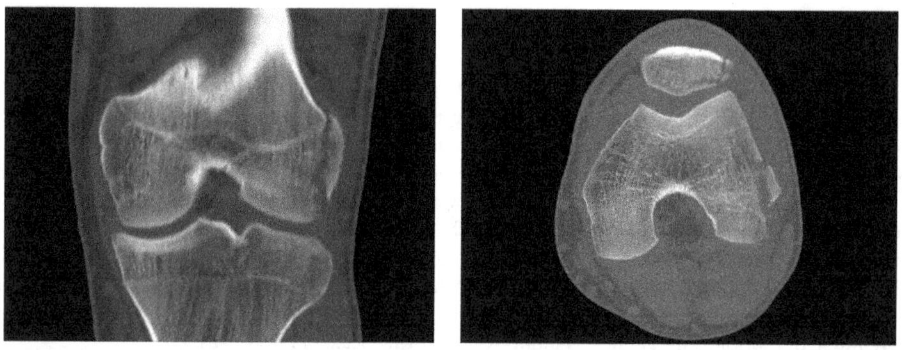

(a) (b)

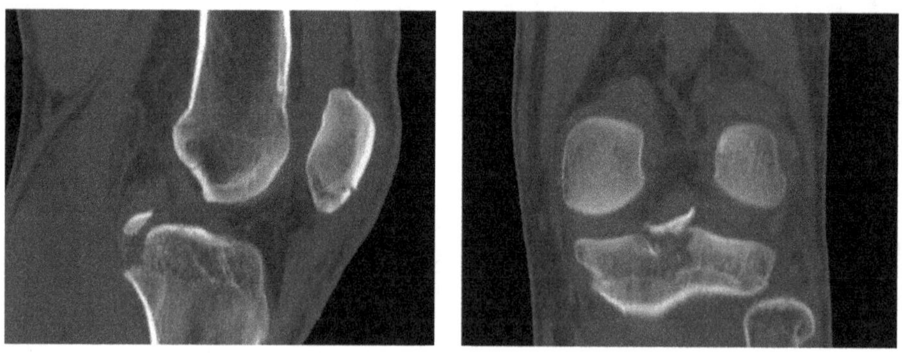

(c) (d)

Figure 2: Coronal (a, d), axial (b), and sagittal (c) CT scan on admission to the Emergency Department.

was immobilized with a cast and the patient was proposed for surgical intervention.

3. Surgical Technique

3.1. Patient Positioning. The patient was positioned supine on the operative table under general anesthesia with the leg flexed at 90°. A tourniquet was used in surgery as there are no contraindications.

3.2. Portals. Two standard arthroscopic portals (anteromedial and anterolateral) and two accessory arthroscopic portals (posteromedial and posterolateral) were used (Figure 4).

3.3. Diagnostic Arthroscopy. The joint was examined through the anteromedial and anterolateral portals: an ACL pseudolaxity was observed; there were no meniscal or cartilage injuries. The arthroscope inserted from the anterolateral portal was advanced through the transcondylar notch to the

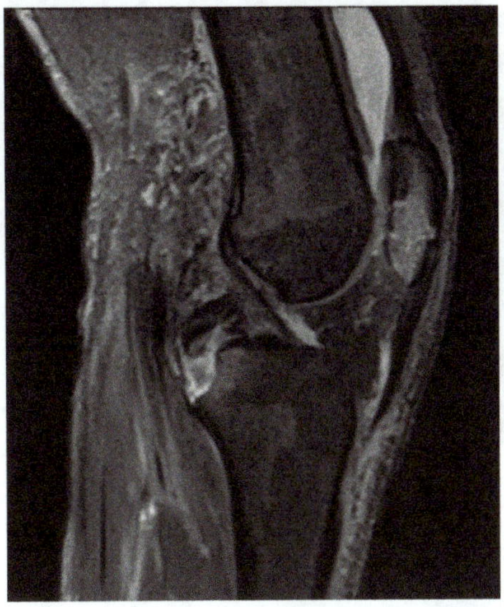

FIGURE 3: MRI (fat-saturated T2-weighted) lateral view showing a displaced avulsion fracture of PCL at tibial attachment.

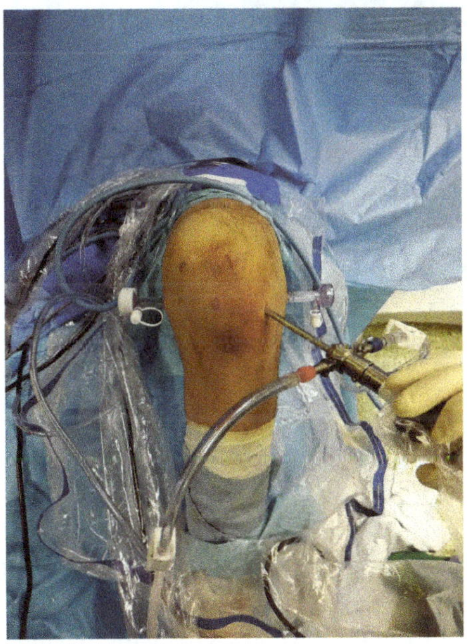

FIGURE 4: Arthroscopic portals used during the procedure (two standard anterior and two accessory posterior).

posteromedial compartment: a tibial avulsion fracture of PCL with a small and comminuted fragment was observed. Under direct visualization, a spinal needle helps to identify the location and direction of the posteromedial portal. The arthroscope inserted from the anteromedial portal was advanced at the same manner to the posterolateral compartment. Under direct visualization, a spinal needle helps to identify the location and direction of the posterolateral portal. Plastic cannulas were kept in both posterior portals during the procedure. The transeptal approach was performed to expose, debride and manipulate accurately the PCL footprint. A Switching Stick was advanced from the posterolateral portal through the posterior septum. Careful orientation and direct visualization

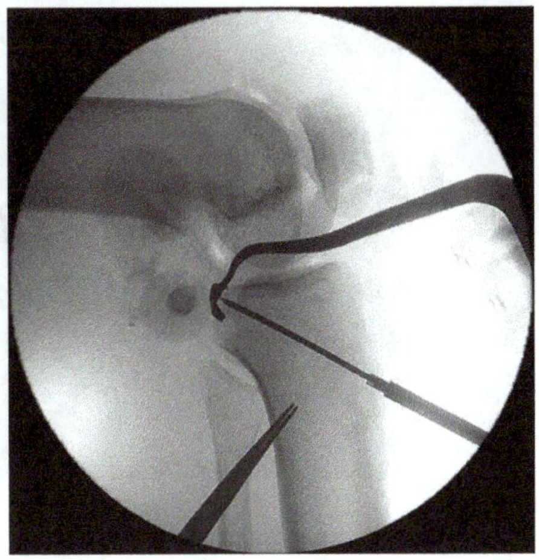

FIGURE 5: Insertion of K-wires to the PCL tibial footprint controlled by fluoroscopy.

were essential in order to not compromise the posterior neurovascular structures. Following, a shaver from posteromedial portal facing anterior was advanced from medial to lateral. At this moment, careful dissection of the PCL footprint and cleaning of the scar tissue were performed with the arthroscope in posterior portals.

3.4. Fixation of PCL Tibial Attachment. The PCL footprint on the tibia was identified by posteromedial portal. The center was raw using a curved rasp by the posterolateral portal. Blood clots, free bony fragments, and soft tissue interposed were debrided using the shaver until the avulsed fragment and tibial bony bed could be clearly released from the posterior capsule. A 2.5 cm longitudinal incision was made just medial to the tibial tubercule, and two parallel 2.5 mm K-wires were inserted through the tibial PCL guide to the medial and lateral borders of the tibial footprint, respectively (Figure 5). A Knee Scorpion loaded with SutureTape was inserted through the posteromedial portal, and a cinch stitch was created in the medial PCL tibial footprint. Similarly, the process was repeated through the posterolateral portal. At this time, the PCL footprint presented two cinch stitches at its medial and lateral portions. A 1.0 mm shuttle suture was inserted via the medial bone tunnel. The procedure was repeated for the lateral tunnel. Each suture crossed the posterior part of the ligament, passed the loop, and pulled to the outside through the contralateral tunnel, creating an interlaced suture configuration (Figure 6). Tensioning was performed with the knee at 90° of flexion, applying an anterior force to the proximal tibia and maintaining tension in both sutures. Arthroscopic reduction was confirmed by the relationship of the condyles and meniscus and the restoration of the articular step-off. The threads were fixed on the tibia using a cortical button fixation.

3.5. Fixation of LCL Femoral Attachment. The leg was flexed at 30° with valgus force. Closed reduction of the fragment of LCL attachment at the lateral femoral condyle was performed under fluoroscopic control. Two percutaneous screws (4.0 mm) were inserted and fixed the fragment (Figure 7).

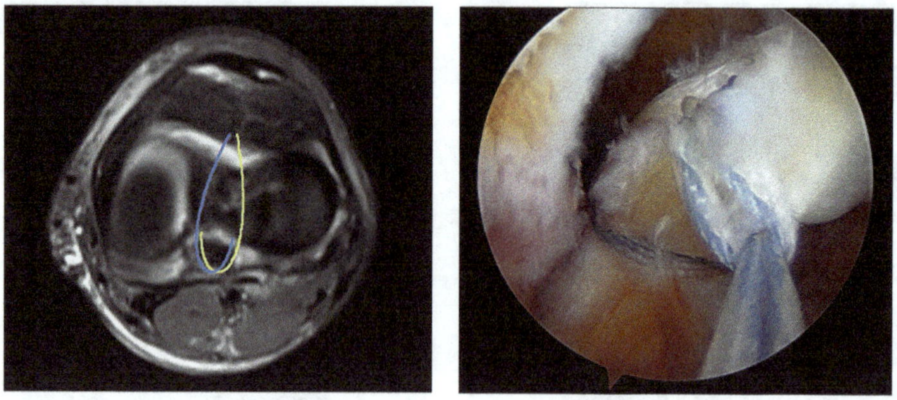

(a) (b)

Figure 6: MRI (T2-weighted) axial view - schematic representation of each suture (yellow and blue lines) crossing the posterior part of the base of the PCL and exiting the contralateral tunnel (a). Arthroscopic posteromedial view - interlaced suture configuration for PCL avulsion fracture (b).

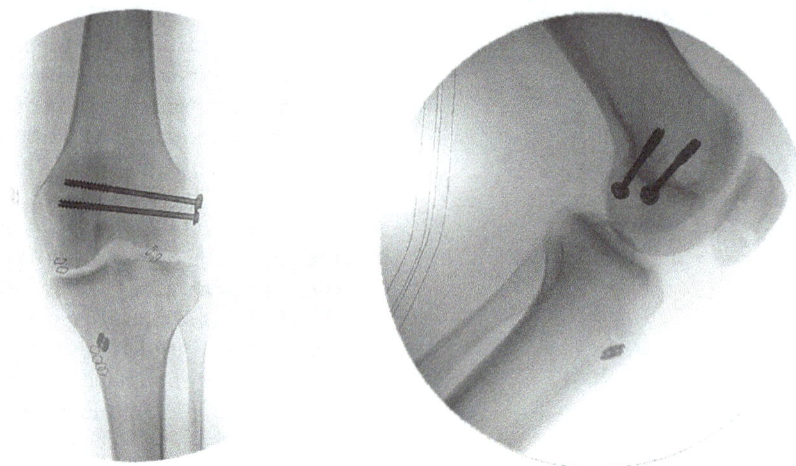

(a) (b)

Figure 7: Coronal (a) and sagittal (b) intraoperative X-ray showing the final reduction and fixation of PCL and LCL avulsion fractures.

3.6. Postoperative Rehabilitation. The limb was immobilized in extension with a cast during 2 weeks. Then, the patient started isometric exercises and passive mobilization with a PCL dynamic brace. Progressive weight bearing and active full range of motion were performed after 2 months postoperative. Three months after surgery, the avulsion fractures of PCL and LCL and the patella fracture were healed (Figure 8). The patient returned to sports 6 months later without limitations or sequelae. After 1 year of follow-up, the TLKSS was 92.

4. Discussion

PCL is the primary restraint to posterior tibial translation and the secondary restraint to external rotation of the knee joint [1]. Its injury varies from 3 to 23% of all knee injuries, and it is more frequent in the younger age group [3, 6]. It is commonly seen as part of multiligament knee injuries and associated to an increase of road traffic accidents and sports injuries [1, 3, 7]. The true incidence of multiligament knee injuries in the skeletally immature population is unknown owing the difficulty to promptly identify it at admission, and there is no consensus regarding the optimal management [6]. In young patients, these injuries mainly manifest as an avulsion fracture due to the strength of the ligamentous structures and weakness of the bone and physis; in contrast, adults are more likely to experience ligamentous failure within the substance of the ligament [7]. PCL rupture can occur at its mid substance, femoral, or tibial attachment, with or without bony avulsion [1, 6].

Conservative treatment is indicated for avulsion fractures with a mild displacement, whereas surgery should be performed in cases of displaced avulsion fracture of PCL >5 mm and injuries with >10 mm of posterior instability [1, 5]. Until recently, the posterior open approach has commonly used but it was thought that it would entail more risks and morbidity. This approach should be reserved for cases of delayed diagnosis because of possible nonunion, which require an adequate and easier exposure of the PCL and tibial avulsion site [8]. Song et al. [4] refers in a meta-analysis that all studies on the posterior approach and arthroscopic

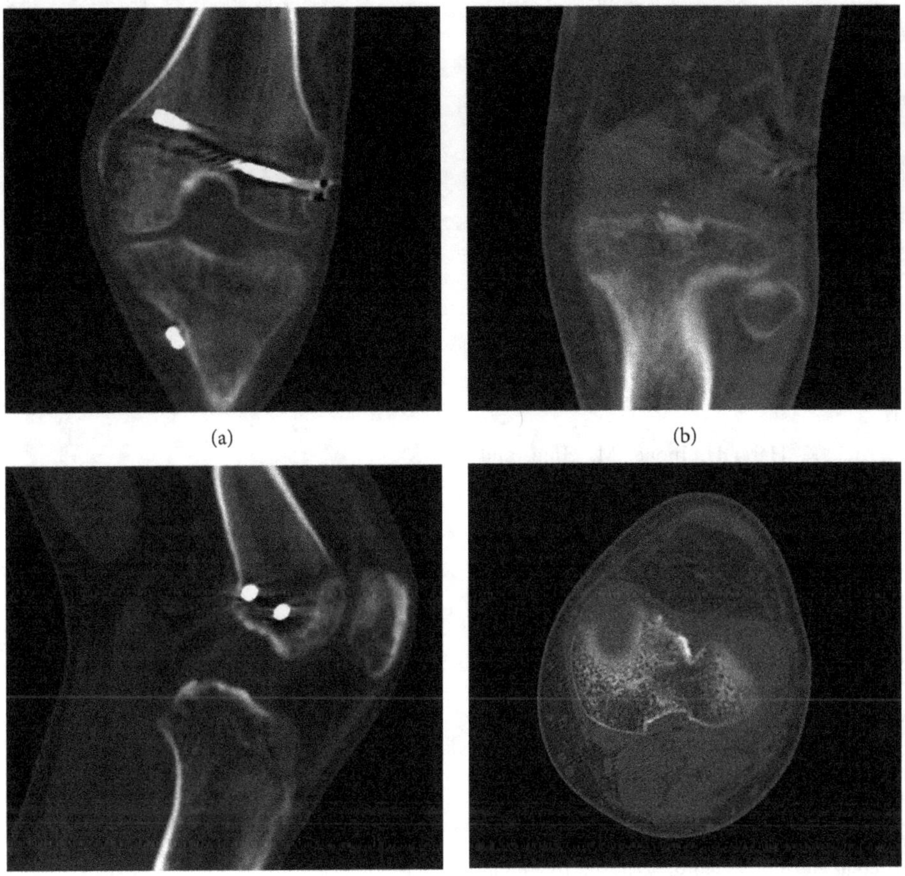

(a) (b) (c) (d)

FIGURE 8: Coronal (a, b), sagittal (c), and axial (d) control CT scan after 3 months postoperative with evidence of fracture healing.

fixation for displaced PCL avulsion fractures have satisfactory results, despite significant heterogeneity among studies with various techniques, fixation devices, and sizes of fracture fragments and follow-up periods. However, the development of the arthroscopic techniques and minimally invasive approaches provides a faster recovery and gives the chance of diagnosis and treatment of concomitant intraarticular injuries [4, 5]. Martinez-Moreno and Blanco-Blanco [9] performed the first arthroscopically assisted fixation of PCL avulsion fractures in cadaveric knees in 1988. The first report of an arthroscopic technique in vivo for PCL fixation using 3 canulated screws was described in 1995 by Littlejohn and Geissler [10]. In the last 20 years, some authors have been enhancing different types of fixation, including cannulated screws, wires or sutures, and these all proven to be effective [3]. The pullout procedure can be a solution to fix small and comminuted fragments to the tibial footprint that would be difficult to reduce through another way. The new configuration described in this case for the PCL avulsion fracture allowed to embrace the ligament and to create a high strength fixation with a large area for support. Despite many authors do not consider the use of the posterolateral portal, the association of posterior portals through a transseptal approach offers a direct view to posterior knee, allowing a better and more secure way for debridement and repair of the structures around the posterior capsule [5].

High rates of concomitant ligament or meniscus lesions are seen in PCL injuries, warranting a thorough knee preevaluation, including clinical examination and imaging studies. Fanelli and Edson [11] reported 96.5% of PCL injuries occurring in combination with other ligaments. In this case, the size of the LCL avulsion fracture allowed an effective osteosynthesis and healing with percutaneous screws, restoring the normal function of the knee. An early surgical repair was also essential to avoid arthrofibrosis and loss of the knee motion, being this the most common long-term complication observed after multiligament knee injury [6, 7].

This surgical procedure is simple and less invasive than previous methods, requiring no additional arthroscopic devices. It allows the repair of the PCL lenght, union of the fragments, and an early range of motion with minimal morbidity.

Acknowledgments

This research received a specific grant from Arthrex for article processing charges.

References

[1] R. Lamoria, D. Goyal, M. Bansal, S. Kaler, and R. Upadhyay, "Clinical experience with arthroscopic suture pull technique

in isolated PCL avulsion injuries," *Journal of Clinical Orthopaedics and Trauma*, vol. 11, Suppl 3, pp. S362–S367, 2020.

[2] W. Zhu, W. Lu, J. Cui et al., "Treatment of tibia avulsion fracture of posterior cruciate ligament with high-strength suture fixation under arthroscopy," *European Journal of Trauma and Emergency Surgery*, vol. 43, no. 1, pp. 137–143, 2017.

[3] L. B. Chen, H. Wang, K. Tie, A. Mohammed, and Y. J. Qi, "Arthroscopic fixation of an avulsion fracture of the tibia involving the posterior cruciate ligament," *The Bone & Joint Journal*, vol. 97-B, no. 9, pp. 1220-1225, 2015.

[4] J.-G. Song, K.-W. Nha, and S.-W. Lee, "Open posterior approach versus arthroscopic suture fixation for displaced posterior cruciate ligament avulsion fractures: systematic review," *Knee Surgery and Related Research*, vol. 30, no. 4, pp. 275–283, 2018.

[5] S. Nakagawa, Y. Arai, K. Hara, H. Inoue, M. Hino, and T. Kubo, "Arthroscopic pullout fixation for a small and comminuted avulsion fracture of the posterior cruciate ligament from the tibia," *Knee Surgery & Related Research*, vol. 29, no. 4, pp. 316–320, 2017.

[6] P. O. Hooper, C. Silko, T. L. Malcolm, and L. D. Farrow, "Management of posterior cruciate ligament tibial avulsion injuries: a systematic review," *The American Journal of Sports Medicine*, vol. 46, no. 3, pp. 734–742, 2018.

[7] R. Badrinath and C. W. Carter, ""Multiligamentous" injuries of the skeletally immature knee: a case series and literature review," *JAAOS: Global Research and Reviews*, vol. 2, no. 10, p. e079, 2018.

[8] T. M. Guimarães, P. V. P. Helito, F. J. Angelini, M. K. Demange, J. R. Pécora, and C. P. Helito, "Delayed treatment of a posterior cruciate ligament tibial insertion avulsion fracture in a child with open physis: a case report with a 4-year follow-up," *Journal of Pediatric Orthopaedics. Part B*, vol. 26, no. 5, pp. 477–481, 2017.

[9] J. L. Martinez-Moreno and E. Blanco-Blanco, "Avulsion fractures of the posterior cruciate ligament of the knee: an experimental percutaneous rigid fixation technique under arthroscopic control," *Clinical Orthopaedics and Related Research*, vol. 237, pp. 204–208, 1988.

[10] S. G. Littlejohn and W. B. Geissler, "Arthroscopic repair of a posterior cruciate ligament avulsion," *Arthroscopy: The Journal of Arthroscopic & Related Surgery*, vol. 11, no. 2, pp. 235–238, 1995.

[11] G. C. Fanelli and C. J. Edson, "Posterior cruciate ligament injuries in trauma patients: part II," *Arthroscopy: The Journal of Arthroscopic & Related Surgery*, vol. 11, no. 5, pp. 526–529, 1995.

31

Neglected Pediatric Osteochondral Fracture Dislocation of the Patella

Ta-Li Hsu[1] **Shang-Ming Lin**[2] **Chih-Hung Chang,**[1,3] **and Tsung-Yu Lan**[1,2]

[1]*Department of Orthopedic Surgery, Far Eastern Memorial Hospital, New Taipei City, Taiwan*
[2]*Department of Materials and Textiles, Oriental Institute of Technology, New Taipei City, Taiwan*
[3]*Yuan Ze University Graduate School of Biotechnology and Bioengineering, Taiwan*

Correspondence should be addressed to Tsung-Yu Lan; gbwsh0130@yahoo.com.tw

Academic Editor: Johannes Mayr

Pediatric osteochondral fracture dislocation of the patella is sometimes difficult to diagnose on the basis of physical examination or plain film radiography. Magnetic resonance imaging plays an important role in its early diagnosis, and early treatment can prevent damage to the articular cartilage as well as decrease the dislocation rate. Currently, many treatment choices have been reported with good results, but there is no consensus on which treatment option may lead to the best outcome. Herein, we describe the case of a 14-year-old girl with neglected osteochondral fracture dislocation of the patella. The outcome was optimal on the basis of a 2-year postoperative follow-up; thus, we believe that fixation with headless screws is a simple and effective method if the fracture fragment is large enough.

1. Introduction

Osteochondral fractures of the femur or patella associated with patellar dislocation are more frequently noted in the pediatric population than in adults and may be accompanied by a spectrum of soft tissue injuries [1, 2]. Because of neglect in the initial phase [2], repositioning of these fractures in skeletally immature patients is important to improve healing capacity [2, 3] and to prevent secondary osteoarthritis with pain and functional limitation. Many treatment options have been developed recently without consensus on which treatment option may lead to the best outcome [3]. Herein, we describe a case of neglected osteochondral fracture dislocation of the patella that was successfully treated with open reduction and internal fixation on the basis of clinical and radiographic results.

2. Case Presentation

A 14-year-old girl without any previous clinical history presented with a painful, swollen right knee joint after playing volleyball. She was first treated conservatively for knee sprain at another institute, but the pain persisted. She was brought to our clinic for a second opinion 2 weeks after the injury.

The physical examination of the right knee showed loss of full extension, swelling during the range of motion, and tenderness. Initial radiographs showed lateral subluxation of the right patella with one fragment in the knee joint (Figures 1(a)–1(c)). Magnetic resonance imaging (MRI) demonstrated an osteochondral defect over the central aspect of the patella with a large loose body (Figures 1(d) and 1(e)). Surgery was suggested.

On the third posttrauma week, open reduction and internal fixation were performed. Under general anesthesia with the patient in the supine position, we performed a medial parapatellar arthrotomy to approach the fractured patella. The patella was flipped laterally, and the articular surface of the patella was exposed. Debridement and irrigation of the fracture site with normal saline were conducted. Finally, reduction was performed, and the fracture was fixed with two headless screws (Acutrak®, Acumed, Beaverton, Oregon) (Figure 2(a)). The medial patellofemoral ligament was also repaired. Intraoperative findings revealed the osteochondral fragment ($30 \times 25 \times 10\,\text{mm}^3$) from the central aspect of the patella (Figure 2(b)), an intra-articular loose body,

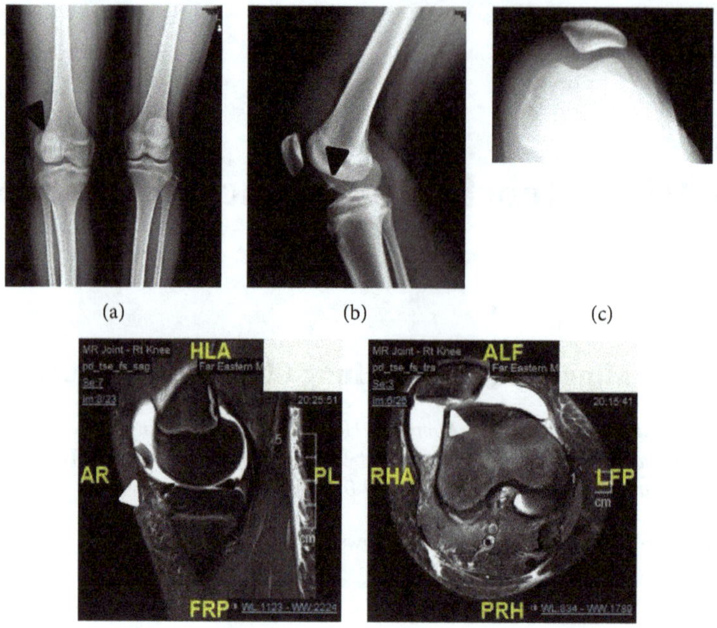

(a) (b) (c)

(d) (e)

FIGURE 1: Preoperative radiographs and magnetic resonance images. (a–c) Preoperative standard radiographs of the patella. (d, e) Preoperative magnetic resonance images. The arrowheads indicate the neglected osteochondral fracture dislocation of the patella.

hemarthrosis, and rupture of the medial patellofemoral ligament, which caused lateral subluxation of the patella. The calculated surgical time from incision to wound closure was 1 hour.

Postoperatively, partial weight bearing was immediately allowed and a dynamic functional knee brace was applied. The knee was fixed in full extension for 2 weeks, gradual knee flexion was allowed, and physical therapy was prescribed.

After 2 months postoperatively, the patient showed good patella gliding without pain. She could do squats and sports activities as well as she could before the injury (Figures 3(a) and 3(b)). Follow-up radiographs also demonstrated healing of the osteochondral fracture (Figures 4(a) and 4(b)). After 1 year, implant irritation was noted, and implant removal was suggested.

Second-look arthroscopy was performed and showed resorption of the cartilage over the screw head. The screw head and some metallosis were found. There were no significant degenerative changes in the cartilage (Figures 5(a)–5(c)). After removal of the implant, her discomfort disappeared.

3. Discussion

Although the exact prevalence of osteochondral fractures is still unknown [1, 2], they still account for 30 to 50% of the acute patellar dislocation rate [2]. The frequent delay in diagnosis naturally affects the healing capacity after repositioning these lesions. The most affected area is located around the medial patellar facet or at the lateral side of the distal femur [4, 5]. To date, the diagnosis of osteochondral fracture dislocation of the patella is difficult to establish on the basis of a physical examination or plain film radiography. Negative radiography results have been reported in about 36% of children with osteochondral fracture [6]. If the patient has any complaint of acute knee pain with or without a history of trauma that is accompanied by knee effusion and major loss of mobility, patellar dislocation associated with osteochondral defect should be highly suspected. Besides, intra-articular injury is highly suspected when hemarthrosis is observed following knee trauma [4, 7, 8]. The correct diagnosis may be very difficult to make without MRI or arthroscopic examination [2–4, 8].

Timely diagnosis is key to preventing damage to the articular cartilage because the development of fibrous tissue at the fracture side will affect proper reduction [7]. The redislocation rate will also increase if it is left untreated, as observed by Hawkins et al. [5, 9]. If the osteochondral fragments are too small to be fixed to the fracture site, removal of the fragment, drilling, microfracture, and chondrocyte implantation should be considered. To avoid possible damage to the cartilage and achieve rigid fixation, fragments smaller than 2 cm^2 should be excised or managed nonoperatively for equivalent or better outcomes if the osteochondral fragment does not involve a weight-bearing surface [4, 10]. However, if the fragment is big enough, many other treatment choices are available to fix osteochondral fractures of the patella, including replacement of the native fragment with internal fixation, resorbable implant fixation, crossing suture technique, allograft replacement, autograft replacement, and autologous chondrocyte transplantation [2, 11–21]. If the osteochondral lesion is $<1.5\,cm^2$, osteochondral cylinder transplantation is recommended, and if the lesion is $>1.5\,cm^2$, autologous chondrocyte implantation plus subchondral bone grafting should be considered, according to Salzmann et al. [10]. The goal is to reproduce a smooth gliding articular surface of the hyaline cartilage, which may prevent secondary osteoarthritis with pain and functional limitation [3]. To date, there is still no consensus on which treatment option may

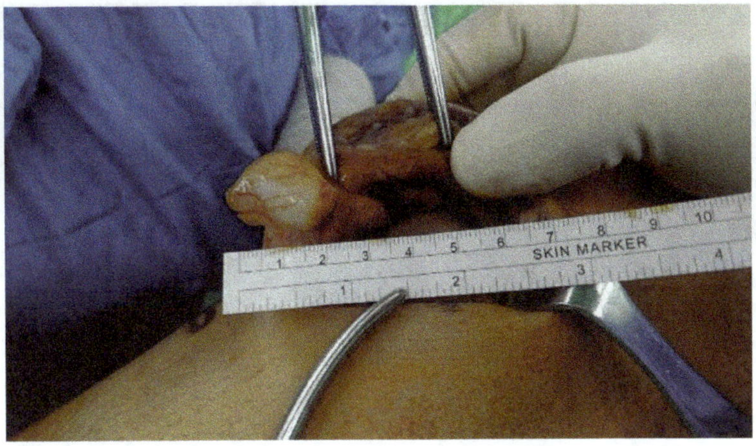

(a)

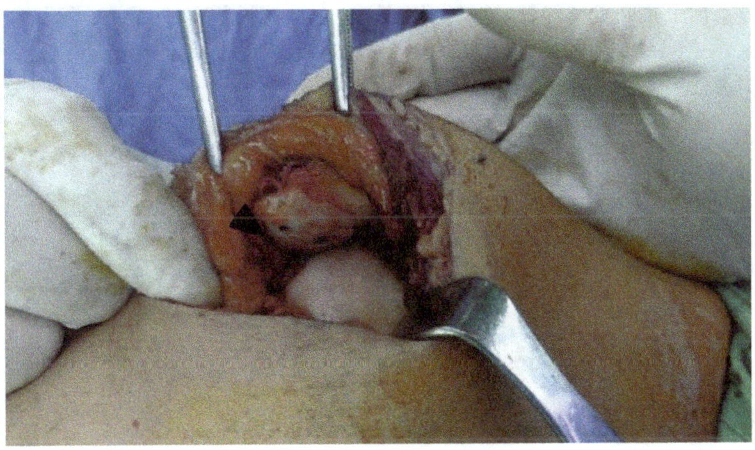

(b)

Figure 2: (a) Intraoperative view of osteochondral fracture dislocation of the patella. (b) The arrowhead indicates the fractured fragment. The fragment is perfectly reduced and fixed by two cannulated screws. The screw head is totally embedded.

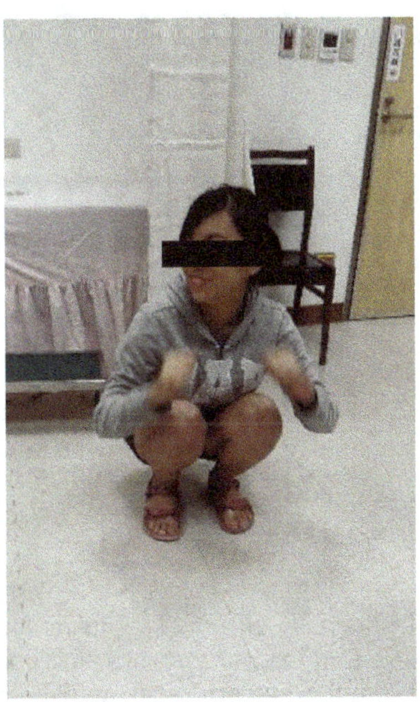

(a)

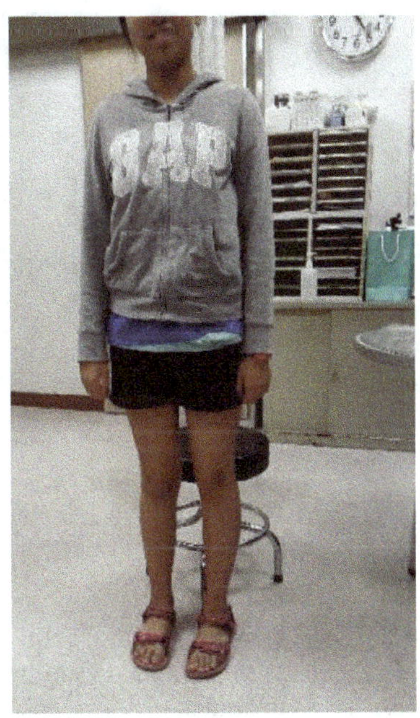

(b)

Figure 3: Postoperative status at 3 months. (a, b) The patient can do squats and sports activities as well as she could before the injury.

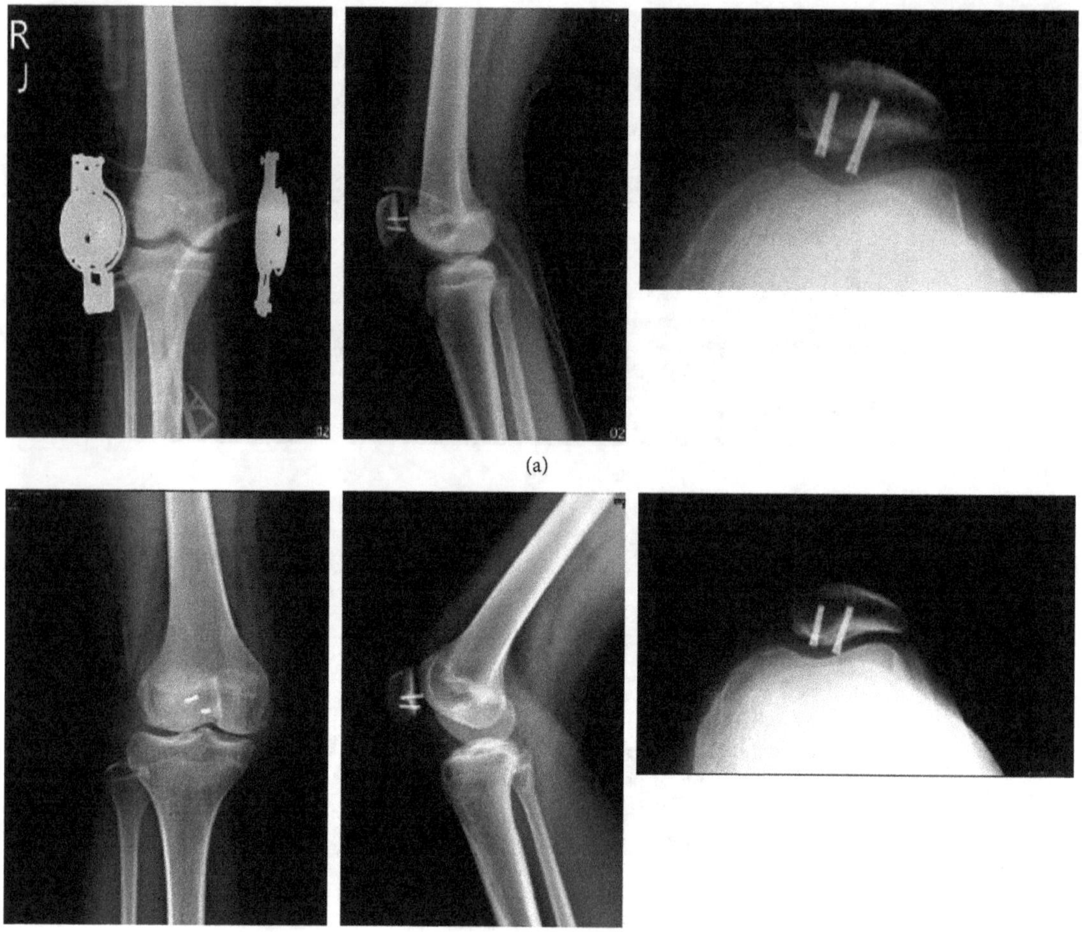

(a)

(b)

Figure 4: (a) Postoperative standard radiographs at the 1-week follow-up. Note that the dislocation and articular surface are corrected. (b) Postoperative standard radiograph showing a healed fracture site and the implant in situ at 9 months.

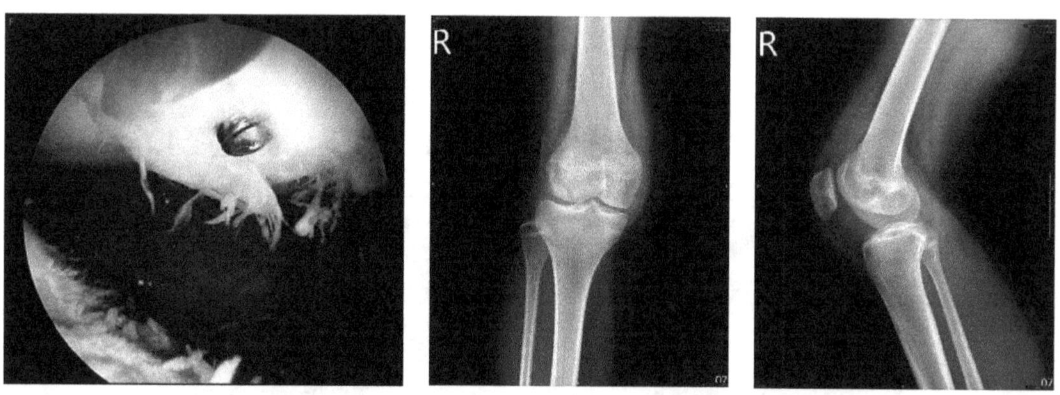

(a) (b) (c)

Figure 5: (a) Postoperative second-look arthroscopy at 1-year follow-up showing blurring of the cartilage and metallosis but no obvious degenerative changes in the cartilage. (b, c) Postoperative radiograph shows the healed fracture.

lead to the best outcomes. For smaller osteochondral fragments, the crossing suture technique with ultrabraid (Smith & Nephew, Memphis, TN) is a treatment choice [6]. Although good long-term functional results have been mentioned with the use of bioabsorbable ultra-high strength poly(L-lactide) pins or absorbable sutures (Vicryl 2, Ethicon, Somerville, NJ) [3, 13], implant breakage, foreign body reaction, and aseptic synovitis have been reported [6, 22]. A two-component fibrin sealant (adhesive system of fibrin) and butyl-2-cyanoacrylate tissue glue (first synthesized in 1949) were both reported to yield good results if the osteochondral fragments were large enough or too thin to be secured with anchors or Herbert screws [19, 20]. Headless cannulated compression screws were also successfully used by Rae and Khasawneh in 1988 to fix fragments that were large enough [16, 17]. Local friction and irritation are thought to be prevented when the screws are completely embedded in the cartilage and bone. Embedding the screw at a depth of 3 mm has been recommended in order to achieve peak compression strength [17]. After a recent review of the literature, we found that no study has recommended which kind of fragment size is better for headless cannulated compression screw fixation. On the basis of our experience, we recommend the use of a fragment size larger than 3 cm^2 for headless cannulated compression screw fixation, as this results in no degenerative changes in the cartilage and a good clinical outcome.

The main limitation of the present study is the small number of patients. Further studies of this technique with more patients are needed to clarify the outcome of this surgical technique.

Early MRI plays an important role in making the correct diagnosis of neglected osteochondral fracture dislocation of the patella. Our case was initially diagnosed as an anterior cruciate ligament avulsion fracture and then diagnosed as neglected osteochondral fracture dislocation of the patella on the basis of the MRI findings. Treatment of osteochondral fracture dislocation of the patella is sometimes challenging. However, internal fixation with headless screws is an effective method for a large osteochondral fragment. The follow-up result was clinically good in our case, but second surgery to remove the implant is sometimes necessary.

References

[1] M. A. Seeley, M. Knesek, and K. L. Vanderhave, "Osteochondral injury after acute patellar dislocation in children and adolescents," *Journal of Pediatric Orthopedics*, vol. 33, no. 5, pp. 511–518, 2013.

[2] F. Chotel, G. Knorr, E. Simian, F. Dubrana, G. Versier, and the French Arthroscopy Society, "Knee osteochondral fractures in skeletally immature patients: French multicenter study," *Orthopaedics & Traumatology: Surgery & Research*, vol. 97, no. 8, pp. S154–S159, 2011.

[3] P. Lüthje and I. Nurmi-Lüthje, "Osteochondral fracture of the knee treated with bioabsorbable implants in two adolescents," *Acta Orthopaedica Belgica*, vol. 74, no. 2, pp. 249–254, 2008.

[4] K. L. Bauer, "Osteochondral injuries of the knee in pediatric patients," *The Journal of Knee Surgery*, vol. 31, no. 5, pp. 382–391, 2018.

[5] A. A. Mashoof, M. D. Scholl, A. Lahav, P. E. Greis, and R. T. Burks, "Osteochondral injury to the mid-lateral weight-bearing portion of the lateral femoral condyle associated with patella dislocation," *Arthroscopy: The Journal of Arthroscopic & Related Surgery*, vol. 21, no. 2, pp. 228–232, 2005.

[6] W. M. Ng, M. Z. M. Al-Fayyadh, J. Kho, T. Seow Hui, and M. R. B. Mohamed Ali, "Crossing suture technique for the osteochondral fractures repair of patella," *Arthroscopy Techniques*, vol. 6, no. 4, pp. e1035–e1039, 2017.

[7] A. Callewier, A. Monsaert, and G. Lamraski, "Lateral femoral condyle osteochondral fracture combined to patellar dislocation: a case report," *Orthopaedics & Traumatology, Surgery & Research*, vol. 95, no. 1, pp. 85–88, 2009.

[8] D. Abbasi, M. M. May, E. J. Wall, G. Chan, and S. N. Parikh, "MRI findings in adolescent patients with acute traumatic knee hemarthrosis," *Journal of Pediatric Orthopedics*, vol. 32, no. 8, pp. 760–764, 2012.

[9] R. J. Hawkins, R. H. Bell, and G. Anisette, "Acute patellar dislocations," *Am J Sports Med*, vol. 14, no. 2, pp. 117–120, 1986.

[10] G. M. Salzmann, P. Niemeyer, A. Hochrein, M. J. Stoddart, and P. Angele, "Articular cartilage repair of the knee," *The Orthopaedic Journal of Sports Medicine*, vol. 6, no. 3, 2018.

[11] J. M. Flynn, M. S. Kocher, and T. J. Ganley, "Osteochondritis dissecans of the knee," *Journal of Pediatric Orthopedics*, vol. 24, no. 4, pp. 434–443, 2004.

[12] S. Ghahremani, R. Griggs, T. Hall, K. Motamedi, and M. Boechat, "Osteochondral lesions in pediatric and adolescent patients," *Seminars in Musculoskeletal Radiology*, vol. 18, no. 5, pp. 505–512, 2014.

[13] J. Bradley and D. J. Dandy, "Results of drilling osteochondritis dissecans before skeletal maturity," *Journal of Bone and Joint Surgery. British Volume*, vol. 71-B, no. 4, pp. 642–644, 1989.

[14] E. L. Cain and W. G. Clancy, "Treatment algorithm for osteochondral injuries of the knee," *Clinics in Sports Medicine*, vol. 20, no. 2, pp. 321–342, 2001.

[15] S. J. Walsh, M. J. Boyle, and V. Morganti, "Large osteochondral fractures of the lateral femoral condyle in the adolescent: outcome of bioabsorbable pin fixation," *The Journal of Bone and Joint Surgery-American Volume*, vol. 90, no. 7, pp. 1473–1478, 2008.

[16] P. S. Rae and Z. M. Khasawneh, "Herbert screw fixation of osteochondral fractures of the patella," *Injury*, vol. 19, no. 2, pp. 116–119, 1988.

[17] S. Aydoğmuş, T. M. Duymuş, and T. Keçeci, "An unexpected complication after headless compression screw fixation of an osteochondral fracture of patella," *Case Reports in Orthopedics*, vol. 2016, Article ID 7290104, 4 pages, 2016.

[18] C. Pascual-Garrido, C. J. Moran, D. W. Green, and B. J. Cole, "Osteochondritis dissecans of the knee in children and adolescents," *Current Opinion in Pediatrics*, vol. 25, no. 1, pp. 46–51, 2013.

[19] T. Visuri and T. Kuusela, "Fixation of large osteochondral fractures of the patella with fibrin adhesive system: a report of two operative cases," *The American Journal of Sports Medicine*, vol. 17, no. 6, pp. 842–845, 1989.

[20] R. Gul, F. Khan, Y. Maher, and D. O'Farrell, "Osteochondral fractures in the knee treated with butyl-2-cyanoacrylate glue," *Acta Orthopaedica Belgica*, vol. 72, no. 5, pp. 641–643, 2006.

[21] H. Kang, J. Li, X. X. Chen, T. Wang, S. C. Liu, and H. C. Li, "Fixation versus excision of osteochondral fractures after patellar dislocations in adolescent patients: a retrospective cohort study," *Chinese Medical Journal*, vol. 131, no. 11, pp. 1296–1301, 2018.

[22] M. G. Friederichs, P. E. Greis, and R. T. Burks, "Pitfalls associated with fixation of osteochondritis dissecans fragments using bioabsorbable screws," *Arthroscopy: The Journal of Arthroscopic & Related Surgery*, vol. 17, no. 5, pp. 542–545, 2001.

32

Two Cases of Morel-Lavallée Lesion Which Resulted in a Wide Skin Necrosis from a Small Laceration

Tadahiro Nakajima, Kaoru Tada, Mika Nakada, Masashi Matsuta, and Hiroyuki Tsuchiya

Department of Orthopaedic Surgery, Graduate School of Medical Science, Kanazawa University, 13-1 Takaramachi, Kanazawa 920-1302, Japan

Correspondence should be addressed to Tadahiro Nakajima; t_nnnkaji@yahoo.co.jp

Academic Editor: George Mouzopoulos

Morel-Lavallée lesion (MLL) is a degloving injury in soft tissues caused by shear force accompanying trauma. Even if it is a small lacrimal wound at the initial visit, there is a range of skin necrosis which is not suitable for it. As a cause of the injury, a shearing force was applied over a wide range, and penetrating blood vessel damage to the skin occurred, resulting in skin necrosis. Attention is required.

1. Introduction

Morel-Lavallée lesion (MLL) is defined as a closed, internal soft tissue degloving injury produced most commonly as a result of a strong, shearing, and tangential force [1]. This lesion is characterized by the development of a fluid collection between the subcutaneous soft tissue and the muscular fascia (Figure 1). Here, we present two cases of MLL that occurred in the distal thigh and lower leg which resulted in a wide skin necrosis.

2. Case Presentation

Case 1 is a 66-year-old female, victim of a traffic accident. Her left thigh was caught in a car tire. She developed swelling and several contusions of her left thigh and sustained laceration of the medial side of her left knee. She underwent washout of her wound on that day. Intraoperatively, a small size of fat masses came out from the wound site (Figure 2(a)). After the washing, she underwent daily dressing changes and local wound care. One month after the injury, however, the wound failed to heal and skin necrosis developed on the anterior medial part of her left thigh (Figure 2(b)). She was admitted and underwent split-thickness skin grafting. After the skin graft, the healing was complete (Figure 2(c)). A computerized tomography (CT) scan performed three months after the injury demonstrated just a small fluid collection between the subcutaneous soft tissue and the muscle fascia (Figure 2(d)).

Case 2 is a 26-year-old male who presented with swelling over the right lower leg. His legs were caught between the rollers during work. He sustained several contusions of the right lower leg and a laceration of the medial side of his right knee. He underwent irrigation and debridement on that day. Intraoperatively, a small size of fat masses came out from the wound site (Figure 3(a)). On the next day after the injury, compartment pressures of the right lower leg were over 40 mmHg. He underwent an emergent fasciotomy to leave the compartment open. Approximately three weeks after the injury, skin ulcer of the right lower leg advanced to necrosis (Figure 3(b)). He required serial debridements and negative pressure wound therapy (NPWT) dressings followed by split-thickness skin graft from his thigh. After the skin graft, the healing was complete (Figure 3(c)).

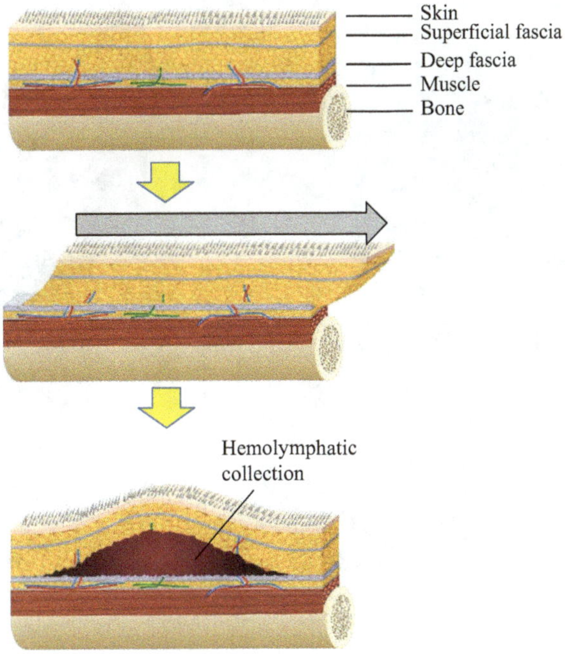

Figure 1: Illustration of Morel-Lavallée lesions. Tangential shearing force causes a closed soft tissue degloving injury, in which the skin and subcutaneous tissue are separated from the underlying fascia. This separation creates the space which can fill with blood and lymph.

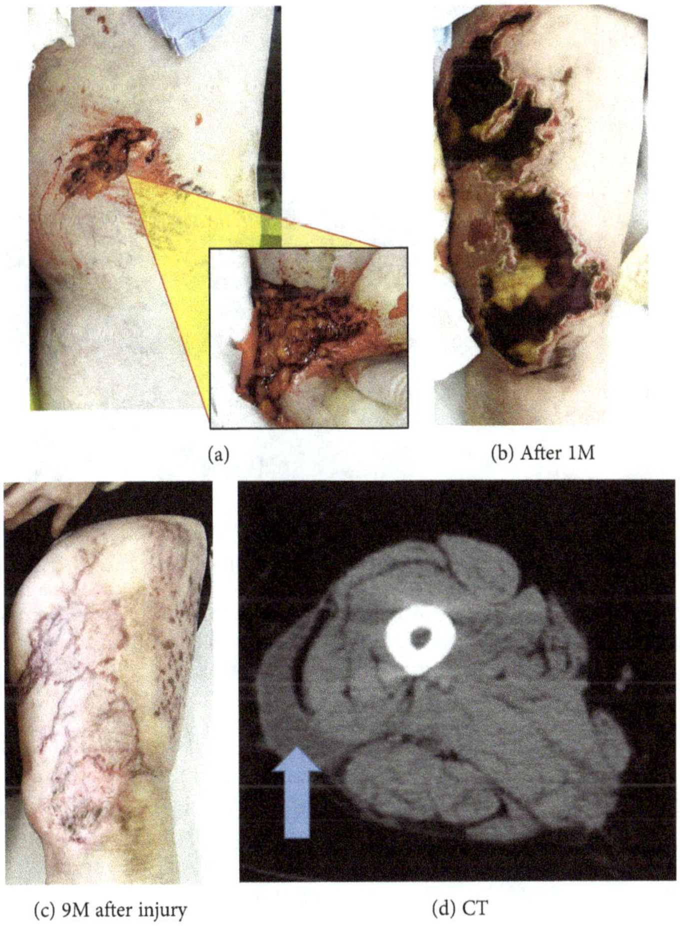

Figure 2: (a) Intraoperative photo. Fat masses came from a small size of wound. (b) Clinical photo. One month after the injury. Skin necrosis develops. (c) Clinical photo. Nine months after the injury. Skin grafts were performed, and the healing was complete. (d) CT scan performed three months after the injury. A small fluid collection between the subcutaneous soft tissue and the muscle fascia is indicated by an arrow.

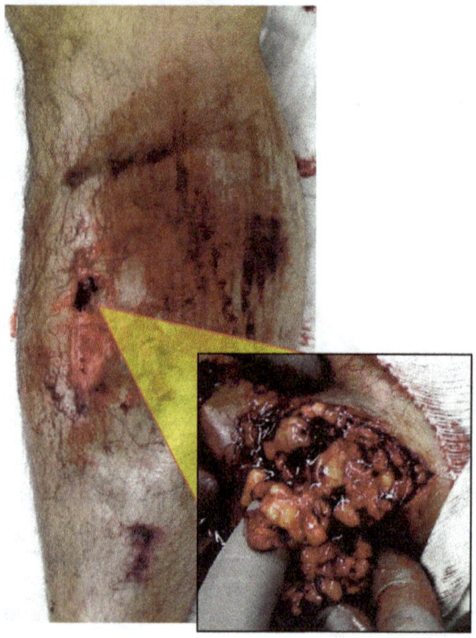

(a)

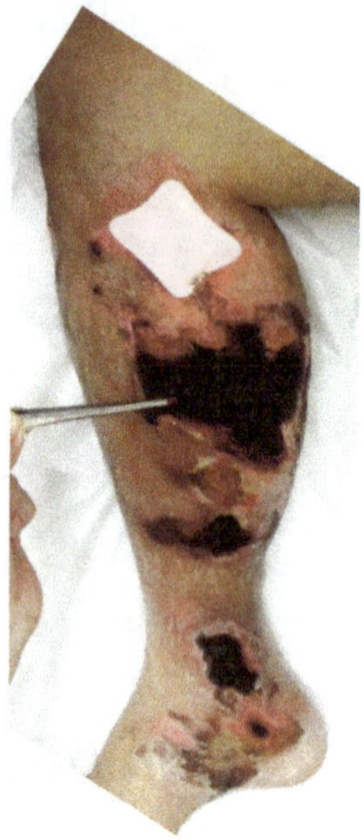

(b) 1M after injury

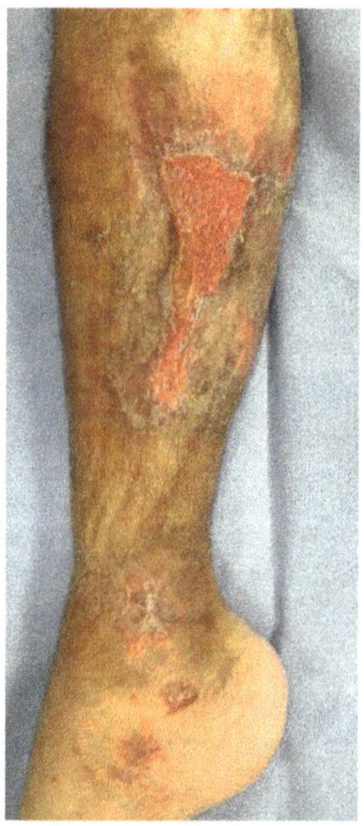

(c) 9M after injury

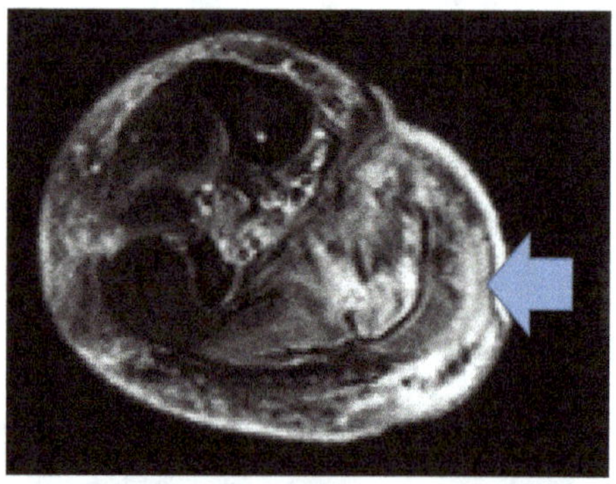

(d) MRI, STIR sequence

FIGURE 3: (a) Intraoperative photo. Fat masses came from a small size of wound. (b) Clinical photo. One month after the injury. Skin necrosis develops. (c) Clinical photo. Nine months after the injury. After the split-thickness skin graft, the healing was complete. (d) MRI performed one month after the injury. A small fluid collection between the subcutaneous soft tissue and the muscle fascia in indicated by an arrow.

Magnetic resonance imaging (MRI) performed one month after the injury showed just a small collection of fluid between the subcutaneous soft tissue and the muscle fascia (Figure 3(d)).

3. Discussion

MLL was first described by Morel-Lavallée in 1848 [2], and it is the sequela of a closed degloving injury involving separation of the skin and subcutaneous fat from the underlying fascia [3]. It has been well described as most commonly occurring in the greater trochanter, other common locations including elsewhere around the pelvis or thigh [4]. Less commonly occurring sites include the gluteal and lumbosacral regions, as well as the lower leg [5]. Moreover, Vanhegan et al. reviewed and identified a rare site of incidence as calf/lower leg (1.5%) [6]. The diagnosis of MLL is based on physical examination and imaging studies. Typical image finding of CT and MRI is a subcutaneous fluid collection [7]. In our two cases though, CT and MRI showed just a small fluid collection between the subcutaneous soft tissue and the underlying fascia. It is considered that fluid collection exuded subcutaneously was discharged from laceration. It is possible that once a shearing force is added and the penetrating branch is damaged, blood flow to the subcutaneous tissue does not recover and the skin falls into necrosis. That is why a wide skin necrosis which is incompatible with the small laceration at the initial examination occurred. It should be noted that in the cases of high-energy trauma, especially due to the shearing force, there may be cases where skin necrosis occurs extensively and healing is prolonged even though the wound is small.

4. Conclusion

A laceration that is thought to have been subjected to shear force may cause extensive skin necrosis afterwards and requires caution.

References

[1] A. Kalaci, S. Karazincir, and A. N. Yanat, "Long-standing Morel-Lavallée lesion of the thigh simulating a neoplasm," *Clinical Imaging*, vol. 31, no. 4, pp. 287–291, 2007.

[2] M. Morel-Lavallee, "Decollements traumatiques de la peau et des couches sousjacentes," *Arch Gen Med*, vol. 1, pp. 20–38, 1863, 172-200, 300-332.

[3] S. Dawre, S. Lamba, S. H, S. Gupta, and A. K. Gupta, "The Morel-Lavallee lesion: a review and a proposed algorithmic approach," *European Journal of Plastic Surgery*, vol. 35, no. 7, pp. 489–494, 2012.

[4] D. J. Hak, S. A. Olson, and J. M. Matta, "Diagnosis and management of closed internal degloving injuries associated with pelvic and acetabular fractures: the Morel-Lavallée lesion," *The Journal of Trauma*, vol. 42, no. 6, pp. 1046–1051, 1997.

[5] D. E. Moran, N. A. Napier, and E. C. Kavanagh, "Lumbar Morel-Lavallee effusion," *The Spine Journal*, vol. 12, no. 12, pp. 1165-1166, 2012.

[6] I. S. Vanhegan, B. Dala-Ali, L. Verhelst, P. Mallucci, and F. S. Haddad, "The Morel-Lavallée lesion as a rare differential diagnosis for recalcitrant bursitis of the knee: case report and literature review," *Case Reports in Orthopedics*, vol. 2012, Article ID 593193, 5 pages, 2012.

[7] S. G. Tejwani, S. B. Cohen, and J. P. Bradley, "Management of Morel-Lavallee lesion of the knee: twenty seven cases in the national football league," *The American Journal of Sports Medicine*, vol. 35, no. 7, pp. 1162–1167, 2007.

33

Lumbar Radiculopathy Caused by Epidural Gas Collection

Dong Hu, Kai Xu, and Songhua Xiao

Department of Orthopedic, Beijing Tsinghua Changgung Hospital, School of Medicine, Tsinghua University, Beijing, China

Correspondence should be addressed to Songhua Xiao; songhua_xiao@163.com

Academic Editor: Eyal Itshayek

Background. Degenerated intervertebral discs in the lumbar spine are commonly found with vacuum phenomenon. In a few cases, gas can migrate into the lumbar spinal canal and compress the nerve root. *Case Presentation.* We report a case of lumbar radiculopathy caused by epidural gas collection in a 59-year-old woman. Originally, the gas was formed in the intervertebral disc and possibly migrated backward because of the motion of lumbar spine, forming a single large gas formation. The nerve root was freed from the gas-filled cyst after needle puncture was performed. Patient's symptoms in the leg were significantly relieved following surgery. *Conclusion.* There is still no satisfactory explanation for the pathogenesis of gas formation in the spinal canal. In our case, the presence of gas in the spinal canal and gas inside a narrowed disc suggests a communication between the two structures.

1. Introduction

It is rare for intraspinal gas to cause lumbar radiculopathy, and there are only a few relevant case reports [1–6]. It is possible that epidural gas may be misdiagnosed as epidural masses or herniated intervertebral discs by magnetic resonance imaging (MRI) [7]. Computed tomographic (CT) scan is the preferred investigation to diagnose it as seen in all cases in literature. We recently encountered a case of lumbosacral radiculopathy caused by epidural gas collection in the lumbar region.

2. Case Presentation

A 59-year-old woman presented with right leg pain that first appeared in January 2019. Axial CT revealed multiple intracannular posterolateral gas bubbles at L5-S1 level (Figure 1). A coexisting vacuum disc phenomenon indicates the presumed origin of the gas bubbles. There was no history of invasive procedures such as epidural injection or surgery. Conservative treatment had been successful. Partial relief of pain had been achieved during the following two years.

Since March 2021, however, patient's ability to walk gradually deteriorated due to recurrence of the symptom. Her symptom had not improved with conservative therapy. A positive straight leg raising test at 45° was found in right leg without any motor weakness on physical examination. According to MRI results, a well-encapsulated low signal intensity lesion was related to gas formation or calcification (Figure 2). An additional CT was performed, revealing a large intraspinal epidural bubble compressing the right S1 nerve root (Figure 3). An ipsilateral percutaneous L5/S1 interlaminar approach endoscopic surgery was performed with enlargement of the lateral recess. At surgery, the S1 nerve root appeared swollen and the gas-containing pseudocyst was observed at the axilla region of the nerve root, covered with a thin capsule. There was no herniated disc around the pseudocyst. The nerve root was freed from the gas-filled cyst after needle puncture was performed. Patient's symptoms in the leg were significantly relieved following surgery. The patient was pain-free 6 months after the surgery.

3. Discussion

Epidural gas is mainly composed of nitrogen and is frequently trapped within a thin layer of nonspecific fibrous tissue membrane that is similar to the posterior longitudinal ligament [8, 9]. Clinical symptoms of epidural gas can be similar to those of other more common causes of lumbar

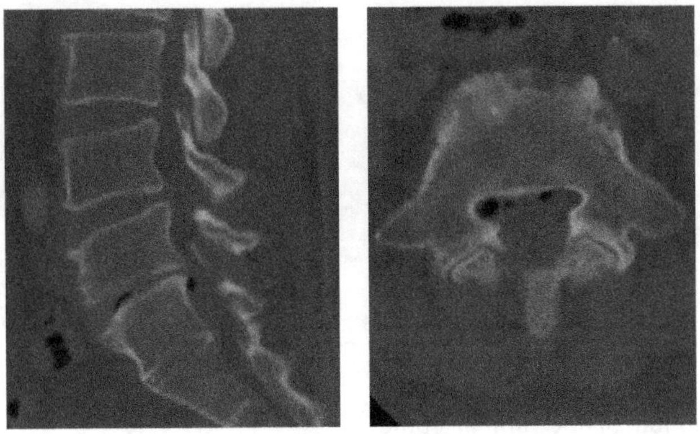

(a) (b)

FIGURE 1: CT scan images revealing multiple gas bubbles at L5/S1 level as shown in axial (a) and sagittal (b) cuts.

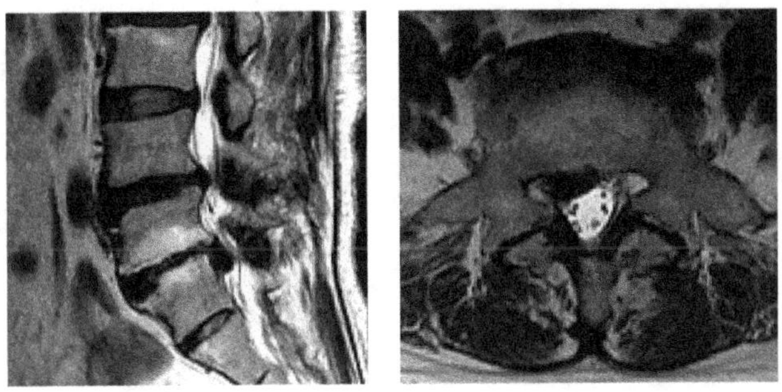

(a) (b)

FIGURE 2: T2 sequences in sagittal (a) and axial orientation (b) illustrate a caudally shifted hypointense mass in the right lateral recessus L5/S1 with contact to the nerve root S1 suspicious of a sequestered disc herniation.

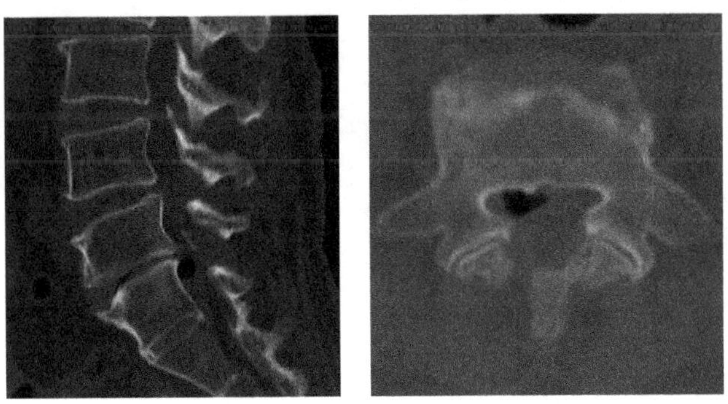

(a) (b)

FIGURE 3: CT reveals a single large epidural gas bubble mimicking disc herniation on MRI as shown in axial (a) and sagittal (b) cuts. A coexisting vacuum disc phenomenon indicates the presumed origin of the gas bubble.

radiculopathy [10]. There have been very few reports in the literature of symptomatic lumbar radiculopathy caused by a gas bubble.

There is still no satisfactory explanation for the pathogenesis of gas formation in the spinal canal. In our case, the presence of gas in the spinal canal and gas inside a narrowed disc suggests a communication between the two structures. Possibly, the motion of the lumbar spine causes a pressure gradient, resulting in a valve-pump mechanism that propels the gas into the spinal canal. Gas in the epidural space usually disappears spontaneously in most patients, so conservative treatment and a period of observation are recommended before surgery [11]. In our case, the patient had multiple gas bubbles at L5/S1 level. The bubbles were not absorbed spontaneously but forming a single large gas formation which leads to surgery two years later. Decompression and fusion surgery could be used in patients with spine instability and spinal canal stenosis, whereas simple microscopic/endoscopic removal of cyst could be sufficient in patients without spine instability and spinal canal stenosis. In this case, we offered different operation options for her to choose from, including fusion surgery, endoscopic surgery, and CT-guided needle puncture. The patient picked endoscopic surgery in consideration of lower cost and less invasive procedure compared with fusion surgery, while lower recurrence rate compared with CT-guided needle puncture. The patient was pain-free 6 months after the surgery, while a longer follow-up period is required to fully observe the long-term recurrence of the cyst lesion in this patient.

4. Conclusion

Intraspinal gas collection is a rare cause of lumbar radiculopathy. We speculate that the motion of the lumbar spine induces a pressure gradient, resulting in a valve-pump mechanism that propels the gas into the spinal canal. Surgery should be considered when conservative therapy failed.

Data Availability

The patient's data used in this study are restricted by the Ethics Board of Tsinghua Changgung Hospital in order to protect patient privacy.

Consent

Consent was obtained from the patient for participation in this study.

Authors' Contributions

SX carried out the operation. DH and KX followed up the patient. DH wrote the manuscript. All authors read and approved the final manuscript.

Acknowledgments

DH and SX were funded by the Precision Medicine Research Program of Tsinghua University (Grant number 10001020115).

References

[1] B. Demierre, A. Ramadan, H. Hauser, A. Reverdin, B. Rilliet, and J. Berney, "Radicular compression due to lumbar intraspinal gas pseudocyst: case report," *Neurosurgery*, vol. 22, no. 4, pp. 731–733, 1988.

[2] H. Yoshida, K. Shinomiya, O. Nakai, Y. Kurosa, and I. Yamaura, "Lumbar nerve root compression caused by lumbar intraspinal gas Report of three cases," *Spine (Phila Pa 1976)*, vol. 22, no. 3, pp. 348–351, 1997.

[3] S. U. Kuh, D. H. Heo, K. S. Kim, and Y. J. Cho, "Lumbar epidural gas-containing pseudocysts as a cause of severe radicular pain," *Joint, Bone, Spine*, vol. 78, no. 4, pp. 398–401, 2011.

[4] H. Yasuoka, O. Nemoto, M. Kawaguti, S. Naitou, K. Yamamoto, and Y. Ukegawa, "An unusual case of nerve root compression by intradiscal gas pseudocyst of the lumbar spine," *Journal of the Royal Army Medical Corps*, vol. 156, no. 1, pp. 47-48, 2010.

[5] G. Ayberk, M. F. Ozveren, and T. Yildirim, "Spinal gas accumulation causing lumbar discogenic disease: a case report," *Acta Orthopaedica et Traumatologica Turcica*, vol. 49, no. 1, pp. 103–105, 2015.

[6] H. Belfquih, B. El Mostarchid, and A. Akhaddar, "Sciatica caused by lumbar epidural gas," *The Pan African Medical Journal*, vol. 18, p. 162, 2014.

[7] E. Hassler, T. Gattringer, U. Wiesspeiner, H. Deutschmann, and F. Fazekas, "Spinal epidural gas mimicking lumbar disc herniation," *Neurology*, vol. 89, no. 14, pp. 1528-1529, 2017.

[8] L. T. Ford, L. A. Gilula, W. A. Murphy, and M. Gado, "Analysis of gas in vacuum lumbar disc," *AJR. American Journal of Roentgenology*, vol. 128, no. 6, pp. 1056-1057, 1977.

[9] F. M. Salpietro, C. Alafaci, D. Collufio et al., "Radicular compression by lumbar intraspinal epidural gas pseudocyst in association with lateral disc herniation. Role of the posterior longitudinal ligament," *Journal of Neurosurgical Sciences*, vol. 46, no. 2, pp. 93–95, 2002, discussion 95.

[10] M. Sakir Eksi, E. Ece Ozcan-Eksi, O. Orhun et al., "Could gas-filled pseudocyst mimick extruded disc herniation?," *Journal of Clinical Neuroscience*, vol. 93, pp. 147–154, 2021.

[11] A. Akhaddar, B. Eljebbouri, O. Naama, and M. Boucetta, "Sciatica due to lumbar intraspinal gas pseudocyst," *Internal Medicine*, vol. 49, no. 23, p. 2647, 2010.

34

Ventral Longitudinal Intraspinal Fluid Collection in Patients with Cervical Disc Herniation: A Report of Two Cases

Rui Hirasawa, Takashi Itabashi, Tsuneji Kita, and Chikato Mannoji

Department of Orthopedic Surgery, Japanese Red Cross Narita Hospital, 90-1, Iidacho, Narita-shi, Chiba 286-8523, Japan

Correspondence should be addressed to Rui Hirasawa; r.hirasawa1221@me.com

Academic Editor: Eyal Itshayek

We encountered two cases of cervical disc herniation, wherein cerebrospinal fluid collection in the ventral epidural space between the cervical spine and the thoracic spine was noted. The patients, two women aged 71 and 43 years, were diagnosed with cervical disc herniation and underwent anterior cervical discectomy and fusion. Unexpected cerebrospinal fluid leakage was observed prior to exposure of the dura mater. Notably, the dura mater was intact following the removal of the herniated disc in both cases. No cerebrospinal fluid leakage symptoms were observed, and relief from the neurological symptoms related to the cervical disc herniation was observed in both cases following the surgery. Findings of preoperative magnetic resonance imaging and computed tomography myelography were carefully reviewed, retrospectively. Both patients presented with similar features including expansion of cerebrospinal fluid collection in the ventral epidural space between the cervical spine and the thoracic spine. These observed features were similar to those of superficial siderosis, which is a form of duropathy—a disease caused by dural defects. Therefore, the patients in this case study might have a subclinical duropathy with associated cervical disc herniation.

1. Introduction

Epidural arachnoid cysts are one of the most common causes of epidural spinal cerebrospinal fluid (CSF) collection. Epidural arachnoid cysts are primarily located on the dorsal side of the dura and can cause spinal cord compression.

A unique pathological condition, in which CSF collection is observed in the ventral epidural space due to dural defects, has been reported in the recent years [1–5]. Dural hypoplasia, history of trauma, and osteophytes are presumed to be the cause of dural defects and CSF collection. This pathological condition can induce superficial siderosis (SS), craniospinal hypovolemia, or spinal cord herniation and result in clinical symptoms [6]. Kumar defined this pathological condition as duropathy [6].

Herein, we report two cases of cervical disc herniation accompanied by CSF collection in the ventral epidural space, with expansion in the ventral epidural space between the cervical spine and the thoracic spine, which may be associated with duropathy.

2. Case Presentation

2.1. Case 1. A 71-year-old woman was referred to our hospital with a two-week history of cervical pain and numbness in the left upper limb. Neurological examination showed that her left upper limb had a slight motor weakness, with a manual muscle test score of 4. Hoffmann and Wartenberg reflexes were positive in both hands, and deep tendon reflexes in all extremities were hyperactive. However, the patient's left hand displayed reduced dexterity. MRI revealed cervical disc herniation, which compressed the left side of the spinal cord primarily at the C5-6 disc level (Figure 1). Analysis of CSF obtained by a lumbar puncture showed no apparent abnormality and normal protein levels. CSF pressure was not measured. A diagnosis of cervical myelopathy due to cervical disc herniation was established, and an anterior cervical discectomy and fusion (ACDF) at C5-6 was performed.

During the surgery, unexpected CSF leakage was observed when the posterior longitudinal ligament was incised with a scalpel. The dura mater was observed to be

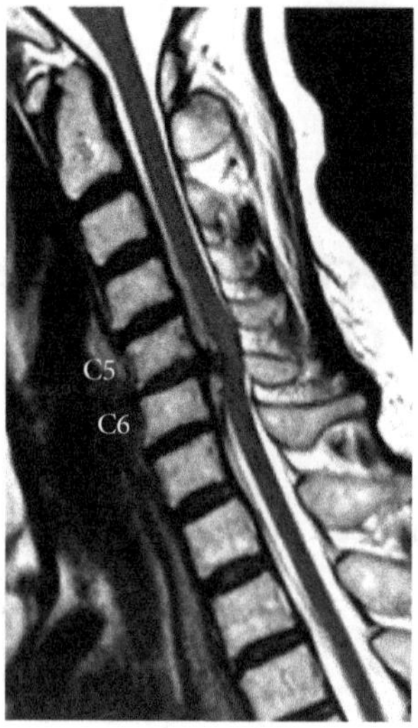

FIGURE 1: Case 1. Preoperative MRI. T2-weighted sagittal view showing cervical disc herniation at C5-C6 compressing the spinal cord.

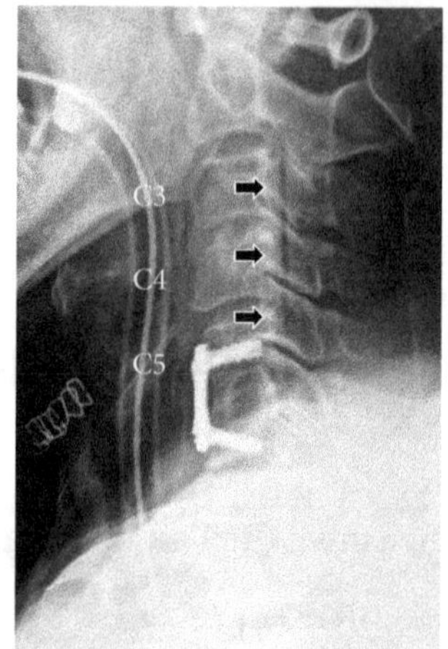

FIGURE 2: Case 1. Postoperative X-ray (lateral view). A black line (possibly air) was observed posterior to the cervical vertebrae between the bottom of the C2 vertebra and the middle of the C5 vertebra (black arrows).

intact after the removal of the herniated disc. Thus, it was determined that the membrane that was incised when the CSF leakage occurred was not the dura mater. Fibrin glue was used on the surface of the dura, and no additional treatment of the CSF leakage was performed. Autologous iliac bone was grafted and fixed with a plate and screws. A postoperative X-ray image of the cervical spine revealed a black line posterior to the cervical vertebrae from the bottom of the C2 vertebra to the middle of the C5 vertebra (Figure 2). Preoperative MRI and CT myelography images were carefully reviewed, and CSF collection on the ventral side of the dura expanding from the C2 vertebra to the T6 vertebra was identified (Figure 3). CT myelography is routinely performed 30 minutes after injection of contrast medium. CT myelography was also performed after the surgery and showed that the CSF collection at the surgical site disappeared. However, the CSF collection persisted in the region between levels T2 and T6. An MRI performed 6 months after the surgery showed continued CSF collection between levels C7 and T6. However, no spinal cord compression was observed. Neurological symptoms were relieved after the surgery, and no symptoms related to the CSF leakage were observed. Although the patient was asymptomatic at one year postsurgery, an MRI of the brain was performed, which did not show signs of siderosis, brain sagging, meningeal thickening, or any other abnormality.

2.2. Case 2. A 43-year-old woman was referred to the hospital with a seven-month history of numbness in both upper limbs and the right lower limb and coldness in the right lower limb. While neurological examination showed no muscle weakness, Hoffmann and Wartenberg reflexes were positive in the left hand. Deep tendon reflexes in all extremities were hyperactive. MRI results showed cervical disc herniation, with compression on the left side of the spinal cord, predominantly at the C4-5 disc level (Figure 4(a)). A diagnosis of cervical myelopathy due to the cervical disc herniation at C4-5 was established. Preoperative MRI and CT myelography images showed CSF collection on the ventral side of the dura mater, similar to that seen in Case 1 (Figure 4(b)). CSF collection was observed between levels C4 and T7 (Figure 5). Analysis of CSF obtained by a lumbar puncture showed no apparent abnormality including normal protein levels. CSF pressure was not measured. ACDF was performed at C3-4 and C4-5. C3-4 was included for investigation, as the preoperative X-ray showed instability during flexion and extension of the cervical spine. During surgery, CSF leakage was observed at C4-5 when the posterior longitudinal ligament was incised with a scalpel. Intact dura mater was observed after the removal of the herniated disc. These findings during the surgery were consistent with those described for Case 1. The tissue on the surface of the dura mater was sent for pathological examination. However, only nucleus pulposus tissue was identified. Neurological symptoms were relieved after the surgery, and no further symptoms related to the CSF leakage have been reported.

3. Discussions

To our knowledge, there have been no reports of epidural CSF leakage related to cervical disc herniation. However, the visual findings in the cases presented here were similar to cases reported by Kumar et al., which involved CSF collection in the ventral epidural space and were associated with SS [1]. SS is a rare disease that causes hemosiderin deposition in the subpial layers of the brain or spinal cord as a result of chronic or repeated bleeding into the subarachnoid space. Hemosiderin deposition typically causes cerebellar ataxia and sensorineural hearing loss [1, 7]. Kumar et al. reported that CSF collection was observed in 14 of 30 patients with SS. These patients with CSF collection were reported to exhibit dural defects. Additionally, it was observed that the CSF collection was longitudinally extensive and ventrally located in the majority of the patients [1]. Accordingly, this CSF collection was named ventral longitudinal intraspinal fluid collection (VLISFC) [6].

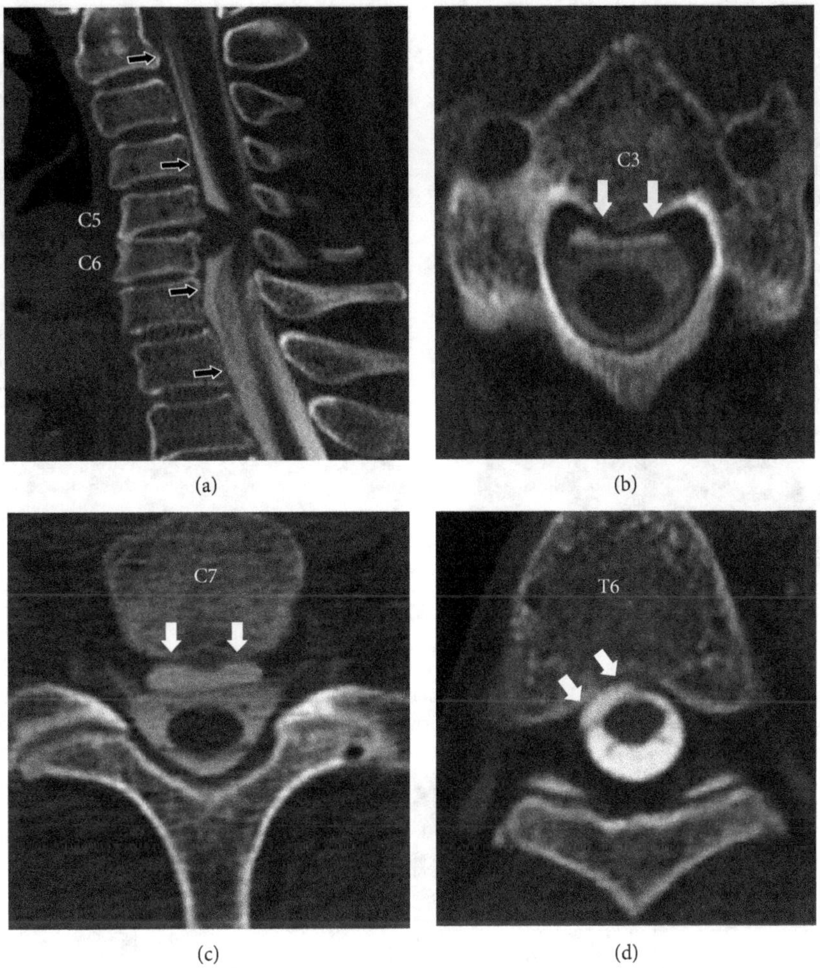

FIGURE 3: Case 1. Preoperative CT myelography. (a) Sagittal view: fluid collection on the ventral side of the dura (black arrows) adjacent to the cervical disk herniation at C5-C6. (b–d) Axial views: ventral longitudinal intraspinal fluid collection (VLISFC) between C2 and T6 (white arrows).

We have reviewed previous reports about VLISFC (Table 1) and found that most VLISFC cases occur between the cervical and thoracic vertebrae. Some reports have attributed VLISFC to dural defects at the same site caused by a protruding disc, osteophytes, a disc-osteophyte complex, or calcification [6, 8]. As a disease associated with dural defects, spinal cord herniation is frequently reported to occur at the thoracic vertebra level, particularly between levels T2 and T8 [9–11]. CSF leakage associated with craniospinal hypovolemia also tends to occur at the thoracic vertebral level and is presumed to be due to dural defects caused by a spondylotic spur or disc herniation [12]. While almost all of the dural defects have been observed at the thoracic spine level in previous reports of VLISFC with associated dural defects (Table 1), there is a possibility that dural defects may also occur at the cervical vertebral level due to osteophytes or disc herniation. However, no dural defects were observed during the anterior cervical surgery in the cases presented herein. With regard to Case 2, protruding osteophytes were observed in CT images at the T2 and T3 vertebral levels. Although the dural defect sites were not identified in the cases presented here, based on previous reports, there is a high possibility that the dural defects existed at the thoracic vertebral level in both cases.

Since the first report by Kumar et al., SS with associated VLISFC has been reported by several institutions [1, 13–15]. In 2012, Kumar et al. also reported cases of VLISFC due to CSF leakage from dural defects in diseases such as SS, craniospinal hypovolemia, and spinal cord herniation [1, 16, 17]. The clinical features of these diseases were reported to overlap and have a common dural lesion [6]. Additionally, a case of SS with associated VLISFC accompanied by spinal cord herniation at the dural defect site was reported by Boncoraglio et al. [9]. Kumar et al. and Holle et al. reported cases of craniospinal hypovolemia related to SS and suggested that craniospinal hypovolemia and SS have similar symptoms, CSF analysis profiles, and imaging findings [18, 19]. Inoue et al. reported a case of spinal cord herniation following craniospinal hypovolemia caused by a dural tear [20]. Kumar has proposed that "duropathy" is a suitable collective term for the group of the diseases caused by these dural lesions [6]. Table 1 shows that VLISFC occur in association with SS, spontaneous intracranial hypotension (SIH) or craniospinal hypovolemia, and spinal cord herniation. Therefore, the pathology of these diseases may overlap due to the presence of similar dural lesions. While previous reports of VLISFC involved symptomatic cases, the two patients in the cases presented here did not experience

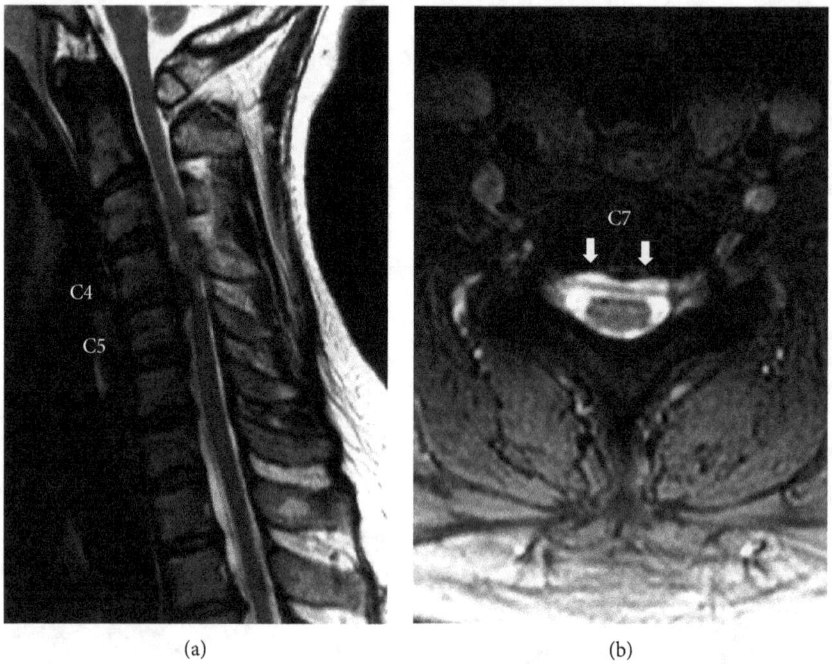

Figure 4: Case 2. Preoperative T2-weighted MRI. (a) Sagittal view: cervical disc herniation compressing the spinal cord was observed at C4-C5. (b) Axial view at the C7 vertebra level: fluid collection was observed on the ventral side of the dura (white arrows).

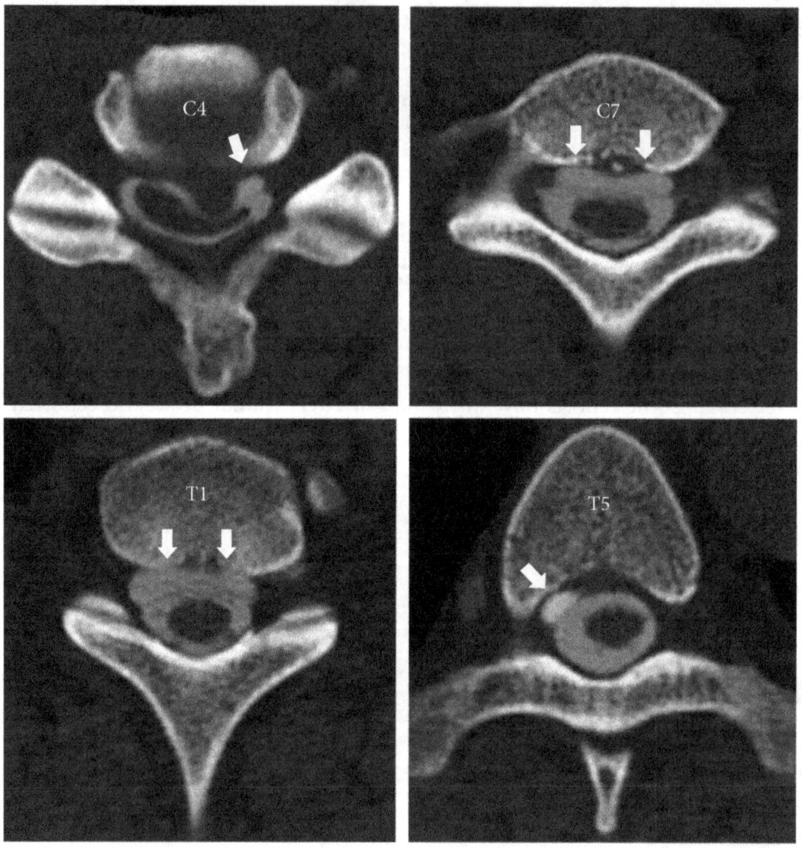

Figure 5: Case 2. Preoperative myelography (axial views): VLISFC (white arrows) between C4 and T5.

headaches, cranial nerve symptoms, or cerebellar ataxia, which are sometimes observed in patients with CSF leakage. To our knowledge, the cases presented herein are the first reported cases of asymptomatic VLISFC. However, it is possible that these two patients described are in the stage preceding duropathy and may develop neurological symptoms related to SS,

Table 1: List of published VLISFC cases.

Author (year)	Patient age/sex	Range of VLISFC	Cause of dural defects (level)	Diagnosis
Rabin et al. (1998) [16]	29/female	Entire spine	Not identified	SIH
	27/female	C6-T3	Not identified	SIH
	37/female	C6-T2	Not mentioned	SIH
Kumar et al. (2007) [22]	77/male	Cervical to thoracic spine	Not mentioned	SS and CH
Holle et al. (2008) [18]	59/male	C5-T6	Thoracic disc herniation (T5-6)	SS and CH
Kumar et al. (2009) [19]	64/male	C3-T11	Calcified disc (T7-8)	SS and CH
Payer et al. (2010) [2]	47/female	Cervical to thoracic spine	Calcification (T4)	SS and ALS
Driver-Dunckley et al. (2010) [23]	54/male	C3-L1	Past spinal injury	SS
Schievink et al. (2011) [3]	35/male	C6-T7	Not mentioned	SS and SIH
	22/male	C2-T12	Not mentioned	SIH
	54/female	C6-T10	Not mentioned	SIH
	63/male	T1-T7	Not mentioned	SIH
	37/female	C6-T11	Not mentioned	SIH
	51/male	C3-L5	Not mentioned	SIH
	15/male	C6-T7	Not mentioned	SIH
Cheng et al. (2011) [4]	53/male	C7-T4	Multilobulated arachnoid cyst	SS
Deluca et al. (2011) [8]	48/male	C2-L4	Unknown (T12-L1)	SS
	40/male	C3-L1	Unknown (T11-12)	SS
	32/male	C2-T12	Not mentioned	SS
Boncoraglio et al. (2012) [9]	69/male	C2-T9	Spinal cord herniation (T6-T7)	SS and spinal cord herniation
Kumar et al. (2012) [24]	58/male	Cervical to lumbosacral spine	Calcified disc (T2-3)	SS and CH
Egawa et al. (2013) [13]	67/male	C2-T8	Unknown (T2-3)	SS
	54/male	C7-T8	Unknown (T1-2)	SS
Toro et al. (2014) [5]	66/male	T3-T8	Thoracic disc herniation (T8-9)	SS
Arishima et al. (2017) [14]	50/male	C2-T12	Unknown (T7-8)	SS
	59/male	C2-T12	Unknown (C7)	SS
Takai et al. (2017) [15]	58/male	Cervical to thoracic spine	Unknown (T3)	SS

SIH: spontaneous intracranial hypotension; SS: superficial siderosis; CH: craniospinal hypovolemia; ALS: amyotrophic lateral sclerosis.

craniospinal hypovolemia, or spinal cord herniation in the future. Therefore, further careful observation is necessary.

There have been reports of patients with VLISFC leading to bibrachial amyotrophy or lower motor neuron weakness. This reported amyotrophy may result from chronic dynamic compression on the spinal cord or nerve conduction block over a tethered motor root segment produced by VLISFC-induced dorsal cord displacement [8]. This proposed mechanism is similar to the pathology of Hirayama disease [21]. In cases presented here, no amyotrophy or lower motor neuron weakness was observed prior to the surgery and preoperative MRI and CT myelography images did not display spinal cord compression due to VLISFC. However, as they still have VLISFC, further careful observation is required.

Although the occurrence of VLISFC may be exceedingly rare, it is notable that it can be identified by MRI or CT myelography. If VLISFC is observed, unexpected CSF leakage may occur during the anterior cervical spine surgery and further careful observation will be required if VLISFC is still observed after surgery.

4. Conclusions

In this study, we reported two cases of cervical disc herniation with asymptomatic VLISFC. This pathological condition could represent a precursory stage of duropathy. Hence, SS, craniospinal hypovolemia, or spinal cord herniation may be experienced by the patients in the future. While the occurrence of VLISFC is exceptionally rare, it can be identified by MRI or CT myelography. If VLISFC is observed, unexpected CSF leakage may occur during anterior cervical spine surgery. These findings indicate that further ongoing observation should be provided if VLISFC is still observed after surgery.

References

[1] N. Kumar, A. A. Cohen-Gadol, R. A. Wright, G. M. Miller, D. G. Piepgras, and J. E. Ahlskog, "Superficial siderosis," *Neurology*, vol. 66, no. 8, pp. 1144–1152, 2006.

[2] M. Payer, C. Sottas, and C. Bonvin, "Superficial siderosis of the central nervous system: secondary progression despite successful surgical treatment, mimicking amyotrophic lateral sclerosis. Case report and review," *Acta Neurochirurgica*, vol. 152, no. 8, pp. 1411–1416, 2010.

[3] W. I. Schievink, M. M. Maya, and M. Nuño, "Chronic cerebellar hemorrhage in spontaneous intracranial hypotension: association with ventral spinal cerebrospinal fluid leaks: clinical article," *Journal of Neurosurgery. Spine*, vol. 15, no. 4, pp. 433–440, 2011.

[4] C. Y. Cheng, M. H. Chen, S. J. Wang, and K. P. Lin, "A proposed mechanism of superficial siderosis supported by surgical and neuroimaging findings," *Medical Hypotheses*, vol. 76, no. 6, pp. 823–826, 2011.

[5] J. Toro, C. Díaz, S. Reyes, V. Jeanneret, and L. E. Burbano, "Superficial siderosis related to a thoracic disc herniation with associated dural injury," *CNS Neuroscience & Therapeutics*, vol. 20, no. 5, pp. 469–472, 2014.

[6] N. Kumar, "Beyond superficial siderosis: introducing "duropathies"," *Neurology*, vol. 78, no. 24, pp. 1992–1999, 2012.

[7] N. Kumar, "Superficial Siderosis," *Archives of Neurology*, vol. 64, no. 4, pp. 491–496, 2007.

[8] G. C. Deluca, C. J. Boes, B. R. Krueger, B. Mokri, and N. Kumar, "Ventral intraspinal fluid-filled collection secondary to CSF leak presenting as bibrachial amyotrophy," *Neurology*, vol. 76, no. 16, pp. 1439-1440, 2011.

[9] G. B. Boncoraglio, E. Ballabio, A. Erbetta, F. Prada, M. Savoiardo, and E. A. Parati, "Superficial siderosis due to dural defect with thoracic spinal cord herniation," *Journal of the Neurological Sciences*, vol. 312, no. 1-2, pp. 170–172, 2012.

[10] A. Darbar, S. Krishnamurthy, J. W. Holsapple, and C. J. Hodge Jr., "Ventral thoracic spinal cord Herniation," *Spine*, vol. 31, no. 17, pp. E600–E605, 2006.

[11] S. Ghostine, E. M. Baron, B. Perri, P. Jacobson, D. Morsette, and F. P. K. Hsu, "Thoracic cord herniation through a dural defect: description of a case and review of the literature," *Surgical Neurology*, vol. 71, no. 3, pp. 362–366, 2009.

[12] B. Mokri, "Low cerebrospinal fluid pressure syndromes," *Neurologic Clinics*, vol. 22, no. 1, pp. 55–74, 2004.

[13] S. Egawa, T. Yoshii, K. Sakaki et al., "Dural closure for the treatment of superficial siderosis," *Journal of Neurosurgery. Spine*, vol. 18, no. 4, pp. 388–393, 2013.

[14] H. Arishima, Y. Higashino, S. Yamada et al., "Spinal endoscopy combined with selective CT myelography for dural closure of the spinal dural defect with superficial siderosis: technical note," *Journal of Neurosurgery. Spine*, vol. 28, no. 1, pp. 96–102, 2018.

[15] K. Takai, T. Komori, M. Niimura, and M. Taniguchi, "Superficial siderosis of the central nervous system associated with intraspinal hemorrhage from ventral thoracic epidural veins and a ventral spinal CSF leak: case report," *Journal of Neurosurgery. Spine*, vol. 26, no. 6, pp. 751–753, 2017.

[16] B. M. Rabin, S. Roychowdhury, J. R. Meyer, B. A. Cohen, K. LaPat, and E. J. Russell, "Spontaneous intracranial hypotension: spinal MR findings," *AJNR. American Journal of Neuroradiology*, vol. 19, no. 6, pp. 1034–1039, 1998.

[17] T. Aizawa, T. Sato, Y. Tanaka, S. Kotajima, M. Sekiya, and S. Kokubun, "Idiopathic herniation of the thoracic spinal cord: report of three cases," *Spine*, vol. 26, no. 20, pp. E488–E491, 2001.

[18] D. Holle, I. E. Sandalcioglu, E. R. Gizewski et al., "Association of superficial siderosis of the central nervous system and low pressure headache," *Journal of Neurology*, vol. 255, no. 7, pp. 1081-1082, 2008.

[19] N. Kumar, J. I. Lane, and D. G. Piepgras, "Superficial siderosis: sealing the defect," *Neurology*, vol. 72, no. 7, pp. 671–673, 2009.

[20] T. Inoue, A. A. Cohen-Gadol, and W. E. Krauss, "Low-pressure headaches and spinal cord herniation. Case report," *Journal of Neurosurgery: Spine*, vol. 98, no. 1, pp. 93–95, 2003.

[21] K. Hirayama and Y. Tokumaru, "Cervical dural sac and spinal cord in juvenile muscular atrophy of distal upper extremity," *Neurology*, vol. 54, no. 10, pp. 1922–1926, 2000.

[22] N. Kumar, A. McKeon, A. A. Rabinstein, P. Kalina, J. E. Ahlskog, and B. Mokri, "Superficial siderosis and CSF hypovolemia: the defect (dural) in the link," *Neurology*, vol. 69, no. 9, pp. 925-926, 2007.

[23] E. D. Driver-Dunckley, J. M. Hoxworth, N. P. Patel, E. P. Bosch, and B. P. Goodman, "Superficial siderosis mimicking amyotrophic lateral sclerosis," *Journal of Clinical Neuromuscular Disease*, vol. 11, no. 3, pp. 137–144, 2010.

[24] N. Kumar, J. L. Fogelson, J. M. Morris, and M. A. Pichelmann, "Superficial siderosis should be included in the differential diagnosis of motor neuron disease," *The Neurologist*, vol. 18, no. 3, pp. 139–145, 2012.

35

Body Builder's Shoulder: Posterior Labrum Periosteal Sleeve Avulsion (POLPSA) and Glenoid Posterior Rim Stress Fracture due to Intense Bench Pressing

Giovanni Bonaspetti, Giovanni Dib, and Flavio Azzola

Department of Orthopaedics and Trauma Surgery, Clinical Institute S. Anna GSD, Via del Franzone 31 25127 Brescia, Italy

Correspondence should be addressed to Giovanni Dib; dib.giovanni@gmail.com

Academic Editor: George Mouzopoulos

Background. Shoulder overuse, both occupational and sports-related, is a major cause of shoulder pain with an estimated incidence of 0.9%-2.5% in the general population and a prevalence of 7%-27% in Europe and United States. We report on a young amateur bodybuilder presenting with a complex shoulder overuse lesion. A posterior labrum periosteal sleeve avulsion (POLPSA) with a chondral lesion of the posterior glenoid cavity and a SLAP lesion was diagnosed. *Case presentation.* A 33-year-old male construction worker complained of 9 months worsening right shoulder pain. He was an amateur body builder who would bench press heavy weights (up to 170 kg). A magnetic resonance arthrogram showed a posterior labrum sleeve avulsion, a stress chondral fracture of the posterior glenoid cavity and a SLAP lesion. Arthroscopic repair of the bicipital anchor, posterior labrum fixation and removal of the chondral fragment, proved successful and allowed the patient to return to his previous sports activity. *Conclusions.* Bench press creates major forces along the anteroposter axis of the upper limbs, pushing the humeral head posteriorly and increasing joint reaction force on the posterior glenoid quadrant considerably as the scapula is locked resting on the bench. This may result in a tendency for the humeral head to subluxate posteriorly which, aggravated by the high number of repetitions, puts the posterior labrum and capsula under very high stress eventually leading to labrum failure. Arthroscopic repair was shown to restore shoulder function in these athletes.

1. Introduction

Shoulder overuse, both occupational and sports-related, is a major cause of shoulder pain with an estimated incidence of 0.9%-2.5% in the general population and a prevalence of 7%-27% in Europe and United States [1–3]. Prolongued exposure to repeated strains and use of heavy weights may put the shoulder joint under considerable stress eventually leading to shoulder dysfunction. This is particularly true for overhead athletes such as baseball pitchers, tennis players, or handball players, with a prevalence as high as 43.5% in these groups [4, 5]. Overuse pathologies involving the wrist and the acromioclavicular joint have been described in body building but this sport is less frequently associated with shoulder joint pathology [6–8]. We report on a young amateur bodybuilder presenting with a complex shoulder overuse lesion. A posterior labrum sleeve avulsion, a stress chondral fracture of the posterior glenoid cavity and a SLAP lesion, was diagnosed.

2. Case Presentation

A 33-year-old male construction worker presented to our clinic complaining of 9 months worsening right shoulder pain. He was an amateur body builder who bench pressed heavy weights (up to 170 kg). However, in the last 9 months, bench pressing became increasingly painful, forcing him to decrease his training load. No previous shoulder trauma was reported. On examination, passive and active shoulder ROM was normal, and shoulder instability tests were negative, while lift-off and biceps load tests were painful. The acromioclavicular joint was not painful on stress or

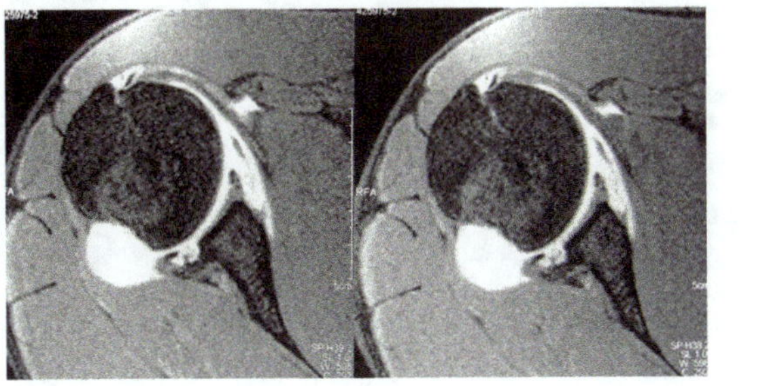

FIGURE 1: FS-PD-TSE MRI sequences depicting posterior labrum avulsion and posterior chondral lesion with a fatigue fracture of the subchondral bone and degenerative cyst.

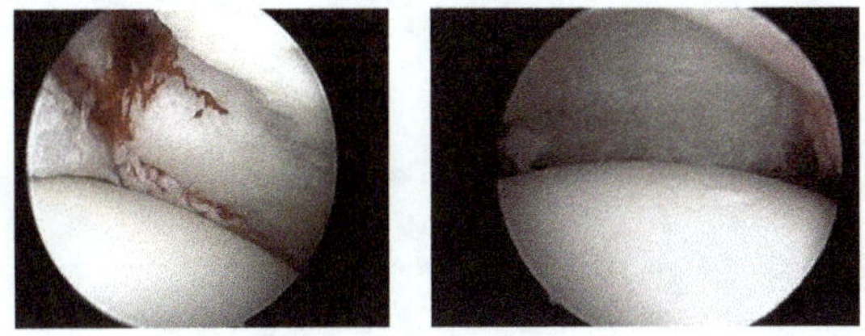

(a) (b)

FIGURE 2: Posterior glenoid labrum avulsion (a) and glenoid chondropathy (b).

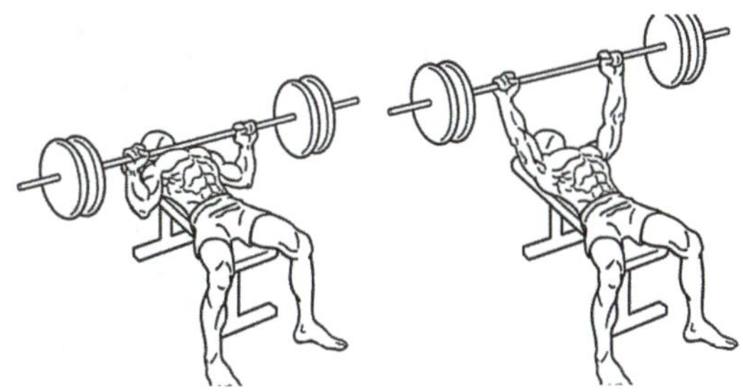

FIGURE 3: Pause and ascent phases of bench pressing.

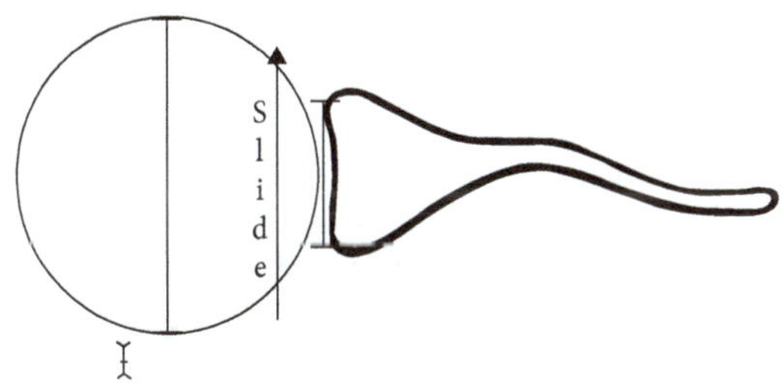

FIGURE 4: Shear forces acting on shoulder during bench pressing.

palpation. The main symptom reported by the patient was a worsening shoulder pain when bench pressing with high loads. He underwent a magnetic resonance arthrogram of his shoulder showing a type 2 SLAP lesion, a large lesion of the posterior glenoid labrum and a glenoid chondropathy (type 2 ICRS) with a stress chondral fracture of the posterior glena progressed into subchondral bone erosion with cyst formation (Figure 1).

He was a candidate to arthroscopic repair: removal of the chondral fragment, repair of the bicipital anchor with a 3.5 mm suture anchor (Twin-Fix ETC Smith & Nephew), refreshing of the posterior glenoid edge, and subsequent posterior labrum fixation with a 5 mm suture anchor (Twin-Fix ETC Smith & Nephew). Notably, the same lesions described on MRI were confirmed on arthroscopy, and no further lesions, such as impact fractures of the humeral head (Hilhyl-sachs or McLaughlin type), were noted (Figure 2).

After 3 months of physical rehabilitation, the patient was able to resume his normal life. Six months postoperatively, he resumed gym training despite medical advice against it. Two years postoperatively, he was still bench pressing his maximal weight.

3. Discussion

Bench pressing biomechanics have been extensively reviewed in the pertinent literature; however, some further considerations are worthy of note.

When bench pressing, the athlete lies flat on his/her back on the bench and holds the weight bar with both hands aligned on the scapular plane. The exercise can be broken down into 5 different phases:

Phase 1: set up: the athlete's body lies on the bench on a 5-points contact position in which the back of the head, the shoulder blades (scapular plane), the gluteals, and the feet remain in contact with the bench or floor.

Phase 2: unrack: grasping the bar with an opposing thumb grip, the athlete lifts the barbell and positions it over his chest.

Phase 3: descent: the athlete lowers the bar to his chest along a straight trajectory, while retracting both scapulae to form a more stable base of support against the bench.

Phase 4: pause: the bar is held still on top of chest, not touching it, preparing to lift.

Phase 5: ascent (and lockout): the athlete pushes the barbell upward until full arm extension, bringing it to the starting position (Figure 3).

Bench pressing creates major forces along the anteroposter axis of the upper limbs. In the first three phases, the weight vector pushes the humeral head posteriorly, increasing the joint reaction force on the posterior glenoid quadrant considerably as the scapula is locked resting on the bench. If the scapula was free to move and not restrained, it could follow the humeral head shift by retracting further backward. A fixed scapula and the posterior push of the humeral head by the barbell weight may result in a tendency for the humeral head to subluxate posteriorly which, aggravated by the high number of repetitions, puts the posterior labrum and posterior capsule under very high stress (Figures 4 and 5).

In the fifth phase, the pectoralis major activates to adducts the humerus against the trunk to lift the barbell, further increasing joint reaction forces on the glenoid cavity. Again, high repetitions may aggravate chondral stress and damage. Higher training weights result in greater posterior humeral head translation, joint hyper pressure, and potential damage. From an anatomical standpoint, the scapula has an angle of 30° with respect to the thoracic cage and is anteverted by 10° (Figure 5). If the hand grip on the bar is wider than shoulder width, this increases the humeral head angle

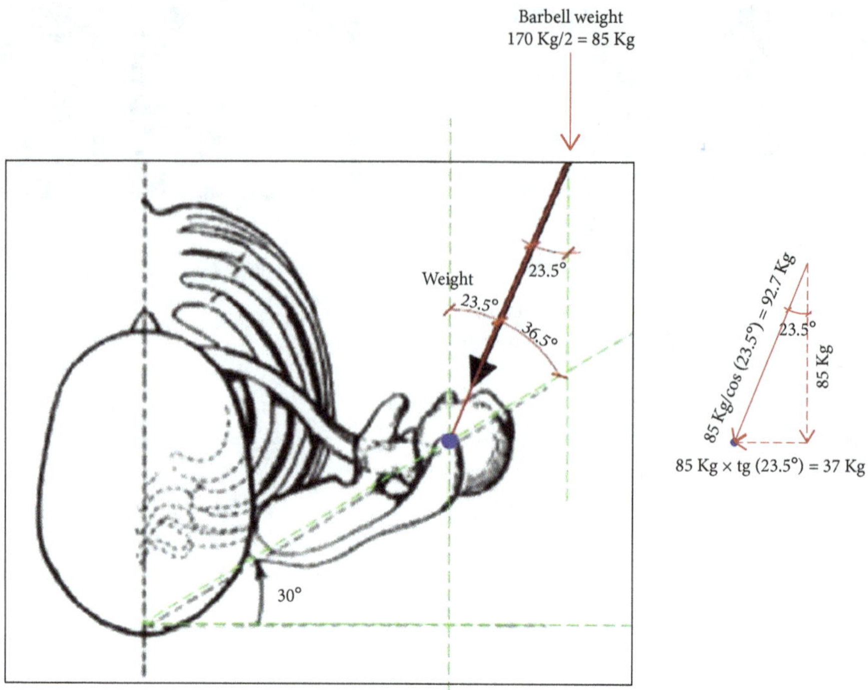

Figure 5: Applied force vectors on shoulder and glenoid articular surface when bench pressing 170 kg.

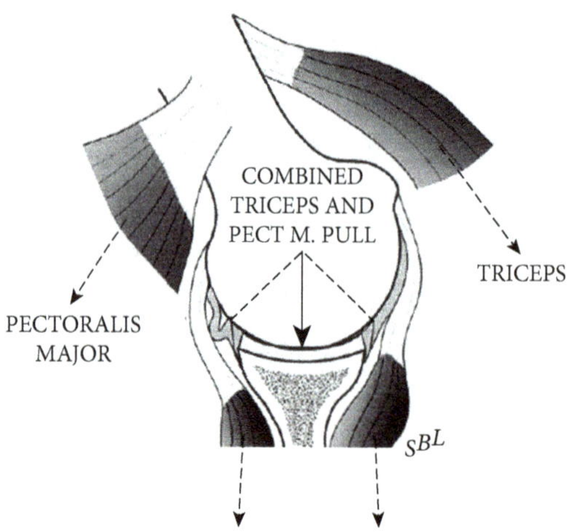

Figure 6: Resulting vector of forces acting on glenohumeral joint by the combined pull of triceps and pectoralis major during cocontraction in the fifth phase of bench pressing.

of incidence with respect to the glenoid cavity, in turn increasing shear forces during posterior translation of the humeral head (Figure 5). In the current case, MRI arthrogram revealed a type 2 SLAP lesion, posterior labrum tear and chondral fracture of the posterior glenoid quadrant with a subchondral degenerative bone cyst. The patient was an amateur body builder who used to bench press up to 170 kg with no history of trauma. Initially, the pain was well managed allowing the patient to maintain his level of training. Thereafter, it gradually worsened to a point where he was unable to keep training to his usual level and sought medical advice. It appears that the mechanism of the lesion was chronic and progressive, consistent with the presence of a degenerative subchondral bone cyst. This explanation would classify such a lesion in the broad spectrum of AIOS (Acquired Instability, Overstressed Shoulder) and posterior shoulder instability. In 2002, Yu et al. described the link between POLPSA and posterior instability but none of these patients had chondral or glenoid damage [9]. In contrast, our patient presented with an avulsion of the posterior labrum together with a stress fracture of the posterior glenoid rim. It is possible that the posterior labrum and capsular damage occurred during the first three phases of bench pressing, when the pectoralis major is not activated and thus not restraining the posterior shift of the humeral head. Instead, chondral glenoid damage and bone cyst formation (secondary to synovial fluid leak) may have occurred during the fifth phase, when cocontraction of the pectoralis major to lift the barbell greatly increases intrarticular pressure and cartilage wear (Figure 6).

Surgical repair proved successful and allowed the patient to return to his previous sports activity. Even though he has managed to continue lifting such heavy weight, it is not in the authors' opinion that a return to such strenuous activities is advisable.

4. Conclusion

To our knowledge, this is the first report of posterior chondral glenoid stress fracture and posterior labrum avulsion in an amateur body builder without a history of shoulder dislocation. Body building and bench pressing put the shoulder under considerable stress, potentially resulting in complex shoulder injury. Arthroscopic repair was shown to restore shoulder function in these athletes.

Data Availability

Data sharing is not applicable to this article as no datasets were generated or analyzed during the current study.

Consent

Written consent was obtained.

Authors' Contributions

GB diagnosed and treated the patient hypothesizing the link between bench press and lesion pathomecanics. GD drafted the work. FA substantively revised the work and was a major contributor in writing the manuscript.

References

[1] J. J. Luime, B. W. Koes, I. J. M. Hendriksen et al., "Prevalence and incidence of shoulder pain in the general population; a systematic review," *Scandinavian Journal of Rheumatology*, vol. 33, pp. 73–81, 2004.

[2] T. Teunis, B. Lubberts, B. T. Reilly, and D. Ring, "A systematic review and pooled analysis of the prevalence of rotator cuff disease with increasing age," *Journal of Shoulder and Elbow Surgery*, vol. 23, pp. 1913–1921, 2014.

[3] H. F. van der Molen, C. Foresti, J. G. Daams, M. H. W. Frings-Dresen, and P. P. F. M. Kuijer, "Work-related risk factors for specific shoulder disorders: a systematic review and meta-analysis," *Occupational and Environmental Medicine*, vol. 74, pp. 745–755, 2017.

[4] V. M. A. de Oliveira, A. C. R. Pitangui, M. R. A. Gomes, H. A. Da Silva, M. H. P. D. Passos, and R. C. Araújo, "Shoulder pain in adolescent athletes: prevalence, associated factors and its influence on upper limb function," *Brazilian Journal of Physical Therapy*, vol. 21, no. 2, pp. 107–113, 2017.

[5] M. G. Saper, L. A. Pierpoint, W. Liu, R. D. Comstock, J. D. Polousky, and J. R. Andrews, "Epidemiology of shoulder and elbow injuries among United States high school baseball players: school years 2005-2006 through 2014-2015," *The American Journal of Sports Medicine*, vol. 46, pp. 37–43, 2018.

[6] S. F. DeFroda, C. Nacca, G. R. Waryasz, and B. D. Owens, "Diagnosis and management of distal clavicle osteolysis," *Orthopedics*, vol. 40, no. 2, pp. 119–124, 2017.

[7] T. Reichel, M. Mitnacht, A. Fenwick, R. Meffert, O. Hoos, and K. Fehske, "Incidence and characteristics of acute and overuse injuries in elite powerlifters," *Cogent Medicine*, vol. 6, article 1588192, 2019.

[8] J. Siewe, G. Marx, P. Knöll et al., "Injuries and overuse syndromes in competitive and elite bodybuilding," *International Journal of Sports Medicine*, vol. 35, pp. 943–948, 2014.

[9] J. S. Yu, C. J. Ashman, and G. Jones, "The POLPSA lesion: MR imaging findings with arthroscopic correlation in patients with posterior instability," *Skeletal Radiology*, vol. 31, pp. 396–399, 2002.

36

Scapular Winging following Sports-Related Injury in a Rugby Player

Shinya Ishizuka, Akinori Kobayakawa, Hideki Hiraiwa, Hiroki Oba, Takefumi Sakaguchi, Masaru Idota, Takahiro Haga, Takafumi Mizuno, Itaru Kawashima, Kanae Kuriyama, and Shiro Imagama

Department of Orthopedic Surgery, Nagoya University Graduate School of Medicine, Nagoya, Japan

Correspondence should be addressed to Shinya Ishizuka; shinyai@med.nagoya-u.ac.jp

Academic Editor: Da sen Li

The most common cause of medial scapular winging is long thoracic nerve palsy (LTN) and subsequent serratus anterior muscle dysfunction. A 16-year-old right-handed male high-school rugby player developed severe right-sided neck and shoulder pain after tackling an opponent while playing rugby. Six weeks after initial injury, the patient observed shoulder muscle weakness when performing his daily activities. On physical examination, limited active elevation of the right shoulder in the scapular plane and scapular winging was observed. Magnetic resonance imaging revealed atrophy of both the SA and subclavius muscles on the right side, and we initially suspected an LTN injury sustained. However, while detailing his history, the patient explained that he also had noted difficulty sucking high viscosity drinks such as shakes and smoothies since childhood. In addition, physical examination showed weakness of the orbicularis oculi muscle. Considering the facial muscle weakness, facioscapulohumeral dystrophy (FSHD) was also suspected, and genetic testing showed chromosome 4q35 deletion with restriction fragments 17 kb and 3 tandem repeated DNA confirming the diagnosis of FSHD. Clinicians should be aware that FSHD could be one of the differential diagnoses of scapular winging after sports injury, and surgeons should rule out the diagnosis of FSHD before performing any surgical treatment for SA palsy.

1. Introduction

The most common cause of scapular winging is long thoracic nerve (LTN) palsy caused by trauma or overuse during sports activity and subsequent serratus anterior (SA) muscle dysfunction [1, 2]. Facioscapulohumeral dystrophy (FSHD), the third most common type of dystrophy, causes asymmetric atrophy of the muscles of the face, upper arm, and shoulder girdle, leading to scapular winging. To the best of our knowledge, there are no case reports of FSHD diagnosed based on scapular winging after a sports-related injury. Herein, we report about an otherwise healthy 16-year-old high school rugby player who presented with complaints of pain and decreased range of motion (ROM) of the right shoulder, as well as unusual scapular winging on the right side for 2 months after a tackle during a rugby game. Clinicians should consider another underlying disorder if the presumed cause does not explain the symptoms sufficiently.

2. Case Presentation

A 16-year-old right-handed male high-school rugby player developed severe right-sided neck and shoulder pain after tackling an opponent while playing rugby. After resting for a few days, the shoulder pain improved, and he began to play rugby again for his high school rugby league. After the initial injury, however, he occasionally experienced similar pain while playing rugby, which resolved after a few days of rest. The primary orthopedist suspected shoulder muscle strain for which the patient was referred to a clinic where he started physical therapy of the shoulder. He underwent 4 weeks of physical therapy, which involved simple strengthening exercises, to

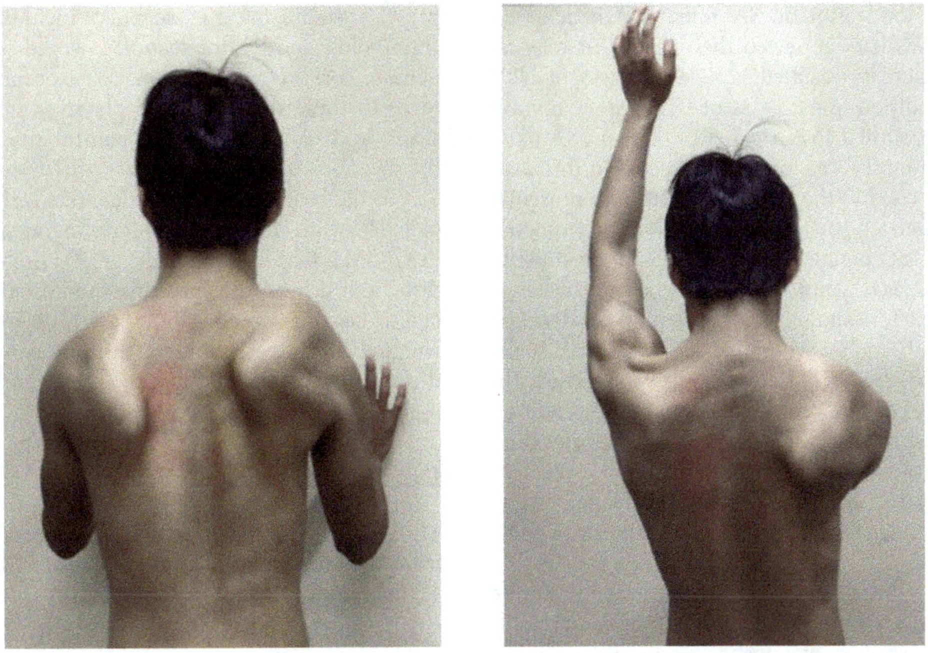

Figure 1: Bilateral scapular winging (right > >left) during (a) wall push test and (b) active shoulder flexion. The patient is unable to elevate his right arm to a horizontal level.

restore his ROM and reduce inflammation; not only pain did not improve, but he also now had persistent shoulder pain—initially, he experienced pain only when moving the shoulder. Six weeks after initial injury, the patient observed shoulder muscle weakness when performing his daily activities. When he was referred to our clinic 2 months after the initial injury, his chief complaint was limited shoulder elevation, not pain. He had no known family history and past history. On physical examination, active elevation of the right shoulder in the scapular plane was limited to 50°, whereas the ROM of his left shoulder was normal. Scapular winging produced by the wall push test and active shoulder elevation was observed bilaterally (right > >left) (Figure 1).

The patient's rotator cuff tests and impingement signs were negative in his right shoulder. Manual muscle testing did not show any weakness of the biceps, triceps, or grip strength. Plain radiographs had no abnormal findings. However, magnetic resonance imaging (MRI) revealed atrophy of both the SA and subclavius muscles on the right side, but no significant pathology was observed in the shoulder joint or cervical spine (Figure 2).

Blood test results showed slight elevations of creatine kinase (CK; 870 U/L), alkaline phosphatase (526 U/L), lactate dehydrogenase (LDH; 370 U/L), and aldolase (10.9 U/L). While detailing his history, the patient explained that he also had noted difficulty sucking high viscosity drinks such as shakes and smoothies since childhood. In addition, physical examination showed weakness of the orbicularis oculi muscle. Initially, we suspected neuralgic amyotrophy or an LTN injury sustained when playing rugby. However, considering the facial muscle weakness, FSHD was also suspected, and genetic testing was ordered to confirm the diagnosis before performing invasive examinations such as electromyography (EMG).

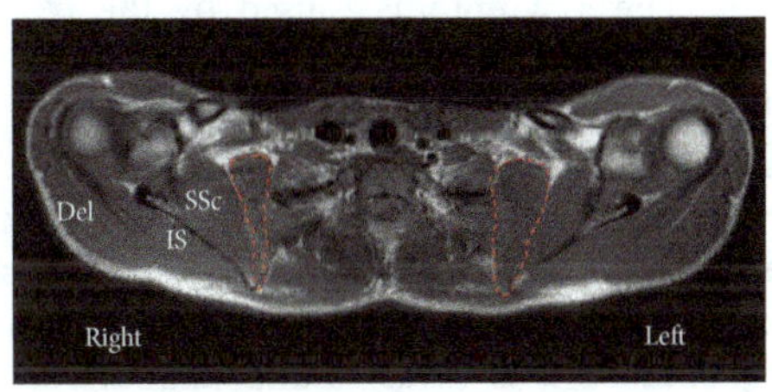

Figure 2: $T1$-weighted magnetic resonance image showing slight atrophy of the serratus anterior muscle (dotted line) on the right side compared with left side in the axial plane. SSc: subscapularis muscle; IS: infraspinatus muscle; Del: Deltoid muscle.

Although he had no family history of muscular dystrophy, genetic testing performed at an outside laboratory showed chromosome 4q35 deletion with restriction fragments 17 kb and 3 tandem repeated DNA (D4Z4) confirming the diagnosis of FSHD. Since the diagnosis of FSHD, he is being followed up periodically to check for any progress of the muscle weakness or development of FSHD-related complications. The patient was informed that data from the case would be submitted for publication and gave their consent.

3. Discussion

In this report, we describe an unusual case of scapular winging in a young patient after he sustained an injury while playing rugby, which was finally diagnosed as FSHD.

Scapular winging causes discomfort, decreased shoulder strength, and ROM [2]. Scapular winging is divided into two types (medial > lateral) [3], and our patient had the medial type. Previous studies reported that the main causes for medial scapular winging are SA dysfunction following

LTN palsy [1, 3] or traumatic SA muscular detachment [4–6]. Other studies have reported that trauma or overuse related to sports activity resulted in 40-90% cases of LTN palsy [7, 8]. In addition, most cases of LTN injury involve the dominant side, similar to our patient [9]. Thus, SA palsy caused by an LTN injury was initially suspected in this case.

FSHD is often cited as the third most common muscular dystrophy characterized by slow progressive asymmetric atrophy of the facial, shoulder, upper arm, and leg muscles [10, 11]. The primary symptoms are scapular protrusion, shoulder pain owing to scapulothoracic instability, or decrease of shoulder strength and ROM. Patients with FSHD usually notice a gradual progression of these chronic symptoms without any inciting events. The slow progression of the condition sometimes makes it difficult for patients to be aware of their own discomfort. Patients with FSHD primarily consult neurologists, pediatricians, and often orthopedists. Hence, FSHD should be widely understood by orthopedists and orthopedic surgeons.

Unfortunately, the diagnosis is often delayed despite symptoms of chronic pain and disability. To avoid a misdiagnosis of FSHD, specific diagnostic questions that focus on facial weakness could be useful, such as "Are you good at whistling?", "Are you good at smiling?", "Do you feel difficult while drinking shakes?", and "Do you sleep with eyes open?" These symptoms caused by the weakness of facial muscles tend to be observed from the early phase of disease. In our case, since the patient experienced some difficulty in drinking shakes and smoothies, he had been avoiding it from childhood. Although an LTN injury can be confirmed using EMG following a medical interview and general examination, we performed genetic testing before the EMG, because it is invasive and painful for patients. FSHD is confirmed by genetic testing which shows the deletion of tandemly repeated DNA (D4Z4 repeats) in chromosome 4q35. In some cases, slight elevations of CK, LDH, or aldolase are observed in blood testing, though these variables are not helpful for the diagnosis [12].

Unfortunately, there is no cure or medical treatment available for FSHD. Most cases of LTN injury recover with conservative management, and recovery can sometimes takes several months to a few years [1, 13–15]. If FSHD had been misdiagnosed and treated conservatively as an LTN injury, it would have resulted in delayed diagnosis or gone undiagnosed. Surgical treatment has some disadvantages as well, for patients. There are several surgical options for SA palsy following an LTN injury, such as LTN release [16], scapulothoracic arthrodesis, and pectoralis major transfer [2, 17]. LTN release has no effect on muscular dystrophy and thus should not be performed for FSDH. The indications of scapulothoracic arthrodesis include both LTN palsy and FSHD [18]. However, pectoralis major transfer for dynamic stabilization of scapula should be avoided in patients with FSHD, because pectoralis major is one of the affected muscles in FSHD.

In our patient diagnosed with FHSD, the cause of neck and shoulder pain following a traumatic event is unclear. The most disabling dysfunction of FSHD is the lack of fixation of the scapula against the thoracic cage during shoulder flexion and abduction [9], and in this situation, the other muscles stabilizing the scapula, including the trapezius, rhomboids, and levator scapulae, would only partially compensate for the SA function. We speculate that excessive force to these muscles while playing rugby caused muscle strain and pain. In fact, the painful sites corresponded to the locations of these muscles.

To the best of our knowledge, this is the first case report of FSHD with unusual scapular winging and limited shoulder ROM after a traumatic event. Physiotherapists, orthopedists, and orthopedic surgeons should be aware that FSHD could be one of the differential diagnoses of scapular winging after sports injury, and surgeons should rule out the diagnosis of FSHD before performing any surgical treatment for SA palsy.

Data Availability

The data that support the findings of this study are available from the corresponding author, [author initials], upon reasonable request.

Consent

Informed consent was obtained from the patient included in this study.

References

[1] M. Vastamaki, L. Ristolainen, H. Vastamaki, and V. Pikkarainen, "Isolated serratus palsy etiology influences its long-term outcome," *Journal of Shoulder and Elbow Surgery*, vol. 26, no. 11, pp. 1964–1969, 2017.

[2] S. Lee, D. D. Savin, N. R. Shah, D. Bronsnick, and B. Goldberg, "Scapular winging: evaluation and Treatment," *Journal of Bone and Joint Surgery*, vol. 97, no. 20, pp. 1708–1716, 2015.

[3] J. T. Didesch and P. Tang, "Anatomy, etiology, and management of scapular winging," *The Journal of Hand Surgery*, vol. 44, no. 4, pp. 321–330, 2019.

[4] K. M. Gaffney, "Avulsion injury of the serratus Anterior," *Clinical Journal of Sport Medicine*, vol. 7, no. 2, pp. 134–136, 1997.

[5] K. Otoshi, Y. Itoh, A. Tsujino, M. Hasegawa, and S. Kikuchi, "Avulsion injury of the serratus anterior muscle in a high-school underhand pitcher: a case report," *Journal of Shoulder and Elbow Surgery*, vol. 16, no. 6, pp. e45–e47, 2007.

[6] J. B. Carr 2nd, Q. E. John, E. Rajadhyaksha, E. W. Carson, and K. L. Turney, "Traumatic avulsion of the serratus anterior muscle in a collegiate rower: a case report," *Sports health*, vol. 9, no. 1, pp. 80–83, 2017.

[7] J. T. Johnson and H. O. Kendall, "Isolated paralysis of the serratus anterior muscle," *The Journal of Bone & Joint Surgery*, vol. 37, no. 3, pp. 567–574, 1955.

[8] A. F. Kaptelin and G. A. Pavlova, "Traumatic paresis of the serratus anterior muscle (diagnosis, clinical aspects, treatment)," *Ortopediia Travmatologiia i Protezirovanie*, vol. 2, pp. 56–59, 1981.

[9] S. M. Friedenberg, T. Zimprich, and C. M. Harper, "The natural history of long thoracic and spinal accessory neuropathies," *Muscle & Nerve*, vol. 25, no. 4, pp. 535–539, 2002.

[10] A. Bergsma, E. H. Cup, M. M. Janssen, A. C. Geurts, and I. J. de

Groot, "Upper limb function and activity in people with facioscapulohumeral muscular dystrophy: a web-based survey," *Disability and Rehabilitation*, vol. 39, no. 3, pp. 236–243, 2017.

[11] K. Mul, S. Lassche, N. C. Voermans, G. W. Padberg, C. G. Horlings, and B. G. van Engelen, "What's in a name? The clinical features of facioscapulohumeral muscular dystrophy," *Practical Neurology*, vol. 16, no. 3, pp. 201–207, 2016.

[12] Y. Matsuzaka, S. Kishi, Y. Aoki et al., "Three novel serum biomarkers, miR-1, miR-133a, and miR-206 for limb-girdle muscular dystrophy, Facioscapulohumeral muscular dystrophy, and Becker muscular dystrophy," *Environmental Health and Preventive Medicine*, vol. 19, no. 6, pp. 452–458, 2014.

[13] M. R. Safran, "Nerve injury about the shoulder in athletes, part 2," *The American Journal of Sports Medicine*, vol. 32, no. 4, pp. 1063–1076, 2004.

[14] S. M. White and C. M. Witten, "Long thoracic nerve palsy in a professional ballet dancer," *The American Journal of Sports Medicine*, vol. 21, no. 4, pp. 626–628, 1993.

[15] J. R. Gregg, D. Labosky, M. Harty et al., "Serratus anterior paralysis in the young athlete," *The Journal of Bone & Joint Surgery*, vol. 61, no. 6, pp. 825–832, 1979.

[16] L. R. Le Nail, G. Bacle, E. Marteau, P. Corcia, L. Favard, and J. Laulan, "Isolated paralysis of the serratus anterior muscle: surgical release of the distal segment of the long thoracic nerve in 52 patients," *Orthopaedics & Traumatology, Surgery & Research*, vol. 100, 4 Supplement, pp. S243–S248, 2014.

[17] G. J. Galano, L. U. Bigliani, C. S. Ahmad, and W. N. Levine, "Surgical treatment of winged scapula," *Clinical Orthopaedics and Related Research*, vol. 466, no. 3, pp. 652–660, 2008.

[18] R. S. Twyman, G. D. Harper, and M. A. Edgar, "Thoracoscapular fusion in facioscapulohumeral dystrophy: clinical review of a new surgical method," *Journal of Shoulder and Elbow Surgery*, vol. 5, no. 3, pp. 201–205, 1996.

37

Massive Osteolysis in a Modern Total Knee Prosthesis

Emmanuel Gibon,[1] Jacquelyn A. Knapik,[2] and Hari K. Parvataneni[1]

[1]*Division of Adult Reconstruction, Department of Orthopedics and Rehabilitation, University of Florida College of Medicine, University of Florida, Gainesville, FL, USA*
[2]*Department of Pathology, Immunology and Laboratory Medicine, University of Florida College of Medicine, University of Florida, Gainesville, FL, USA*

Correspondence should be addressed to Emmanuel Gibon; emmanuel.gibon@gmail.com

Academic Editor: Robert U. Ashford

Case. An 82-year-old woman underwent right total knee replacement with a sequentially irradiated and annealed highly cross-linked polyethylene insert. At 9 years, she was found to have a massive femoral osteolysis with an impending fracture. *Conclusion.* This case demonstrates a rare occurrence of massive femoral osteolysis, requiring revision surgery, with a sequentially irradiated and annealed highly cross-linked polyethylene.

1. Introduction

Total knee arthroplasty is a highly reliable and reproducible procedure to treat end-stage knee osteoarthritis. The Australian registry shows a survivorship of 91.4% at 18 years [1].

First-generation highly cross-linked polyethylene (HXLPE) was first introduced clinically in 2001 for total knee arthroplasty (TKA) [2]. However, due to concern for the potential risk of early fracture, its implementation has been more gradual than for total hip arthroplasty (THA). There remain concerns about transitioning from UHMWPE to HXLPE due to the reduction in ductility and fracture resistance associated with cross-linking. Nevertheless, in vitro studies have shown significant reduction of wear with first-generation HXLPE tibial inserts [3–5]. HXLPE tibial inserts are now predominantly used in Australia and represents 64.2% of all the PE inserts [1].

The X3® (Stryker, Mahwah, NJ) is a second-generation HXLPE, which was widely introduced in 2005. It is produced by gamma irradiating compression-molded GUR 1020 with 30 kGy of gamma irradiation followed by annealing to 130°C. These steps are repeated three times, and then, gas plasma sterilization occurs. The rationale behind this manufacturing technique for X3® was to remove enough free radicals to provide oxidation resistance while retaining the advantage of the UHMWPE mechanical properties. Wang et al. showed this process to be effective at dramatically eliminating free radicals equivalent to the level of virgin UHMWPE [6]. Accelerated aging studies showed similar results [7]. Knee simulator investigations reported wear reduction ranging from 64% to 86% compared to conventional UHMWPE [8–10]. Registry data shows a survivorship of the Triathlon® with X3® of 96.2% at 10 years [1]. Meneghini et al. [11] reported no radiographic osteolysis or mechanical failure of the tibial polyethylene at 5-year follow-up. Minoda et al. [12] showed a 58% reduction of the number of in vivo X3® wear particles compared to conventional PE in TKA.

Here, we present a case of catastrophic femoral osteolysis following a TKA with sequentially annealed highly cross-linked polyethylene, which is, to the best of our knowledge, the first report of this mode of failure in this modern design. The patient was informed that data concerning the case would be submitted for publication, and she provided consent.

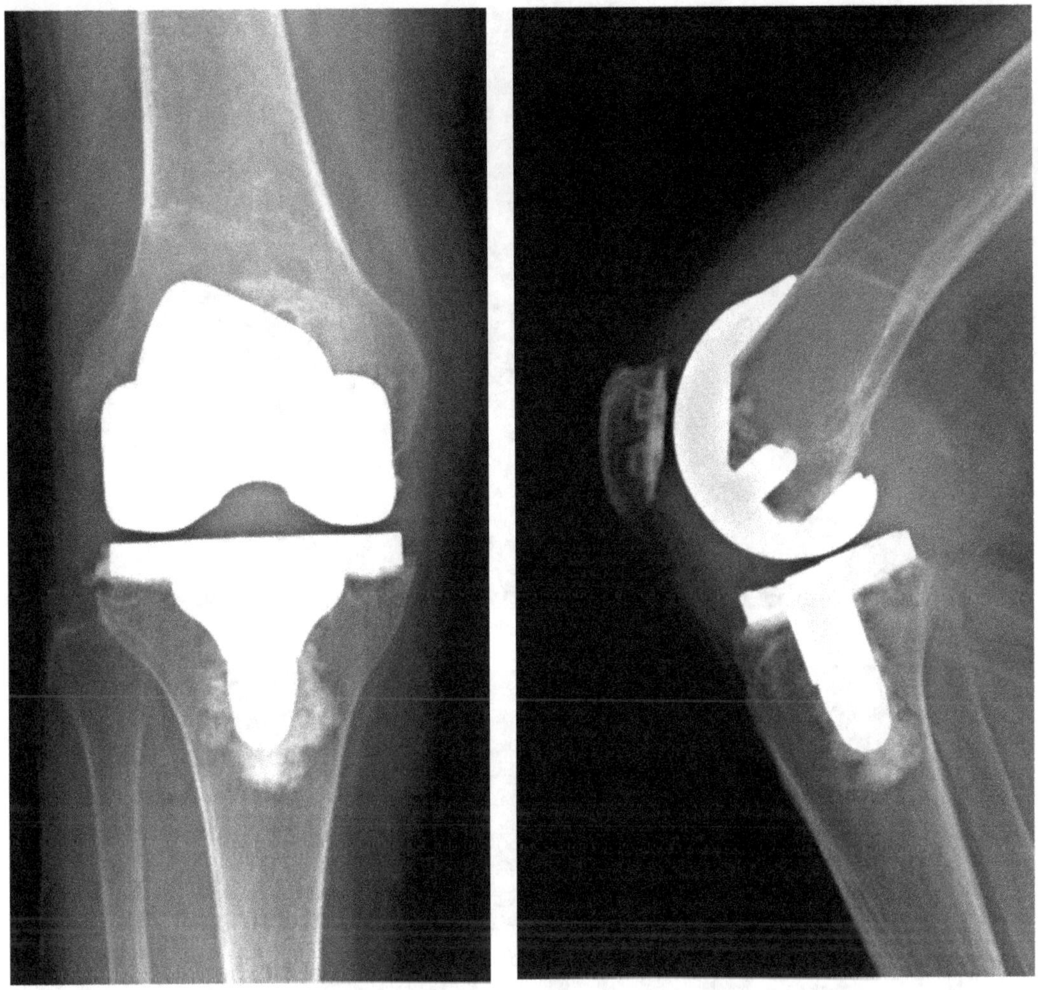

(a) (b)

FIGURE 1: Right knee: (a) AP and (b) lateral radiographs at the time of presentation (February 2019).

2. Case Report

An 82-year-old woman presented to our institution for evaluation of her right TKA, which was performed in 2009 at an outside hospital. Her past medical history was significant only for rheumatoid arthritis (RA) for which she usually took adalimumab biweekly, methothrexate and celecoxib but reported this was well controlled.

Per her outside operative records, implants used at the initial surgery were a cemented Triathlon® CR femoral component, a 9 mm size 3 X3® CS insert, a size 3 Triathlon® universal tibial baseplate, and a 10 mm asymmetric Triathlon® X3® patella.

The patient was initially referred by the primary surgeon to our oncology clinic in February 2019 due to findings of a distal femur lesion in her right knee discovered on follow-up X-rays (Figure 1) and better seen in a noncontrast MRI. At that time, the patient was pain-free but reported feelings of instability. The physical exam showed a well-healed midline surgical incision for TKA without complication. No obvious instability with varus/varus testing or drawer testing was found.

MRI with IV contrast was performed to further characterize this mass in the right distal femur and rule out a malignant lesion (Figure 2). The MRI report showed "post-surgical changes of right TKA with findings typical for osteolysis secondary to particle disease and knee joint effusion with synovitis." The orthopedic oncologist then referred the patient to our adult reconstruction clinic with very low suspicion for a neoplastic process.

The patient was assessed again in April 2019 and mentions occasional knee buckling but without pain. Her X-rays showed a focal well-circumscribed lucent lesion with thin geographic mineralized margin along the distal diametaphysis and deep to the cemented femoral component. There was thinning and weakening of the cortices in several areas. At that time, we recommended surgery due to the fracture risk. The patient declined but was agreeable to close surveillance. She was assessed two months later and did not want to consider surgery, again and refused X-rays due to

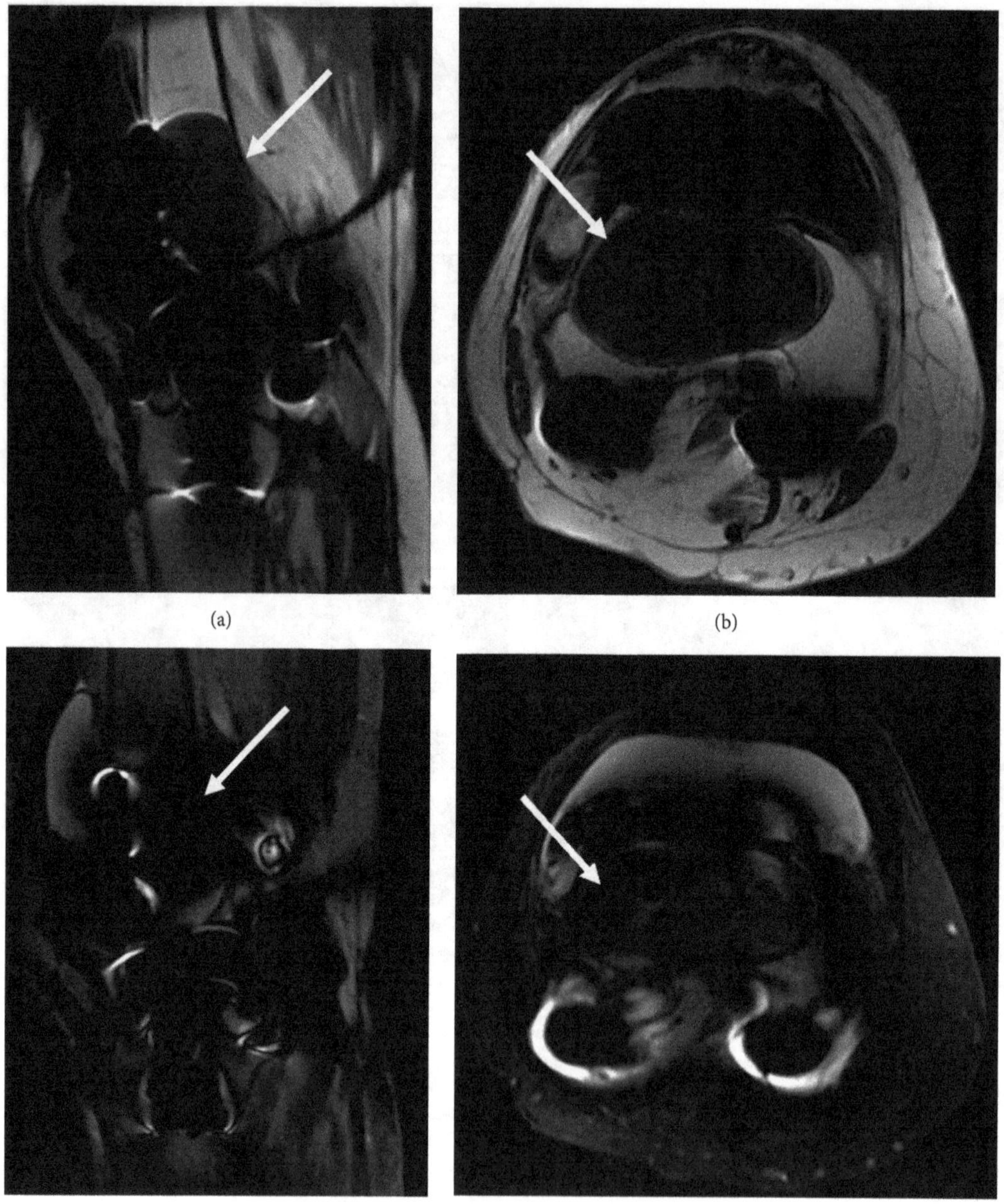

(a) (b) (c) (d)

FIGURE 2: MRI of the right knee with IV gadolinium. In the distal femur, there is low T1 signal in the sagittal (a) and axial (b) views and heterogeneously predominantly low T2 signal in the sagittal (c) and axial (d) views with a sharp rim and thin peripheral enhancement (white arrows) that is in continuity with the prosthesis and typical for osteolysis secondary to particle disease (MRI machine: Titan 3T (Toshiba)).

absence of pain. She returned back a month later with mild knee pain and opted to proceed with a revision TKA for the diagnosis of massive femoral osteolysis and impending femoral fracture. The patient was later seen preoperatively, and the pain and X-rays remained stable (Figure 3).

We utilized the prior incision and entered the join through a medial parapatellar arthrotomy. Clear synovial fluid was seen and sent for culture. The patella and tibia were mobilized and found to be well fixed, although the tibia had some osteolysis. The polyethylene was found to have minor oxidation, but no significant wear was found. We found no third bodies or other debris. We removed the insert and found no backside wear or any other explanation for this massive osteolysis. There was visual appearance of diffuse in vivo oxidation. Based on the extent of the osteolysis, we decided to revise the femur with a stem to bypass the defect. The femoral component was then removed with minimal bone loss. There were massive cystic changes with some debris that we sent for pathology (Figure 4). After refreshing the cuts, we proceeded with reconstruction. The femoral

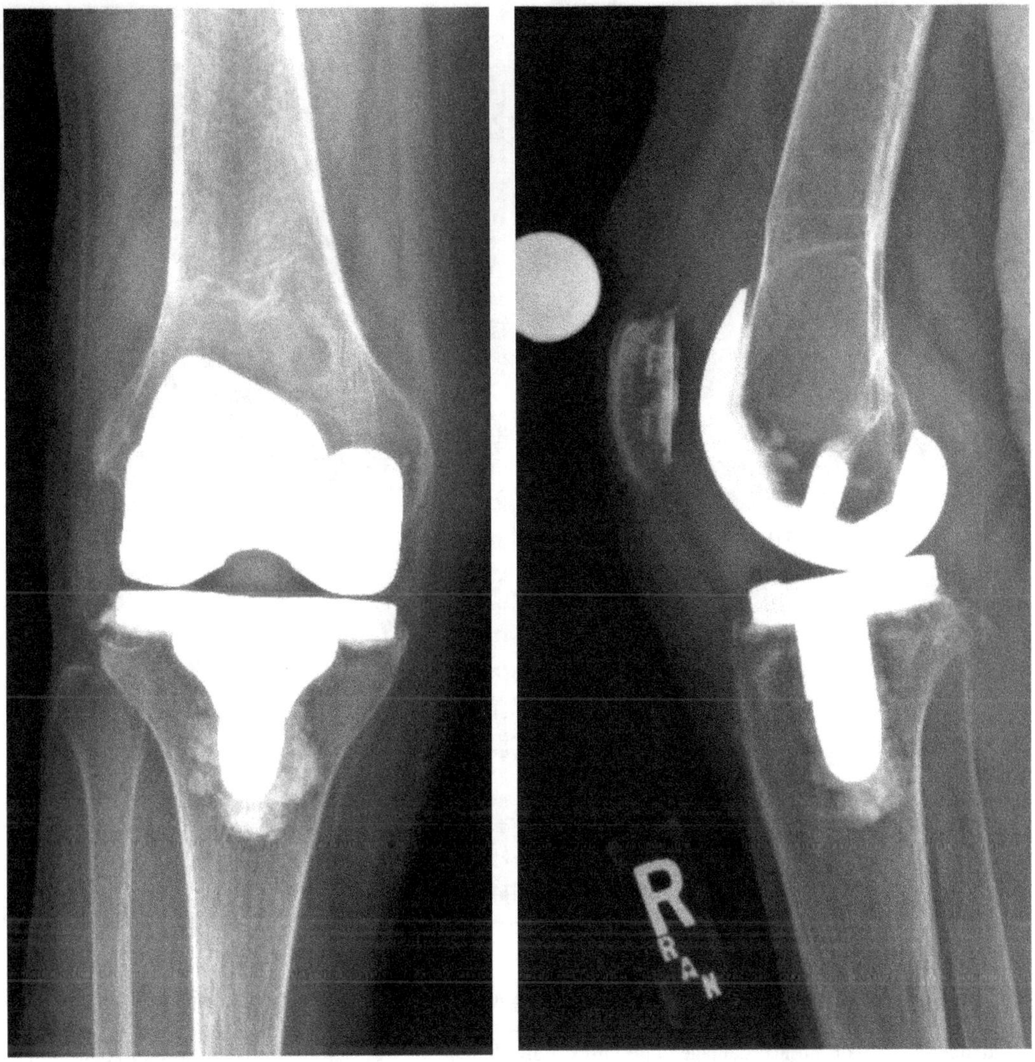

(a) (b)

Figure 3: Right knee: (a) AP and (b) lateral radiographs six months later (October 2019).

reconstruction was performed using a size A Tritanium® metaphyseal cone and Triathlon® femoral component with a 15 mm × 100 mm cemented stem extension and a 16 mm posterior stabilized X3® insert.

All the cultures resulted negative. Microscopic evaluation (Figure 5) of the periprosthetic tissue revealed features typically observed when implant failure has taken place. Numerous multinucleated foreign body giant cells can be seen filled with debris from breakdown products. Some of the giant cells had empty spaces where engulfed methyl methacrylate cement was present but dissolved during tissue processing. Other foreign body giant cells contained shards of refractile debris and fragmented refractile particles. Macrophages also infiltrated the tissue and are filled with phagocytosed microparticles. Chronic inflammatory cells were present but there was no acute inflammation supporting that this was an aseptic process.

At one-year clinical follow-up, the patient was noted to be doing well with no changes in her radiographic examination (Figure 6). Her incision healed uneventfully. The patient was pain free and ambulating without walking aids. At the last follow-up, her right knee range of motion was 0-130°.

3. Discussion

Osteolysis is now an uncommon reason for late failure of modern TKA and has been shown to represent 9% [13]. Our case is unique because it is the first report of a catastrophic femoral osteolysis at just under 10 years in an otherwise well-functioning TKA using a modern HXLPE insert which has an excellent track record. There are only a very limited number of case reports of previous failure of the X3® in TKA, and the failure modes were different than this report. Sonn and

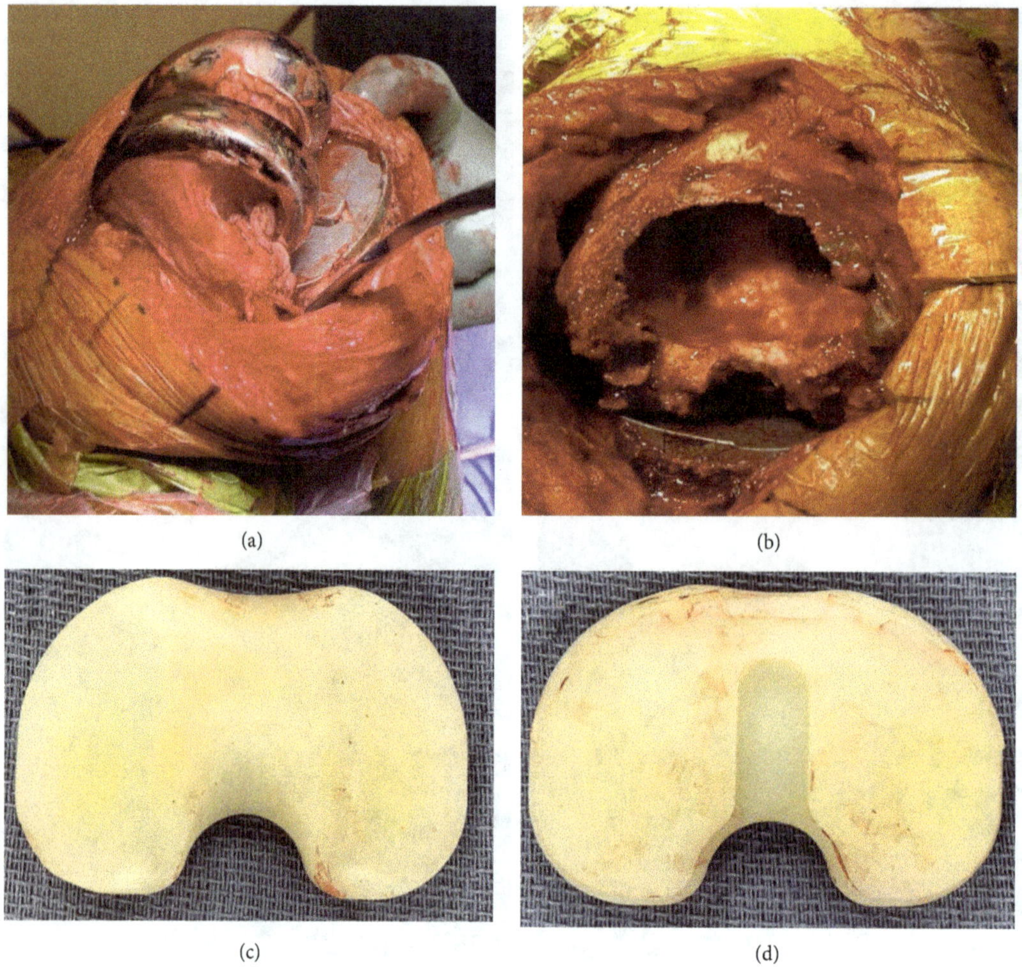

FIGURE 4: Intraoperative findings. (a) Lateral view of the distal femur showing massive osteolysis of the lateral condyle. (b) Top-down view of the distal femur after implant removal showing extension of the osteolysis into the canal. (c) Top view and (d) backside view of the X3® insert with no evidence of wear or surface damage. The entire polyethylene surface demonstrated yellow discoloration consistent with oxidation.

Meneghini [14] discussed an early failure of X3® at 5 years. The mechanism of failure was a completely worn through polyethylene. Kop et al. [15] investigated 15 implants from revision surgeries at a mean of 3 years. Of note, none of the revision was performed for isolated osteolysis. Furthermore, 4 of the 15 bearings exhibited signs of oxidation. MacDonald et al. [16] assessed the in vivo performance of X3® retrieved tibial inserts ($n = 345$) and compared them to gamma inert sterilized PE tibial inserts. The authors found that the X3® inserts had similar oxidation levels when compared to gamma inert controls. Moreover, they had 6 cases of posterior fracture in the X3® cohort and none in the control group.

In our case, one could propose that RA could have resulted in the bony changes. However, the patient's disease was well controlled and the pathology analysis did not notice any microscopic tissue modification pointing toward RA. Pathology also ruled out a neoplasm. Polyethylene-induced osteolysis was further confirmed by histological analysis. Examination of our retrieval PE insert showed signs of burnishing, which is not an uncommon finding for tibial bearings. We did not observe any fracture or delamination of the implant but significant oxidation was seen.

Typical risk factors for osteolysis associated with TKA are malalignment of the mechanical axis and improper ligament balancing, early-generation PE sterilization techniques, back-side wear, third-body abrasion, young age, increased activity level, and elevated body mass index. In our case, the patient was a low-demand 82-year-old woman with a BMI of 23.8 kg/m^2. In this present case, one potential explanation could be an isolated issue with a batch from manufacturing since this is such an unusual case.

The Manufacturer and User Facility Device Experience (MAUDE) database captures failure patterns with certain FDA cleared medical devices in a timely manner. We reviewed this database between 2005 and 2020 and found 15 reported cases related to the X3® insert, and 10 of them were about the tibial inserts. None of them were related to osteolysis.

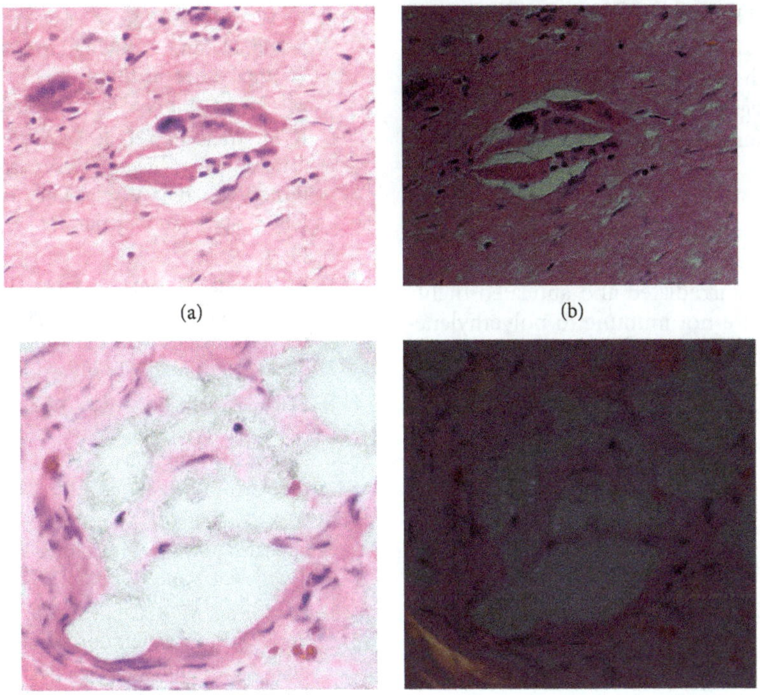

(a) (b)

(c) (d)

FIGURE 5: Histological analysis. (a, c) Multinucleated foreign body giant cells with engulfed shards of PE debris (H&E 40x). (b, d) H&E under refractile light.

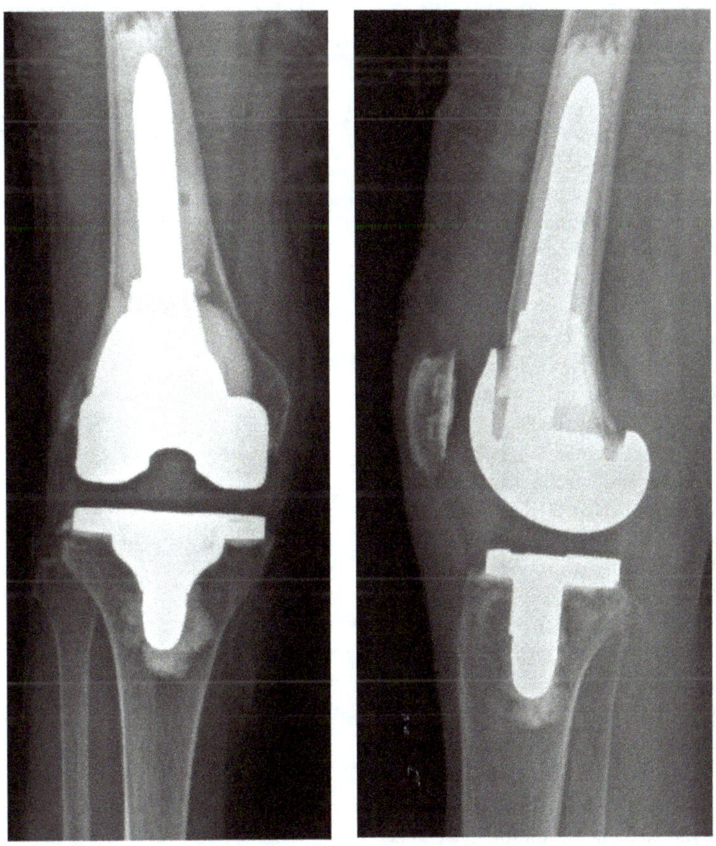

(a) (b)

FIGURE 6: Right knee: (a) AP and (b) lateral radiographs at one-year follow-up.

The use of HXLPE in TKA is still controversial. A recent study by Partridge et al. [17] that combined registries from England, Wales, and Northern Ireland showed that conventional polyethylene had significantly lower aseptic revision rates than HXLPE, except for a very specific subset of patients.

4. Conclusion

In summary, this case demonstrates that primary TKA performed with sequentially irradiated and annealed highly cross-linked polyethylene are not immune to polyethylene-induced osteolysis. Although X3® shows excellent survivorship at 10 years for TKA, routine surveillance of patients might be warranted especially around the first decade after implantation.

Data Availability

The data used to support the findings of this study are included within the article.

References

[1] "Australian National Joint Replacement Registry, Annual Report 2019," 2020, Available at: https://aoanjrr.sahmri.com/annual-reports-2019.

[2] J. T. Hodrick, E. P. Severson, D. S. McAlister, B. Dahl, and A. A. Hofmann, "Highly crosslinked polyethylene is safe for use in total knee arthroplasty," *Clinical Orthopaedics & Related Research*, vol. 466, no. 11, pp. 2806–2812, 2008.

[3] O. K. Muratoglu, C. R. Bragdon, D. O. O'Connor, R. S. Perinchief, M. Jasty, and W. H. Harris, "Aggressive wear testing of a cross-linked polyethylene in total knee arthroplasty," *Clinical Orthopaedics and Related Research*, vol. 404, pp. 89–95, 2002.

[4] O. K. Muratoglu, A. Mark, D. A. Vittetoe, W. H. Harris, and H. E. Rubash, "Polyethylene damage in total knees and use of highly crosslinked polyethylene," *The Journal of Bone and Joint Surgery. American Volume*, vol. 85, Suppl 1, pp. 7–S13, 2003.

[5] S. Utzschneider, N. Harrasser, C. Schroeder, F. Mazoochian, and V. Jansson, "Wear of contemporary total knee replacements - A knee simulator study of six current designs," *Clinical Biomechanics*, vol. 24, no. 7, pp. 583–588, 2009.

[6] A. Wang, H. Zeng, S. S. Yau, A. Essner, M. Manely, and J. Dumbleton, "Wear, oxidation and mechanical properties of a sequentially irradiated and annealed UHMWPE in total joint replacement," *Journal of Physics D: Applied Physics*, vol. 39, no. 15, pp. 3213–3219, 2006.

[7] J. H. Dumbleton, J. A. D'Antonio, M. T. Manley, W. N. Capello, and A. Wang, "The basis for a second-generation highly cross-linked UHMWPE," *Clinical Orthopaedics and Related Research*, vol. 453, pp. 265–271, 2006.

[8] M. A. Kester, L. Herrera, A. Wang, and A. Essner, "Knee bearing technology: where is technology taking us?," *The Journal of Arthroplasty*, vol. 22, no. 7, pp. 16–20, 2007.

[9] R. Tsukamoto, P. A. Williams, H. Shoji et al., "Wear of sequentially enhanced 9-Mrad polyethylene in 10 million cycle knee simulation study," *Journal of Biomedical Materials Research Part B: Applied Biomaterials*, vol. 86B, no. 1, pp. 119–124, 2008.

[10] A. Wang, S.-S. Yau, A. Essner, L. Herrera, M. Manley, and J. Dumbleton, "A highly crosslinked UHMWPE for CR and PS total knee arthroplasties," *The Journal of Arthroplasty*, vol. 23, no. 4, pp. 559–566, 2008.

[11] R. M. Meneghini, L. R. Lovro, S. A. Smits, and P. H. Ireland, "Highly cross-linked versus conventional polyethylene in posterior-stabilized total knee arthroplasty at a mean 5-year follow-up," *The Journal of Arthroplasty*, vol. 30, no. 10, pp. 1736–1739, 2015.

[12] Y. Minoda, K. Hata, K. Goto, T. Itohara, and H. Nakamura, "Sequentially annealed highly cross-linked polyethylene reduced in vivo wear particle generation in total knee arthroplasty," *Journal of Orthopaedic Surgery*, vol. 25, no. 2, 2017.

[13] D. H. Le, S. B. Goodman, W. J. Maloney, and J. I. Huddleston, "Current modes of failure in TKA: infection, instability, and stiffness predominate," *Clinical Orthopaedics and Related Research*, vol. 472, no. 7, pp. 2197–2200, 2014.

[14] K. A. Sonn and R. M. Meneghini, "Early failure of sequentially annealed polyethylene in total knee arthroplasty," *Arthroplasty Today*, vol. 6, no. 1, pp. 18–22, 2020.

[15] A. M. Kop, M. B. Pabbruwe, C. Keogh, and E. Swarts, "Oxidation of second generation sequentially irradiated and annealed highly cross-linked X3™ polyethylene tibial bearings," *The Journal of Arthroplasty*, vol. 30, no. 10, pp. 1842–1846, 2015.

[16] D. W. MacDonald, G. B. Higgs, A. F. Chen, A. L. Malkani, M. A. Mont, and S. M. Kurtz, "Oxidation, damage mechanisms, and reasons for revision of sequentially annealed highly crosslinked polyethylene in total knee arthroplasty," *The Journal of Arthroplasty*, vol. 33, no. 4, pp. 1235–1241, 2018.

[17] T. C. J. Partridge, P. N. Baker, S. S. Jameson, J. Mason, M. R. Reed, and D. J. Deehan, "Conventional versus highly cross-linked polyethylene in primary total knee replacement," *The Journal of Bone and Joint Surgery. American Volume*, vol. 102, no. 2, pp. 119–127, 2020.

38

Infected Nonunion of the Distal Femur in the Elderly with Bone Loss: Case Report and Treatment Options

Neven Starčević[1] and Andrija Karačić[2]

[1]Traumatology Department, University Hospital Sveti Duh, Sveti Duh, 64 Zagreb, Croatia
[2]Department of General Surgery, University Hospital Sveti Duh, Sveti Duh, 64 Zagreb, Croatia

Correspondence should be addressed to Andrija Karačić; karacic.andrija@gmail.com

Academic Editor: Johannes Mayr

The management of infected nonunion associated with bone loss in long bones is both a time-consuming and challenging procedure for the orthopedic and trauma surgeon. In this paper, we present the case of a 75-year-old woman with infected nonunion of the distal femur associated with bone loss after plate osteosynthesis for a distal femur fracture. The patient was referred for nonunion of the distal femur after plate fixation (nonlocking "classic" plate) and was treated with a locking compression plate (LCP) and autologous cancellous bone transplant. During the follow-up, the patient was ambulatory without pain; however, the nonunion failed to heal, therefore, the induced membrane technique (Masquelet procedure) was performed in two stages, tissue samples were taken and revealed a bacterial infection (*S. epidermidis*), and antibiotic treatment was started. Due to infection, fracture healing was slowed, but did commence. Unfortunately, the LC plate failed before union occurred, the nonunion was treated with a femoral nail and blocking (Poller) screws, and the bony defect was filled with Ca-P cement. The patient was operated one last time for cement dislocation when not only the dislocated cement was removed but also the femoral nail dynamized. After one year after treatment completion, the fracture healed, and leg length discrepancy was 1.5 cm shorter on the left side. The patient experienced significant pain relief and can walk with the help of crutches. Our paper demonstrates the application of different techniques in fracture surgery as they are required can result in fracture healing even in very adverse circumstances.

1. Background

Distal femoral fractures account for less than 1% of all adult fractures and between 3% and 6% of all femur fractures [1]. Their frequency among age groups is bimodally distributed: on one side, young patients after high-energy trauma, and on the other older, osteoporotic patients after low-energy trauma [2].

Due to their high severity, even today, distal femur fractures pose a great challenge even to the experienced trauma and orthopedic surgeons [3]. They are difficult to manage, and their treatment often leads to unsatisfactory results with nonunion rates as high as 34% [4].

Although there are several treatment options, there are no standard guidelines for the treatment of distal femur fractures. Possible treatment options are open reduction and internal fixation (ORIF) using locking compression plates (LCP), dynamic condylar screws, angled blade plates, and closed reduction and fixation with retrograde intramedullary nails (RIMN). The great diversity of treatment options merely reflects the great challenges associated with this type of fracture [1]. Surgeons often decide on the modality of treatment depending on their experience and knowledge and the tools and implants they have available.

The most feared complication in fracture surgery is nonunion which is associated not only with bone loss and deformity but also frequently with infection [5]. Risk factors for nonunion are not only patient dependent such as gender, age, and comorbidities but also features of the fractures itself: open fractures, intraarticular, or comminuted fractures [3].

The management of an infected nonunion in the distal femur remains one of the greatest challenges in fracture surgery [6]. Not only for the surgeon: distal femur fracture nonunion has a devastating impact on the patient's function and quality of life. We present a case report of a patient whose infected nonunion of distal femur fractures had been treated with different novel techniques such as the Masquelet procedure and revision of a failed locked plate with a locked femoral nail complicated by Ca-P cement dislocation. After a thorough literature review, we could not find any similar cases which mark our case as a technical novelty.

The following case report has been reported in line with the SCARE criteria [7].

2. Case Presentation

The study was conducted in accordance with the principles of the Declaration of Helsinki. The patient has signed informed consent about the treatment she was subjected to and the processing of her personal information.

We present the case of a 75-year-old woman who presented to our outpatient office in a tertiary care facility looking for a second opinion. The patient had been operated on 6 months before, presenting with a left distal femur fracture. Her comorbidities that included diabetes type 2 (well-regulated, on oral medication), arterial hypertension, sideropenic anemia, and medical history show cataracts and varicose vein surgery. Her medical history did not include any diagnostic work-up for osteoporosis. Clinically, the distal left thigh appeared normal on inspection, and palpation revealed tenderness of the delayed union. The range of motion was normal. X-ray showed an atrophic nonunion after "classic" plate fixation of the distal femur fracture with bone loss (Figures 1 and 2).

A reosteosynthesis with autologous cancellous bone transplant was recommended. Unfortunately, a month after the visit, the patient was presented to the emergency room with acute onset pain and instability in the left lower extremity after walking. Classic X-ray showed plate failure and fragment dislocation (Figure 3).

The patient was admitted to the hospital, and surgery was performed after written/informed consent: the first plate was removed, a reosteosynthesis with a titanium locking compression plate was performed, and the defect was filled with an autologous cancellous bone graft from the iliac crest. The postoperative recovery was uneventful, and classic X-ray showed proper plate position (Figures 4 and 5).

Six months after the procedure, on a follow-up visit, the patient complained about pain around the knee. X-rays showed a halt in bone healing (Figure 6), and another procedure was recommended. The first stage of the induced membrane technique (operation of Masquelet) with a poly-methyl methacrylate (PMMA) cement spacer was performed: the fracture fragments were debrided, and the now widened fracture site was filled with cement (PMMA) (Figure 7).

The second stage was scheduled in two months. During the second stage, PMMA bone cement was extracted from the fracture site, and one screw was removed from the plate

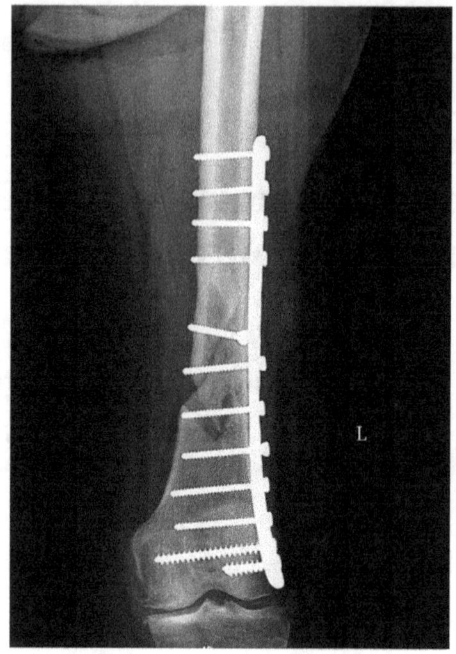

Figure 1: The visible nonunion with the classic plate in AP view.

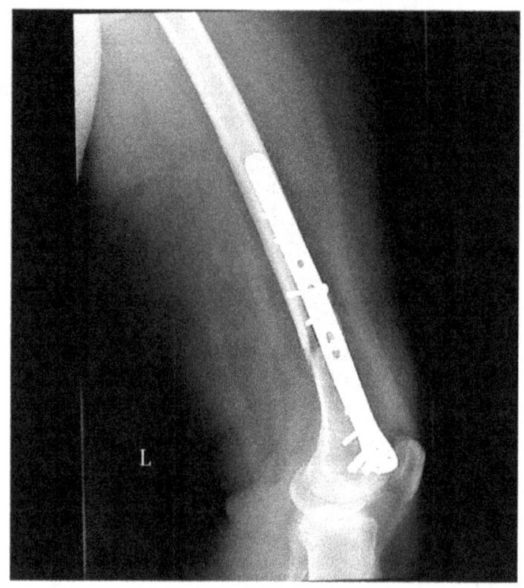

Figure 2: The visible nonunion with the classic plate in LL view.

to lengthen the segment of the plate which is able to bend and therefore prevent breakage. Additionally, an autologous cancellous graft from the proximal tibia mixed with calcium phosphate (Ca-P) cement (Innotere GMBH) was placed in the interfragmentary space.

Tissue samples from the nonunion site were taken. The postoperative recovery was complicated by an episode of fever and elevation of laboratory inflammation markers which was treated successfully with antibiotics. The microbial analysis of the intraoperative fracture site samples confirmed the presence of coagulase-negative *Staphylococcus*, which was treated with antibiotics: ciprofloxacin and clindamycin. Ten months after the last procedure, the was patient presented in our emergency room. She complained about the sudden onset of pain in the left femur during walking, and X-ray confirmed plate breakage (Figure 8).

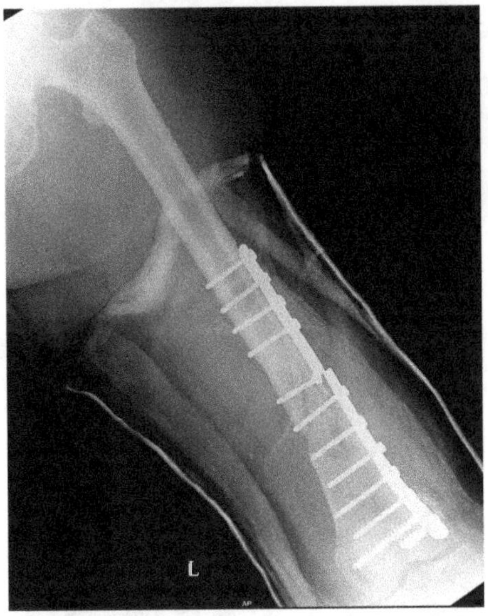

Figure 3: The nonunion with the failed classic plate in AP view.

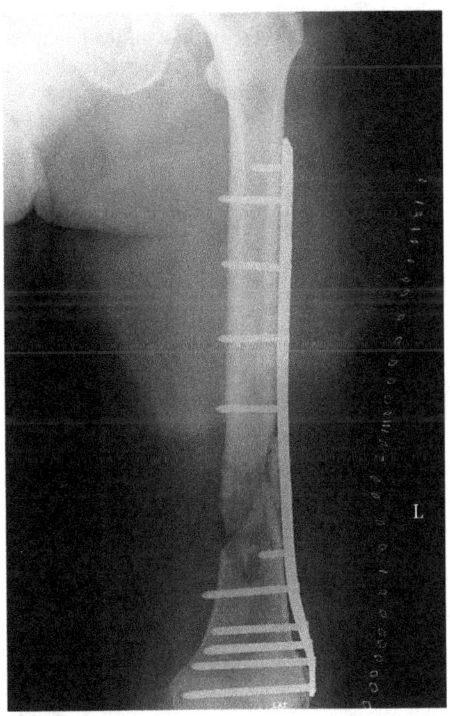

Figure 4: The debrided nonunion with autologous cancellous bone graft stabilized with an LCP in AP view.

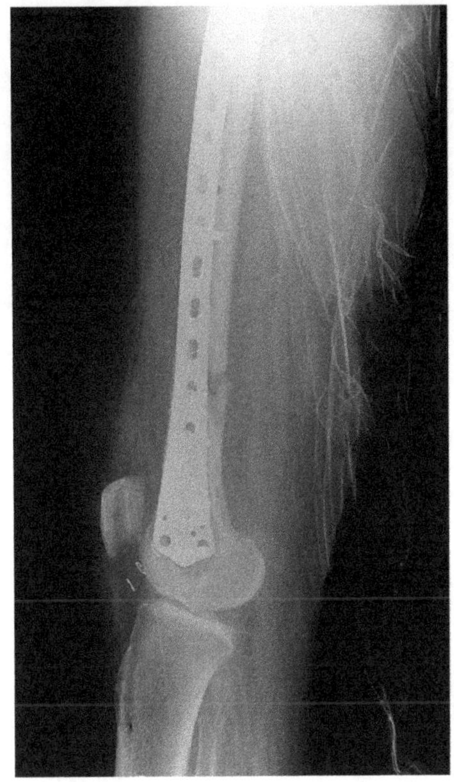

Figure 5: The debrided nonunion with autologous cancellous bone graft stabilized with an LCP in LL view.

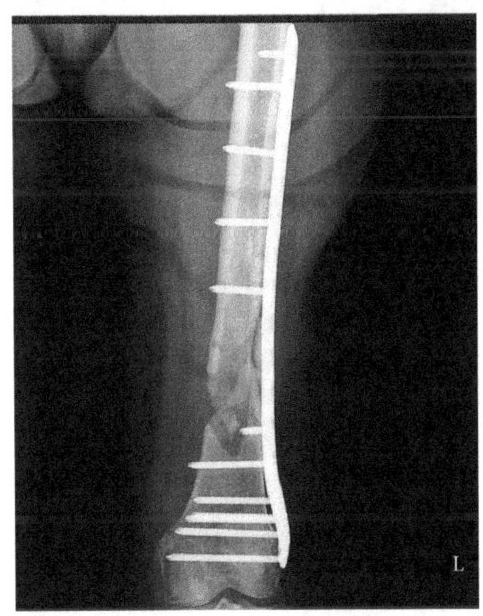

Figure 6: The nonunion is widened, with the plate providing stability in AP view.

The patient was admitted to the hospital again and prepared for surgery: during surgery, the broken plate was extracted, and a locked femoral nail (Stryker) was inserted guided by blocking (Poller) screws. The defect was filled with calcium phosphate cement (Innotere GMBH) (Figure 9).

Again, microbial samples were taken, and *Corynebacterium macginleyi* was detected which was treated with targeted antibiotic therapy. The surgical wound showed signs of infection in the form of minimal serous secretion. The wound was dressed weekly. In one of the regular follow-ups, the patient presented with a tumefaction in the lateral thigh at the site of the surgical wound. A puncture was performed, serous fluid was evacuated, and a sample was sent for microbial analysis. Classic X-ray detected the cause of the tumefaction: a part of the cement dislocated from the fracture site into the surrounding tissue.

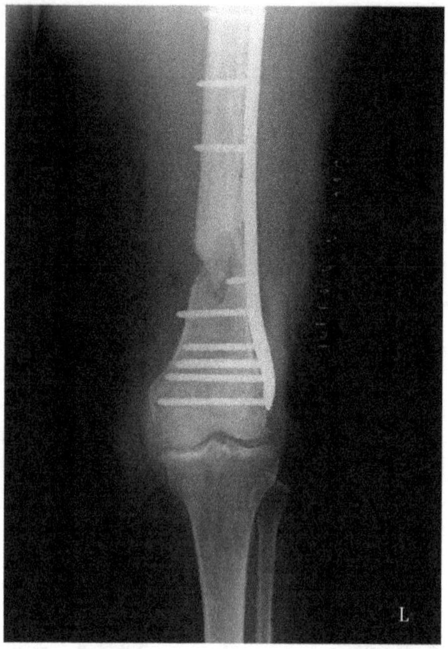

FIGURE 7: The first stage of the induced membrane technique (IMT), the nonunion is partially filled with PMMA cement. The cement is encircled.

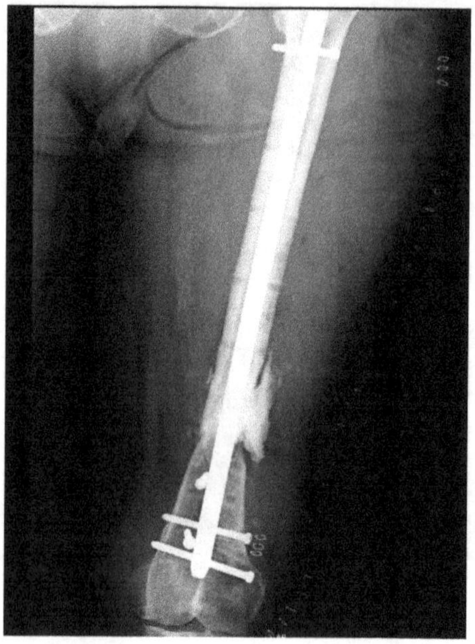

FIGURE 9: The plate was removed, the nonunion was stabilized with a locked intramedullary nail (the position of the nail is secured with Poller blocking screws (marked by arrows)), and the defect was filled with a mixture of cancellous bone graft and Ca-P cement (encircled).

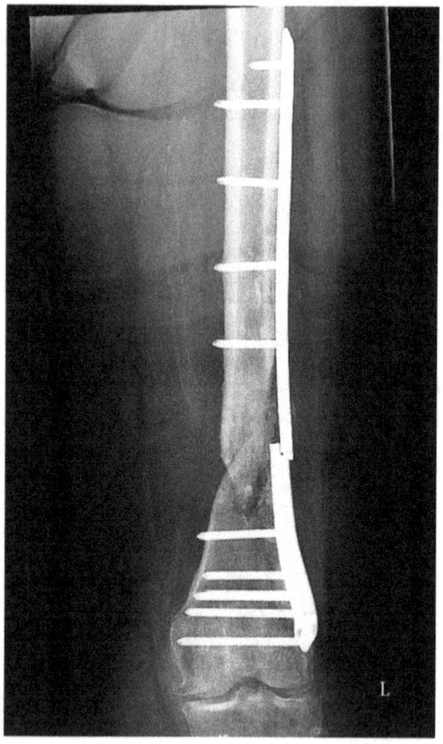

FIGURE 8: The nonunion is readily visible, and the LCP has failed in AP view.

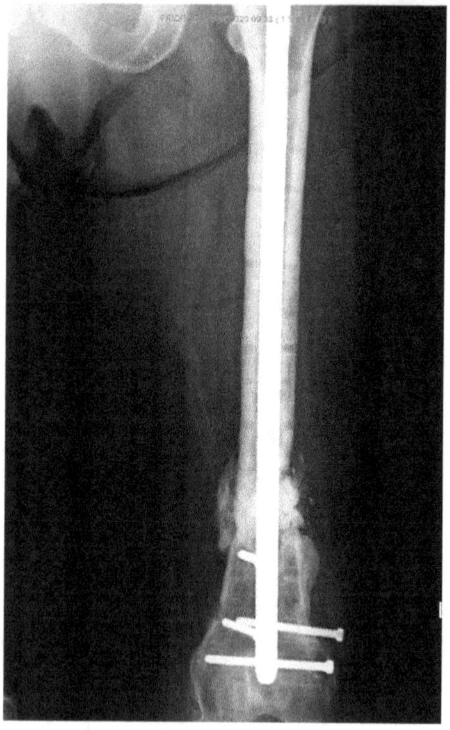

FIGURE 10: Healing of the nonunion after nailing and dynamization in a favorable position is evident, AP view.

Again, the patient was hospitalized for surgery. Secondary dynamization of the femoral nail was performed, and the dislocated cement was removed from the soft tissue. Follow-up was regular, and bone healing was uneventful (Figures 10–12).

One year after the last procedure and three and a half years after the first procedure for the distal femoral fracture, the patient has much less pain and can walk without assistance. Leg length discrepancy was 1.5 cm shorter on the left side.

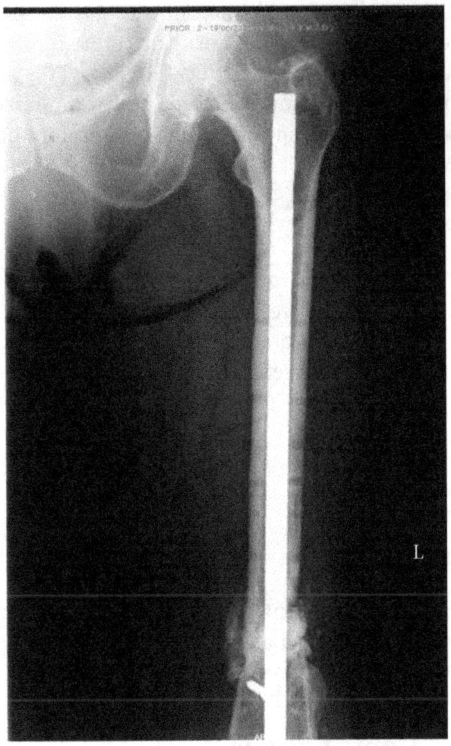

FIGURE 11: Healing of the nonunion after nailing and dynamization in a favorable position is evident, and the tip of the nail does not protrude into the abductor muscles, AP view.

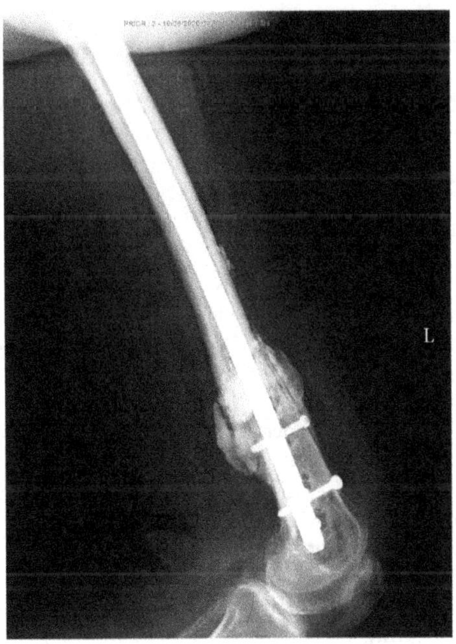

FIGURE 12: Healing of the nonunion after nailing and dynamization in a favorable position is evident, LL view.

3. Discussion

The allure of distal femur fracture surgery is the multiple options the surgeon can deploy for a particular case, while knowing that out of the many options, only one is usually the most appropriate.

This paper demonstrates our approach to this very complex case and how we managed all the problems we encountered along the way with the resources and implants we had at our disposal.

Historically, from the 1960s, onward distal femur fractures were treated conservatively with fracture bracing and traction with success rates up to 67-90% [8]. Only with the development new surgical techniques and technologies the approach has shifted from conservative to surgical stabilization. Especially advances in the understanding of the anatomy and biology of distal femur fractures have led to the introduction of new techniques optimizing surgical treatment.

The fundamental goal of surgical stabilization is to achieve the best as possible reduction and maximal stability. If the risk of nonunion is clearly present, it is recommended to use autologous bone grafts to improve stability and optimize the healing process [9].

Today, the most popular surgical options for distal femur fractures are locking plating (LCP) and retrograde intramedullary nailing (RIMN) with our without a bone graft [3]. These two methods have shown better results than nonlocking plates [10] with minimal differences between each other [11]. Nevertheless, both procedures have nonunion rates from 0% to 34% [1, 4].

In this case report, the following risk factors for nonunion were present: female sex, old age, and diabetes, as well as inappropriate surgical techniques. The authors think that the initial treatment should be criticized for implant selection. Complex cases such as this with an established risk for nonunion call for a fixation system that renders absolute stability while avoiding excessive rigidity of the system itself, for which the "classic" plate fixation is known for. Additionally, we believe that the shortness of the plate and screw positioning compromised the stability of the implant which led to the nonunion and fatigue failure of the implant.

In retrospect, the authors believe that the LCP was also not an appropriate option for the same reason as the "classic" plate fixation. Gautier and Sommer recommend LCP only as bridging plates in achieving relative stability [12] which when analyzing our case makes perfect sense. LCPs have become the predominant treatment option of distal femur fractures because of the high stability afforded, and the minimal amount of periosteal stripping makes the technique less disruptive and invasive but also less technically demanding [13]. Another advantage is their ability to gain fixation in the very distal articular fragments [14]. Despite the advantages, distal femoral fractures treated with LCPs are associated with significant complications: from implant failure to delayed and eventually nonunion [15]. Different reviews with up to 31 cases of distal femur fracture nonunion have shown that LCPs are unfortunately rarely the definitive treatment option [16–18].

After the failure of the LCP technique, one option was the ring external fixator first developed by Ilizarov to achieve bone transport [19]; however, we do not have access to the Ilizarov external fixator. Another possible approach was to use a fibular strut either autogenous or from a bone bank which provides a degree of immediate stability while being osteoinductive and osteoconductive.

Eventually, the decision in our case fell for the Masquelet technique, which in our case has been found to be effective in achieving union. The Masquelet technique, first reported by Masquelet in 2000 [20], is also called the induced membrane technique (IMT). It has been used to reconstruct larger diaphyseal defects. It is a two-stage procedure. During the first stage procedure, an extensive debridement of the site and stabilization of the fracture is performed. The next step is the insertion of a poly-methyl methacrylate (PMMA) spacer into the bone defect. The spacer is thought to act as a foreign body, and its goal is to induce the formation and maturation of a biological membrane encapsulating the bone defect. In the second stage, preferably after 4-8 weeks, the spacer is removed through a longitudinal incision to preserve the biological membrane; and in its place, an autologous cancellous bone graft is placed. The key of the procedure is the induced membrane akin to the periosteum. It is highly vascularized and contains osteogenic cells and growth factors [21]. It forms a closed environment stimulating bone regeneration while at the same time limiting the resorption of autologous bone graft when present. Additionally, it acts as a physical barrier preventing the intrusion of soft tissue and providing a degree of mechanical stability. Today, no clear consensus exists on the optimal approach for this technique, while many different modifications and advancements have been reported [22]. Likewise, outcomes differ largely between those variations [23]. But it is, in general, an effective technique to achieve infection eradication and bone union in around 80% of cases [24].

In this particular case, the authors believe that the combination of the induced membrane technique (Masquelet procedure) as a biological stimulus and the stability provided by the locked intramedullary femoral nail was crucial in obtaining bone healing. The authors believe that we have accomplished the goal to restore the axis of the lower limb when weight bearing without disruption of the extensor apparatus [25].

We would like to draw attention to the Ca-P cement dislocation that developed postoperatively. This rare complication was not reported earlier in the literature after the Masquelet procedure which makes our case even more unique. It is important to perform an X-ray for tumefactions at the operation wound to rule out this very rare complication.

This brief summary explores the alternatives that could have been used and illustrates the aforementioned multiple options the surgeon has when dealing with this challenge.

Another very important aspect of patient management in these cases is the antibiotic regimen, and the duration of treatment which is beyond the orthopedic and trauma surgeon and consultation with an infectious disease specialist is paramount. The same is true for dealing with complications of antibiotics.

4. Conclusion

This paper illustrates the significance of adequate primary surgery because revisions are always much more complicated; however, even in these challenging circumstances, the basic principles are still true. A solid grasp of these principles allows the surgeon to tailor the treatment plan according to the patient and technical abilities to achieve a satisfactory end result and overcome any complications that may arise in this long and difficult journey for the patient and the surgeon.

Abbreviations

RIMN: Retrograde intramedullary nailing
LCP: Locking compression plate
IMT: Induced membrane technique
PMMA: Poly-methyl methacrylate cement.

Data Availability

Not applicable.

Consent

Written informed consent for the publication of this study has been given by the patient. Written informed consent has been given by the patient.

Authors' Contributions

Neven Starcevic performed all surgical procedures on the patient at our institution. Both authors wrote the case report manuscript and performed the literature review together.

Acknowledgments

The authors thank Zarko Rasic (Professor and Chief of Department of General Surgery, University Hospital Sveti Duh).

References

[1] F. W. J. Gwathmey, S. M. Jones-Quaidoo, D. Kahler, S. Hurwitz, and Q. Cui, "Distal femoral fractures: current concepts," *The Journal of the American Academy of Orthopaedic Surgeons*, vol. 18, no. 10, pp. 597–607, 2010.

[2] O. Martinet, J. Cordey, Y. Harder, A. Maier, M. Bühler, and G. E. Barraud, "La epidemiologia de las fracturas del femur distal," *Injury*, vol. 31, pp. 62–94, 2000.

[3] F. Pogliacomi, C. Artoni, F. Calderazzi et al., "Distal femur nonunion treated with retrograde intramedullary nailing and RIA: a case report," *Acta Bio-Medica*, vol. 91, no. 4-S, pp. 259–266, 2020.

[4] W. M. Ricci, P. N. Streubel, S. Morshed, C. A. Collinge, S. E. Nork, and M. J. Gardner, "Risk factors for failure of locked plate fixation of distal femur fractures: an analysis of 335 cases," *Journal of Orthopaedic Trauma*, vol. 28, no. 2, pp. 83–89, 2014.

[5] A. Salduz, Ö. Kaya, H. İ. Balci et al., "Surgical treatment of an infected nonunion of the middle third of the femur associated with femoral shortening in a hemophilia patient," *Case Reports in Orthopedics*, vol. 2016, Article ID 3045262, 4 pages, 2016.

[6] N. A. Ebraheim, G. S. Buchanan, X. Liu et al., "Treatment of distal femur nonunion following initial fixation with a lateral

locking plate," *Orthopaedic Surgery*, vol. 8, no. 3, pp. 323–330, 2016.

[7] R. A. Agha, M. R. Borrelli, R. Farwana et al., "The SCARE 2018 statement: Updating consensus Surgical CAse REport (SCARE) guidelines," *International Journal of Surgery*, vol. 60, pp. 132–136, 2018.

[8] A. Sain, V. Sharma, K. Farooque, M. V, and K. Pattabiraman, "Dual plating of the distal femur: indications and surgical techniques," *Cureus*, vol. 11, no. 12, article e6483, 2019.

[9] A. K. Gangavalli and C. O. Nwachuku, "Management of Distal Femur Fractures in Adults: An Overview of Options," *Orthopedic Clinics of North America*, vol. 47, no. 1, pp. 85–96, 2016.

[10] R. M. Meneghini, B. J. Keyes, K. K. Reddy, and D. C. Maar, "Modern retrograde intramedullary nails versus periarticular locked plates for supracondylar femur fractures after total knee arthroplasty," *The Journal of Arthroplasty*, vol. 29, no. 7, pp. 1478–1481, 2014.

[11] H. Magill, N. Ponugoti, A. Selim, and J. Platt, "Locked compression plating versus retrograde intramedullary nailing in the treatment of periprosthetic supracondylar knee fractures: a systematic review and meta-analysis," *Journal of Orthopaedic Surgery and Research*, vol. 16, no. 1, pp. 1-9, 2021.

[12] E. Gautier and C. Sommer, "Guidelines for the clinical application of the LCP," *Injury*, vol. 34, pp. 63–76, 2003.

[13] E. N. Kubiak, E. Fulkerson, E. Strauss, and K. A. Egol, "The evolution of locked plates," *The Journal of Bone and Joint Surgery*, vol. 88, supplement 4, pp. 189–200, 2006.

[14] E. K. Rodriguez, C. Boulton, M. J. Weaver et al., "Predictive factors of distal femoral fracture nonunion after lateral locked plating: a retrospective multicenter case-control study of 283 fractures," *Injury*, vol. 45, no. 3, pp. 554–559, 2014.

[15] C. E. Henderson, L. L. Kuhl, D. C. Fitzpatrick, and J. L. Marsh, "Locking plates for distal femur fractures: is there a problem with fracture healing?," *Journal of Orthopaedic Trauma*, vol. 25, Supplement 1, pp. S8–14, 2011.

[16] M. J. Gardner, J. B. Toro-Arbelaez, M. Harrison, C. Hierholzer, D. G. Lorich, and D. L. Helfet, "Open reduction and internal fixation of distal femoral nonunions: long-term functional outcomes following a treatment protocol," *Journal of Trauma and Acute Care Surgery*, vol. 64, no. 2, pp. 434–438, 2008.

[17] C. Bellabarba, W. M. Ricci, and B. R. Bolhofner, "Results of indirect reduction and plating of femoral shaft nonunions after intramedullary nailing," *Journal of Orthopaedic Trauma*, vol. 15, no. 4, pp. 254–263, 2001.

[18] M. W. Chapman and C. G. Finkemeier, "Treatment of supracondylar nonunions of the femur with plate fixation and bone graft," *The Journal of Bone & Joint Surgery*, vol. 81, no. 9, pp. 1217–1228, 1999.

[19] R. Bhardwaj, J. Singh, R. Kapila, and R. S. Boparai, "Comparision of Ilizarov ring fixator and rail fixator in infected nonunion of long bones: a retrospective followup study," *Indian journal of orthopaedics*, vol. 53, no. 1, pp. 82–88, 2019.

[20] A. C. Masquelet, F. Fitoussi, T. Begue, and G. P. Muller, "Reconstruction of the long bones by the induced membrane and spongy autograft," *Annales de chirurgie plastique et esthetique*, vol. 45, no. 3, pp. 346–353, 2000.

[21] P. Pelissier, A. C. Masquelet, R. Bareille, S. M. Pelissier, and J. Amedee, "Induced membranes secrete growth factors including vascular and osteoinductive factors and could stimulate bone regeneration," *Journal of orthopaedic research*, vol. 22, no. 1, pp. 73–79, 2004.

[22] P. V. Giannoudis, O. Faour, T. Goff, N. Kanakaris, and R. Dimitriou, "Masquelet technique for the treatment of bone defects: Tips-tricks and future directions," *Injury*, vol. 42, no. 6, pp. 591–598, 2011.

[23] I. Morelli, L. Drago, D. A. George, E. Gallazzi, S. Scarponi, and C. L. Romanò, "Masquelet technique: myth or reality? A systematic review and meta-analysis," *Injury*, vol. 47, pp. S68–S76, 2016.

[24] B. Fung, G. Hoit, E. Schemitsch, C. Godbout, and A. Nauth, "The induced membrane technique for the management of long bone defects," *The Bone & Joint Journal*, vol. 102-B, no. 12, pp. 1723–1734, 2020.

[25] J. A. Ryan, K. N. Meyers, P. DiBenedetto, T. M. Wright, and S. B. Haas, "Failure of the patellar tendon with the patella everted versus noneverted in a matched-pair cadaver model," *HSS Journal*, vol. 6, no. 2, pp. 134–137, 2010.

Complications after Dynamic Hip Screw Osteosynthesis of Proximal Femoral Fractures at Army Instructional Hospital-Libreville

F. M. Bombah,[1] **M. Diawara**,[2] **B. Y. Ekani**,[3] **T. Nana**,[3] **and A. Mikiela**[2]

[1]*Department of Surgery, Faculty of Medicine and Pharmaceutical Sciences, University of Douala, Cameroon*
[2]*Orthopedic and Traumatologic Surgery Department, Army Instructional Hospital, Libreville, Gabon*
[3]*Department of Surgery, Faculty of Medicine and Pharmaceutical Sciences, University of Buea, Cameroon*

Correspondence should be addressed to F. M. Bombah; bombahstick@hotmail.fr

Academic Editor: George Mouzopoulos

The DHS system is an effective means of open reduction and internal fixation of proximal femur fractures. Postoperative complications are little described and deserve to be studied for better preventive and curative treatment. We report the observations of five (5) patients who presented postoperative complications specific to the DHS system at army instructional Hospital-Libreville. These described complications are related to deterioration of internal fixation leading to callus, nonunion, or infection. Those found are the cut out phenomenon, avascular necrosis of the femoral head, and the fracture of the DHS system. All these complications required surgical revision without functional repercussions at the last follow-up. Complications of internal fixation by the DHS system can be avoided by rigorous asepsis, adequate indications for surgery, and rigorous surgical techniques. Good management can restore hip function.

1. Introduction

The DHS system is an effective means of open reduction and internal fixation of proximal femur fractures [1]. It was developed from 1980 by Richards Manufacturing and has been the subject of numerous studies [2, 3]. It has very precise indications and requires practical experience. Postoperative complications are poorly described [4] and deserve to be studied for better preventive and curative treatment. We report the observations of five (5) patients who presented postoperative complications specific to the DHS system.

2. Observations: (Table 1)

2.1. Case 1. 42-year-old patient, motorcycle driver, was a victim of a blunt trauma to the right thigh after a road traffic accident on his motorcycle. The diagnosis of subtrochanteric fracture classified 32C3 according to AO/OTA (Figure 1(a)) is made and a dynamic compressive plate osteosynthesis performed in a clinic. The patient is referred to us 2 weeks postoperatively for posttraumatic plate removal (Figure 1(b)). The plate was deposited, and an osteosynthesis by the DHS system was performed. The evolution after six (6) postoperative months is marked by atrophic pseudarthrosis and a rupture of the plate in the 8th month (Figure 1(c)). The management consisted of a cure of nonunion, a spongy graft, and the internal fixation by a locking plate for proximal femur (Figure 1(d)). At the last follow-up (9 months), the functional [5] and radiological results (presence of callus) were very good.

2.2. Case 2. A 64-year-old trader was brought in an hour after trauma to the right hip in a car accident. The clinical and paraclinical examination made it possible to make the diagnosis of transcervical fracture of the femoral neck classified 31B2.3 according to AO/OTA (Figure 2(a)). The DHS was applied 5 days after the trauma under image intensifier. The course is marked by pain in the hip, pseudarthrosis of

Table 1: Case series.

Cases	Age	Sex	Diagnostic	AO/ OTA	Complication			Treatment
					Disturbed healing	Mechanical	Vascular	
1	42	M	Subtroch	32B2a	Subtrochanteric pseudarthrosis	DHS plate fracture	/	Plate
2	64	M	Transcervical	31B2.3	Neck pseudarthrosis	Cut out phenomenon	Cephalic avascular necrosis	PHRA
3	56	F	Pertroch.	32A2	Neck pseudarthrosis	Cut out phenomenon	Cephalic avascular necrosis	THRA
4	65	M	Pertroch.	31A1.3	Malunion	Cut out phenomenon, DHS sliding screw fracture	/	Remove of DHS system
5	46	M	Pertroch.	31A1.2	Infection	/	/	Necrosectomy, washing drainage

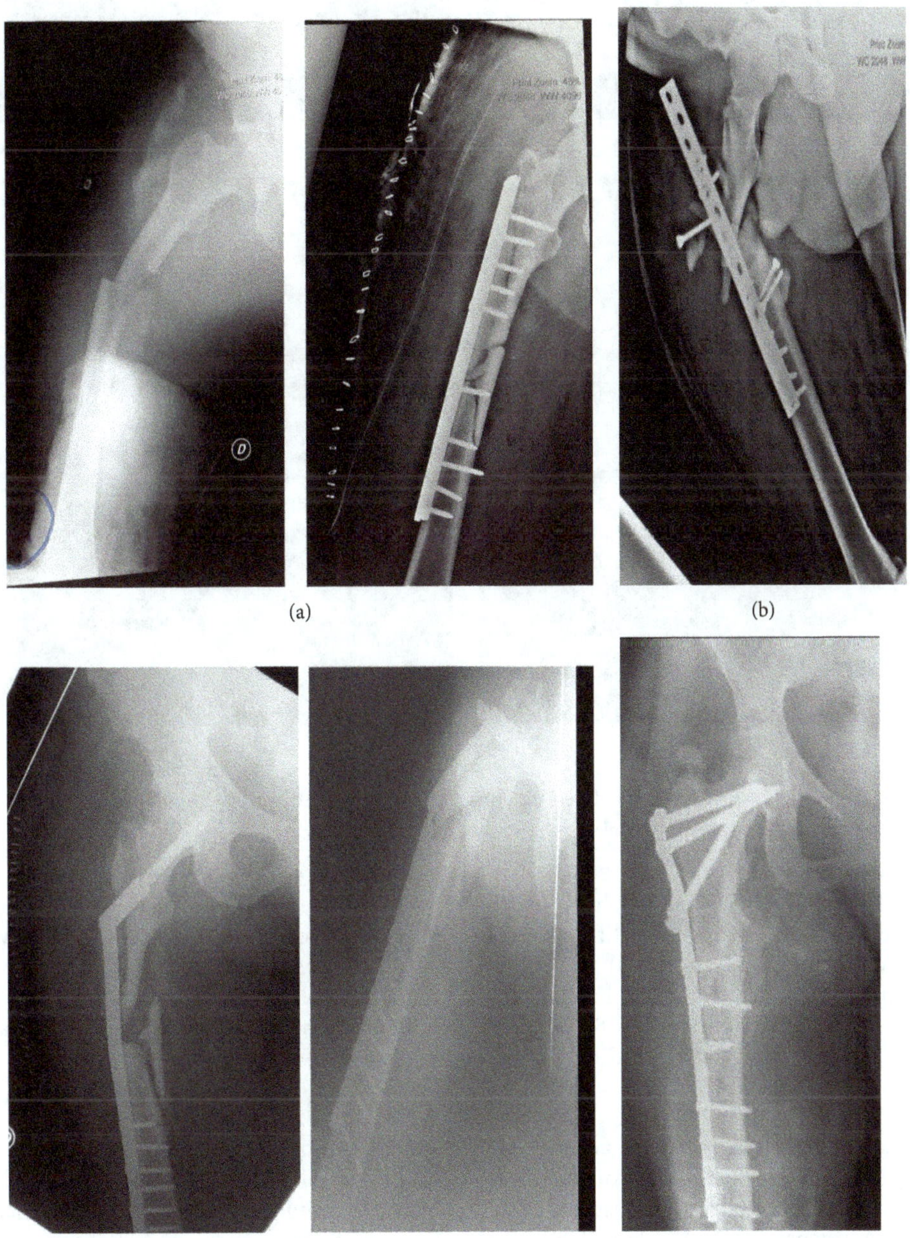

(a) (b) (c) (d)

Figure 1: X-ray of case 1: ((a) subtrochanteric fracture; (b) missed fixation of DCP; (c) atrophic nonunion with fracture of the DHS system; (d) locked plate osteosynthesis).

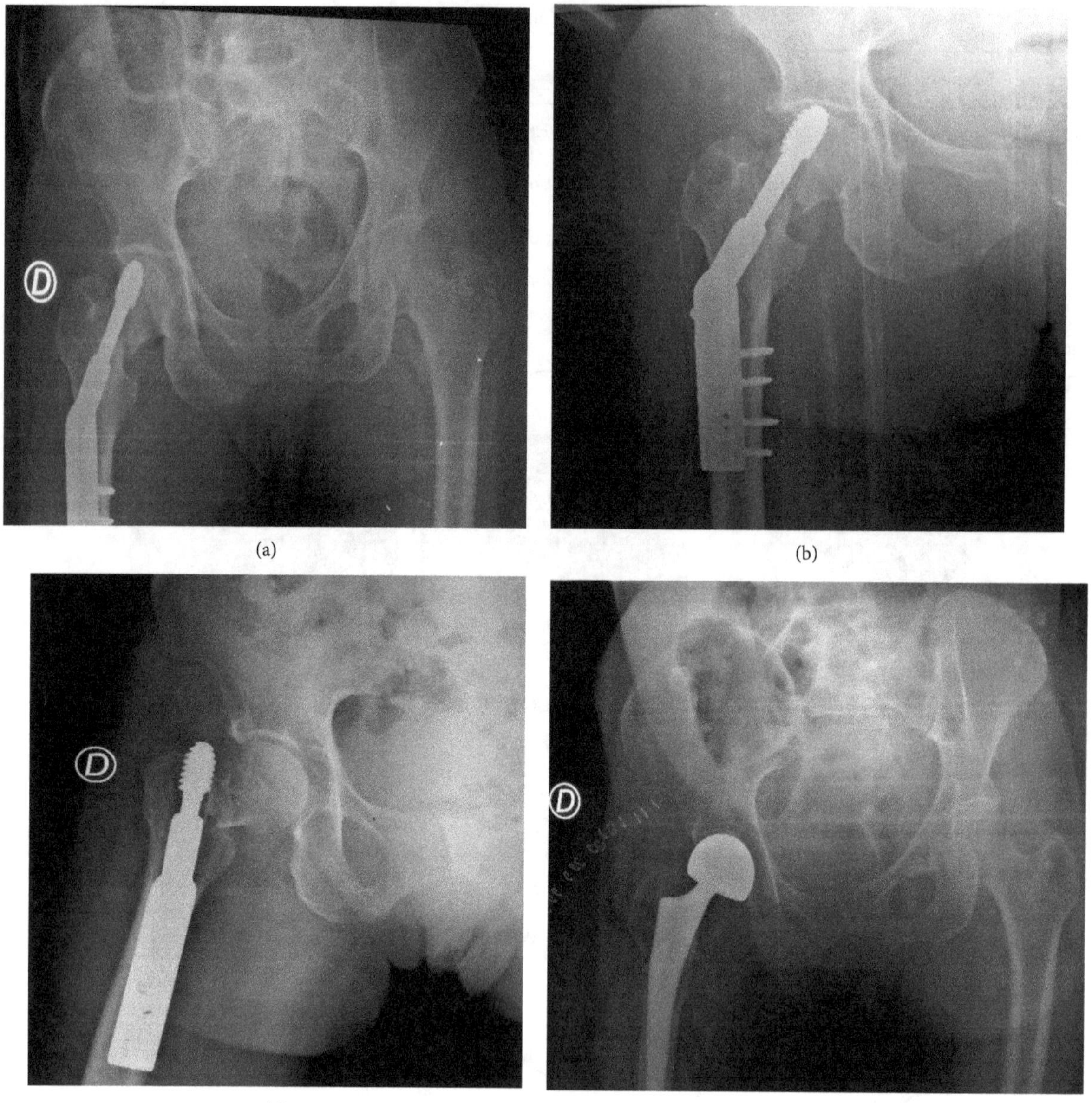

Figure 2: X-rays of patient 2. (a) DHS osteosynthesis of neck fracture. (b) Neck pseudarthrosis with phenomenon. (c) Cut out phenomenon with cephalic osteonecrosis. (d) Right hemiarthroplasty.

the fracture site, and necrosis of the femoral head and a gradual migration of the DHS system objectified in the 4th (Figure 2(b)) and 6th month (Figure 2(c)) postoperatively. The management consisted of a hip hemiarthroplasty (Figure 2(d)). At the last follow-up (18 months), the functional result was very good according to the PMA scale [5].

2.3. Case 3. A 56-year-old female farmer was received one hour from trauma to her right hip after falling from a motorcycle. The diagnosis of a basicervical fracture classified 32A2 according to AO/OTA (Figure 3(a)). A 7-hole DHS was installed. The evolution is marked by a vicious callus in the subtrochanteric region in the 4th postoperative month and pseudarthrosis of the femoral neck (Figure 3(b)). In the 6th postoperative month, osteonecrosis of the femoral head and dynamic screw migration is observed (Figure 3(c)). The DHS was removed, and an uncemented total hip prosthesis was placed. At the last follow-up (24 months), the functional and radiological results were satisfactory according to the PMA scale [5].

2.4. Case 4. A 65-year-old male farmer sustained injuries when a motorbike hit him onto his right hip. At presentation, he was hemodynamically stable, and radiographs confirmed a minimally displaced pertrochanteric fracture of the right hip class 31A1.3 according to AO/OTA (Figure 4). The fracture was stabilized using DHS system after 72 h. The patient had an uneventful peri-operative period and was allowed partial weight bearing. At his six

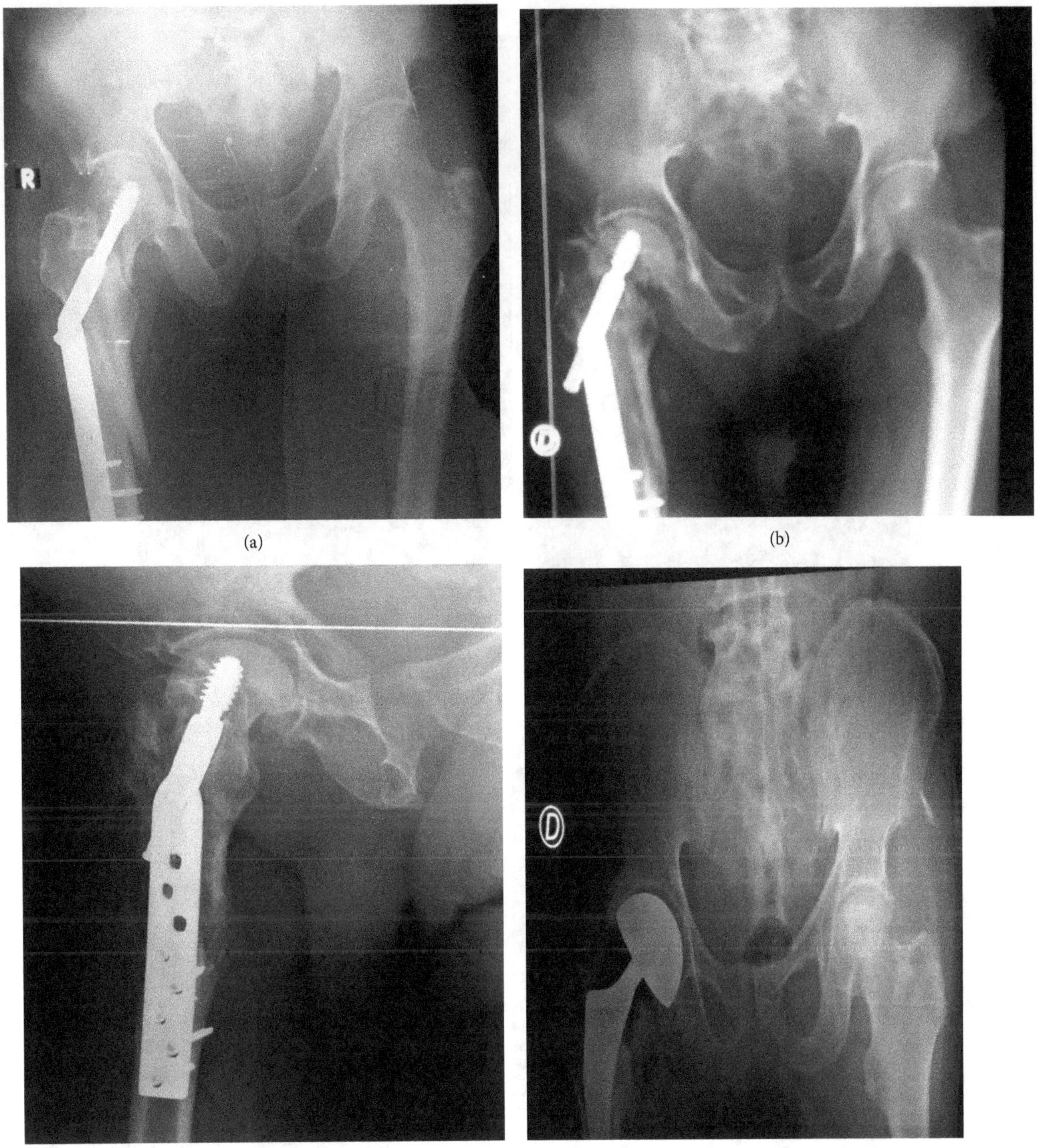

(a) (b) (c) (d)

FIGURE 3: X-rays of patient 3. (a) Osteosynthesis y DHS. (b) Subtrochanteric malunion with pseudarthrosis of femur neck. (c) Cut out phenomenon. (d) Hemiarthroplasty.

week outpatients' clinic appointment, radiographs showed callus and sliding screw fracture. He was therefore permitted full weight bearing after the removed of DHS system. One year after surgery, radiographs showed vicious callus with very good functional result [5]. He has returned to full-time work and is able to participate in low-impact recreational sporting activity.

2.5. Case 5. A 46-year-old male driver was involved in a high-speed motorbike accident in which he sustained injuries onto his right hip. At presentation, he was hemodynamically stable, and radiographs confirmed a minimally displaced pertrochanteric fracture of the left hip class 31A1.2 according to AO/OTA (Figure 5). The fracture was stabilized using the DHS system (Figure 4(b)) after 3 days. The patient had an uneventful peri-operative period and was allowed partial weight bearing. At his nine month outpatients' clinic appointment, suppuration next to the operative scar is the objective, and radiographs showed callus at the proximal femoral fracture. Staphylococcus

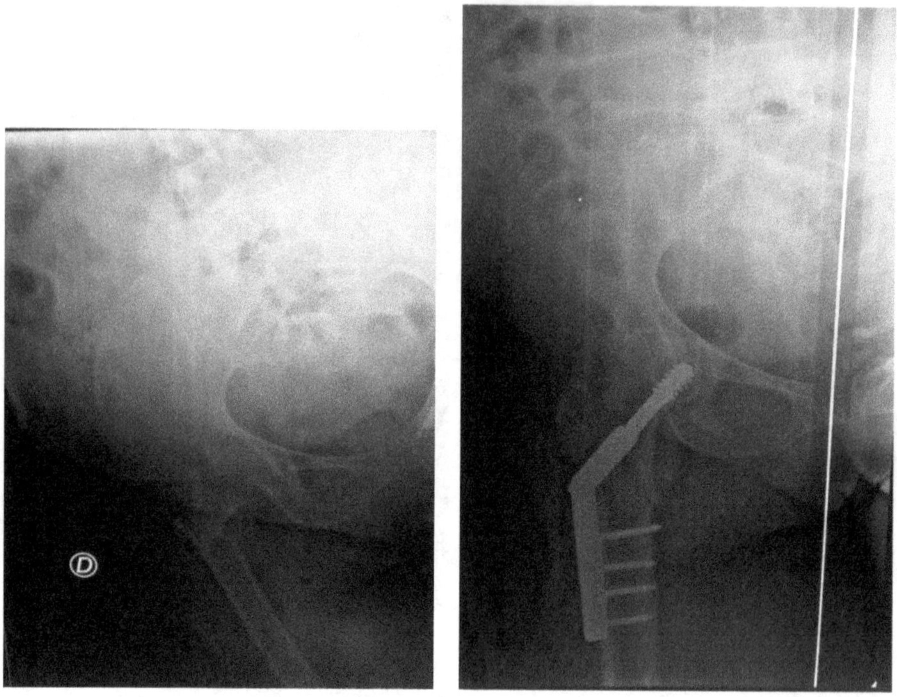

(a) (b)

FIGURE 4: X-rays of patient 4. (a) Pertrochanteric fracture type 31A1.3 AO/OTA. (b) Osteosynthesis by DHS.

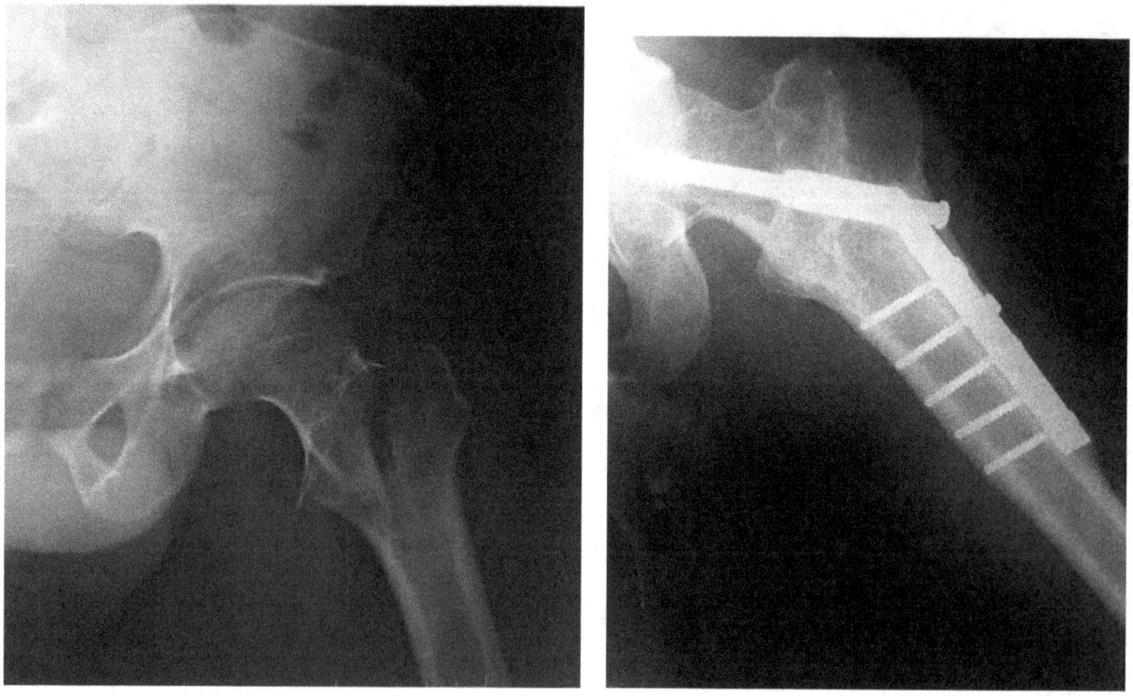

(a) (b)

FIGURE 5: X-rays of patient 5. (a) Pertrochanteric fracture of the left hip class 31A1.2 according to AO/OTA. (b) Osteosynthesis by DHS.

aureus has been identified. The DHS system was removed followed by necrosectomy, washing, and drainage. He has returned to full-time work and is able to participate in recreational sporting activity.

3. Discussion

Postoperative complications of DHS are rare and not enough described [4]. The various complications described are linked to deterioration of internal fixation leading to vicious callus, nonunion, or infection [1]. These complications are the cut out phenomenon, avascular necrosis of the femoral head, fracture of the DHS system, femoral plate fracture, and progression of coxarthrosis [4]. They represent a rate of 6% (22/367) according to Hrubina et al. [4]. We found 5 (6.5%) cases out of 77 internal fixation by DHS. We will discuss the indications, complications, and end treatments of our patients in light of the literature.

The DHS system is indicated mainly for trochanteric fractures. It is easy to set up and gives good results. However, it has limitations in cases of fracture of the lateral pillar of the upper extremity of the femur and comminution of the greater trochanter (case 3) [1].

Infection, although late, is a rare and serious complication. It can involve the vital and functional prognosis of the patient. We find 1 case of infection with Staphylococcus aureus. It is comparable with other relevant studies [6].

Malunion is a frequent complication of trochanteric osteosynthesis 12% for Decoulx and Lavarde [7] and lavender and 5% for Hrubina et al. [8]. It is due to an overestimation of bone quality and/or a technical error. We found 3/77 (3.9%) vicious calluses, one in the trochantero-diaphyseal region (patient 3) and 2 on the trochanteric mass in patient 4 and patient 5. These vicious calluses were tolerable and were not need a secondary realignment.

Pseudarthrosis is rare in the trochanteric mass because the vascularization is excellent [1]. On the femoral neck, there is a risk of cervical nonunion, whether or not associated with cephalic necrosis [9]. We noted 2 cases of nonunion of the cervix with avascular necrosis of the femoral head in patient 2 and patient 4. Hrubina et al. found 2 (0.5%) cases of nonunion in a series of 367 osteosynthesis by the DHS system.

Cut out phenomenon is a complication described in cases of osteoporosis in the elderly [1, 4]. It is also described in cases of targeting errors or progressive impaction of the fracture site. We find 3 cases (case 2, case 3, and case 4) in elderly patients with progressive impaction of the fracture site [10].

There are few articles about the metal breakage after the DHS osteosynthesis. For Hrubina et al. [8], there is metal breakage of K-wire, cortical screws, and sliding screw. We have seen a metal breakage of plate (case 1) and sliding screw (case 4).

4. Conclusion

Postoperative complications from internal fixation by DHS are at army instructional Hospital in Libreville. They are sometimes result from the failings of surgeons. They can be avoided by rigorous asepsis, adequate surgical indications, and rigorous surgical techniques. Good management of its complications can restore hip function.

Authors' Contributions

Freddy Mertens Bombah did the conceptualization, data curation, and writing-original draft. Mohamadou Diawara did the conceptualization and writing-review and editing. Théophile Nana and Boukar Yannick Ekani did the writing-review and editing. Anicet Mikiela did the editing and supervision.

References

[1] A. Morvan, J. Boddaert, J. Cohen-Bittan, H. Picard, H. Pascal-Mousselard, and F. Khiami, "Risk factors for cut-out after internal fixation of trochanteric fractures in elderly subjects," *Orthopaedics & Traumatology: Surgery & Research*, vol. 104, no. 8, pp. 1183–1187, 2018.

[2] P. Oger, V. Katz, N. Lecorre, and P. H. Beaufils, "Fracture of the great trochanter treated by dynamic hip screw plate: measure of impaction according to fracture type," *Revue de Chirurgie Orthopedique et Reparatrice de l'appareil Moteur*, vol. 84, no. 6, pp. 539–545, 1998.

[3] Y. H. Cha, J. I. Yoo, S. Y. Hwang et al., "Biomechanical evaluation of internal fixation of pauwels type III femoral neck fractures: a systematic review of various fixation methods," *Clinics in Orthopedic Surgery*, vol. 11, no. 1, pp. 1–14, 2019.

[4] M. Hrubina, M. Skotak, and J. Behounek, "Complications of dynamic hip screw treatment for proximal femoral fractures," *Acta Chirurgiae Orthopaedicae et Traumatologiae Cechoslovaca*, vol. 77, no. 5, pp. 395–401, 2010.

[5] D.'a. R. Merle, "Cotation chiffrée de la fonction de hanche," *Revue de Chirurgie Orthopédique et Réparatrice de l'appareil Moteur*, vol. 56, pp. 481–486, 1970.

[6] M. Hrubina, M. Skotak, and J. Behounek, "DHS osteosynthesis for proximal femoral fractures: infectious complications," *Acta Chirurgiae Orthopaedicae et Traumatologiae Cechoslovaca*, vol. 80, no. 5, pp. 351–355, 2013.

[7] P. Decoulx and G. Lavarde, "Les fractures de la région trochantérienne," in *71e congrès français de chirurgie*, Masson, Paris, 1969.

[8] M. Hrubina, M. Skotak, O. Krumpl, and P. Mika, "Osteosynthetic material breakage in patients treated with DHS for proximal femoral fracture," *Rozheledy v Chirurgii: Mesicnik Ceskolovenske Chirurgicke Spolecnosti*, vol. 91, pp. 146–150, 2012.

[9] P. Simon, F. Gouin, D. Veillard et al., "Femoral neck fractures in patients over 50 years old," *Revue de Chirurgie Orthopedique et Reparatrice de l'appareil Moteur*, vol. 94, no. 6, pp. 108–132, 2008.

[10] D. V. Prasad, S. Kumar, Y. Rabari, N. Bhatt, N. Suri, and A. Jadhav, "Comparative study between DHS and PFN in management of trochanteric an subtrochanteric femoral fractures," *International Journal of Orthopaedics*, vol. 3, pp. 106–108, 2017.

Acute Attack of Pseudogout with the Wide Lesion in Lumbar Spondylolytic Spondylolisthesis

Hironari Kaneyama,[1] Yuichiro Morishita,[1] Osamu Kawano,[1] Takuaki Yamamoto,[2] and Takeshi Maeda[1]

[1]*Department of Orthopedic Surgery, Spinal Injuries Center, Iizuka, Japan*
[2]*Department of Orthopedic Surgery, Fukuoka University, Fukuoka, Japan*

Correspondence should be addressed to Yuichiro Morishita; uchiro1968@mac.com

Academic Editor: Taketoshi Yasuda

Objective. To report a rare case of an acute attack of calcium pyrophosphate dihydrate (CPPD) deposition disease in a patient with lumbar spondylolytic spondylolisthesis, which demonstrated widespread lesion with neurological deficit. *Methods.* An 86-year-old woman presented with high fever and bilateral neurological deficit of the lower extremities. *Results.* CRP was elevated (20.9 mg/dl). Plain radiographs and computed tomography images showed bilateral L4 spondylolytic spondylolisthesis. Sagittal magnetic resonance (MR) images revealed effusion at the L3-4 interspinous space, and a gadolinium- (GD-) enhanced epidural mass was observed at the level of L4 vertebral body. Axial MR images showed an intra- or epidural lesion at L2-3. Moreover, epidural GD-enhanced masses compressed the dural sac in the shape of a cross at the L3-4 and L4-5 segments. The patient was suspected of having pyogenic arthritis of the lumbar spine in initial diagnosis. A total of 1.2 ml of fluid with a murky, pus-like synovial effusion was aspirated from the L3-4 interspinous space under the fluoroscopic image. Smear speculum of synovial fluid tested negative for bacteria and fungi; however, a number of crystals were seen. Based on the result of smear speculum, we suspected the pathology as crystal deposition disease. Based on polarized light microscopy, which revealed monocle or triclinic intracellular crystals with a positive birefringence, the patient was diagnosed with pseudogout of the lumbar spine. Nonsteroidal anti-inflammatory drugs (NSAIDs) were administered by intravenous drip injection for 3 days, and local and systemic inflammatory signs, as well as neurological deficits, dramatically improved. *Conclusions.* We encountered the rare case of an acute attack of pseudogout with the wide lesion in the lumbar spondylolytic spondylolisthesis. Multiple culture of the effusion provided a definitive diagnosis, which allowed for appropriate, minimally invasive treatment for 8 weeks of NSAID administration that provided the satisfactory recovery from the symptoms.

1. Introduction

Calcium pyrophosphate dihydrate (CPPD) deposition disease is known as "pseudogout" because of the clinical similarity to gouty arthritis [1]. According to the European League Against Rheumatism, four different clinical presentations can be observed: (1) asymptomatic CPPD, (2) osteoarthritis with CPPD, (3) acute CPP crystal arthritis, and (4) chronic CPP inflammatory crystal arthritis.

CPPD deposition disease commonly involves the major peripheral joints. Although CPPD deposition disease of the spine is less common, it can involve the ligamentum flavum; the longitudinal, supraspinous, and interspinous ligaments; the intervertebral discs; and the sacroiliac and apophyseal joint [2–14]. The definitive diagnosis of CPPD deposition disease is suspected on the basis of the clinical picture and radiographic/laboratory findings. The reference standard for the diagnosis of CPPD is based on the

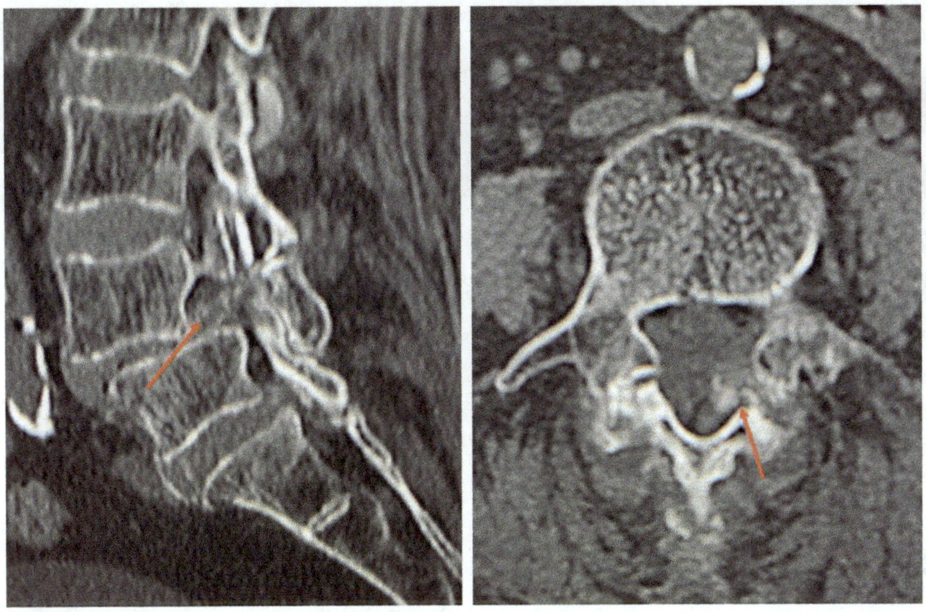

FIGURE 1: A nodular calcification mass was observed from the location of left L4 spondylolysis to the intraspinal canal in plain CT images.

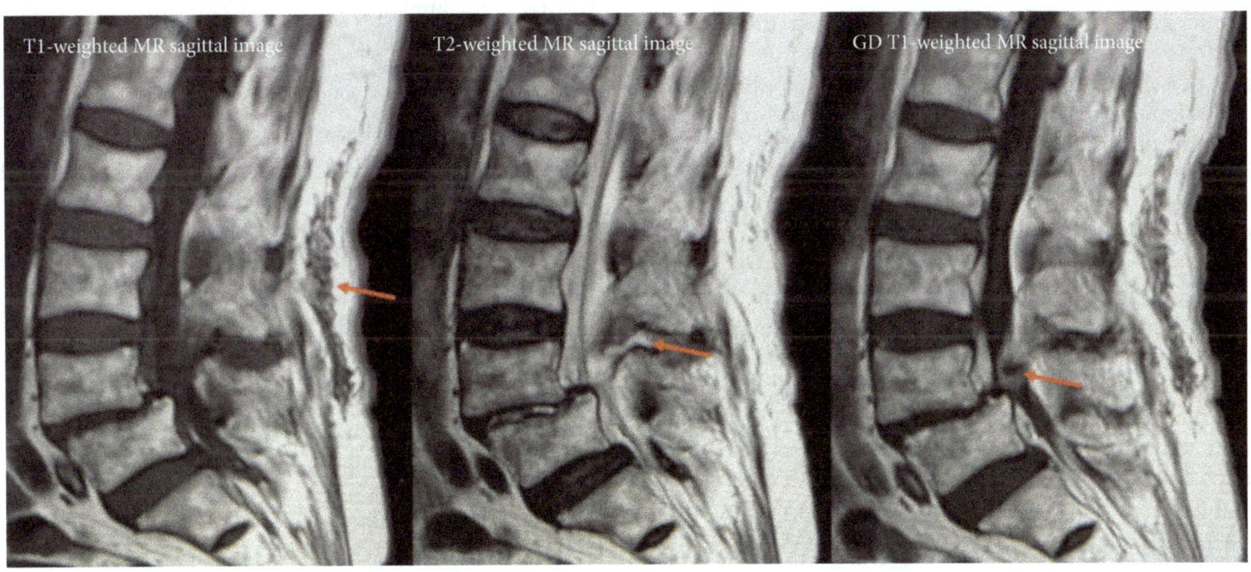

FIGURE 2: An intensity change of the L1-4 supraspinal ligament in T1-weighted images, effusion at the L3-4 interspinous space in T2-weighted images, and a GD-enhanced epidural mass at the level of L4 vertebral body.

identification of CPP crystals in synovial fluid by light microscopy, compensated polarized light microscopy, or phase contrast microscopy [15].

To the best of our knowledge, few reports have thus far referred to an acute attack of pseudogout in the lumbar spine. In our case, there was a large extent of CPPD crystal deposition in the L2-3-4 ligamentum flavum, the L4 spondylolysis, the L3-4 facet joints, and the L3-4 interspinous space. There are no known reports of such widespread related to CPPD crystal deposition in the lumbar spine. We hereby report an acute attack of pseudogout in L4 spondylolytic spondylolisthesis, which demonstrated widespread lesion with neurological deficits.

2. Case Report

An 86-year-old woman presented with sudden low back pain and bilateral lower extremity muscle weakness with numbness. The patient could neither stand alone nor walk unaided. She had bronchitis, with a heavy cough and high fever, a week before the onset of neurological symptoms. The patient had no history of peripheral pseudogout arthritis.

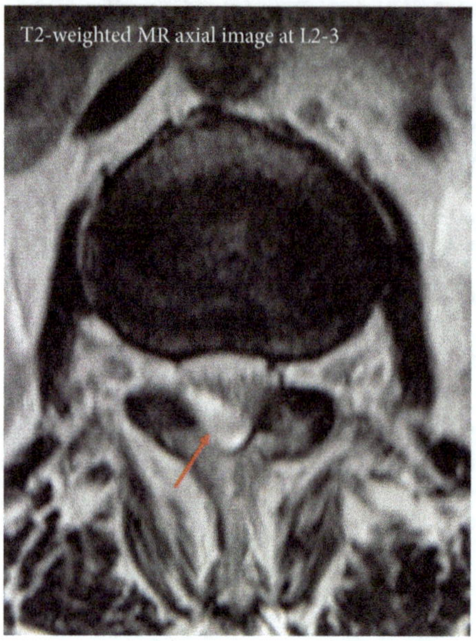

Figure 3: An intra- or epidural lesion at L2-3.

On admission, her body temperature was 37.6°C and she had localized heat and tenderness on her lower back. C-reactive protein (CRP) value was elevated (20.9 mg/dl). Neurological examination was normal for objective sensory evaluation; however, motor function below the iliopsoas was 3 to 4 in manual muscle testing. There were no abnormalities in her deep tendon reflex or pathological reflex.

Plain radiographs of the lumbar spine showed L4 spondylolisthesis without dynamic instability. Plain computed tomography (CT) images showed bilateral L4 spondylolytic spondylolisthesis. The nodular calcifications were observed at the L3-4 interspinous space, the L2-3 and L3-4 ligamentum flavum, the bilateral L3-4 facet joints, and the location of left L4 spondylolysis (Figure 1). Sagittal magnetic resonance (MR) images (Figure 2) showed an intensity change of the L1-4 supraspinal ligament in T1-weighted images and effusion at the L3-4 interspinous space in T2-weighted images. A gadolinium- (GD-) enhanced epidural mass was observed at the level of L4 vertebral body, which compressed the dural sac. Axial T2-weighted MR images showed an intra- or epidural lesion at L2-3 (Figure 3). Moreover, epidural GD-enhanced masses compressed the dural sac in the shape of a cross at the L3-4 (Figure 4) and L4-5 segments.

The patient was suspected of having pyogenic arthritis of the lumbar spine with intra- or epidural abscess in initial diagnosis. Therefore, aspiration of the effusion was performed for the bacterium identification. A total of 1.2 ml of fluid with a murky, pus-like synovial effusion (Figure 5(a)) was aspirated from the L3-4 interspinous space under the fluoroscopic image. Smear speculum of synovial fluid tested negative for bacteria and fungi; however, a number of crystals were seen. Based on the result of smear speculum, we suspected the pathology as crystal deposition disease. Polarized light microscopy revealed monocle or triclinic intracellular crystal with a positive birefringence (Figure 5(b)). The patient was diagnosed as having a pseudogout attack of the lumbar spine.

Flurbiprofen axetil (nonsteroidal anti-inflammatory drugs) was started immediately by intravenous drip injection and continued for 3 days. Local and systemic indications of inflammation, as well as neurological deficit, dramatically improved within 3 days. Loxoprofen sodium hydrate was administered orally for 8 weeks (Figure 6).

A follow-up evaluation 8 and 12 months after treatment showed complete resolution of symptoms. MR images revealed no abnormal lesion.

3. Discussion

Most reported cases of spinal CPPD involve nodular deposition in the ligamentum flavum or atlanto-occipital ligament rather than in the fibrocartilage of a disc [13]. In the lumbar spine region, chronic radiculopathy or cauda equina syndrome by nodular CPPD crystal deposition in the lumbar ligamentum flavum or facet joint has been observed. Most patients are usually treated surgically for conventional lumbar spinal stenosis.

In a search of clinical articles, based on PubMed, since the year 2000, only a few case reports [5, 7, 8, 10, 12, 13] of CPPD crystal deposition involving the lumbar spine were found. Specifically, only 2 case reports described acute CPPD crystal arthritis of the lumbar spine (Table 1) [8, 13].

In our case, there was a large extent of CPPD crystal deposition in the L2-3-4 ligamentum flavum, the L4 spondylolysis, the L3-4 facet joints, and the L3-4 interspinous space. Moreover, calcification in major peripheral joints, right elbow, bilateral hips, left knee, and left ankle, was seen in plain radiographs retrospectively. Although the association with an acute pseudogout attack in the lumbar spine is not confirmed, the patient had a respiratory infection before the onset of neurological symptoms. Generally, CPPD patients are asymptomatic before an acute episode. Acute attacks are typically triggered by intercurrent internal events [15–17]. We hypothesized that the respiratory infection might be one of the initiating factors that activated preexisting asymptomatic CPPD. CPPD crystal arthritis can present as an acute monoarthritis that affects a large joint and produces systematic symptoms such as fever, chills, and malaise. Therefore, septic arthritis must be always ruled out.

The therapeutic modalities for an acute attack of CPPD crystal arthritis were controversial [18]. In our case, multiple cultures of the spinal effusion led to a definitive diagnosis, and 8 weeks of NSAID administration provided the satisfactory recovery from the symptoms.

4. Conclusions

We encountered the rare case of an acute attack of pseudogout with the wide lesion in the lumbar spondylolytic spondylolisthesis. Multiple culture of the effusion provided a definitive diagnosis, which allowed for appropriate, minimally invasive treatment for 8 weeks of NSAID administration that provided the satisfactory recovery from the symptoms.

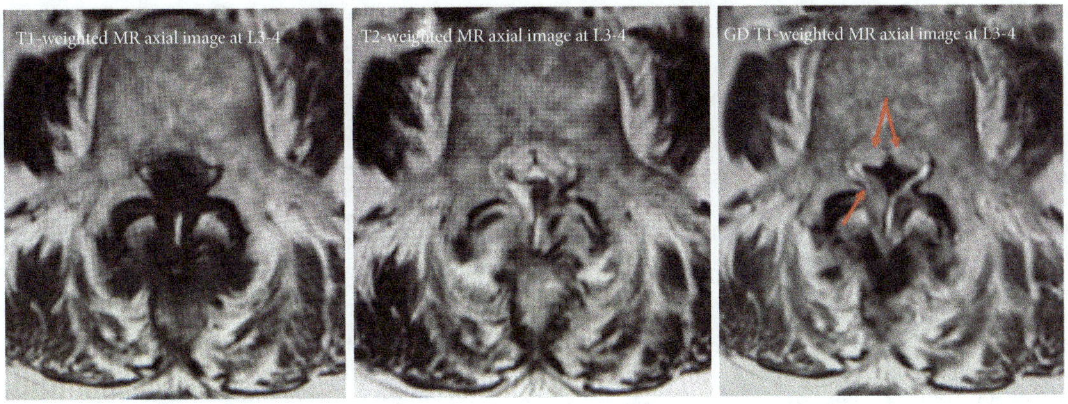

FIGURE 4: Epidural GD-enhanced masses compressed the dural sac in the shape of across at the L3-4.

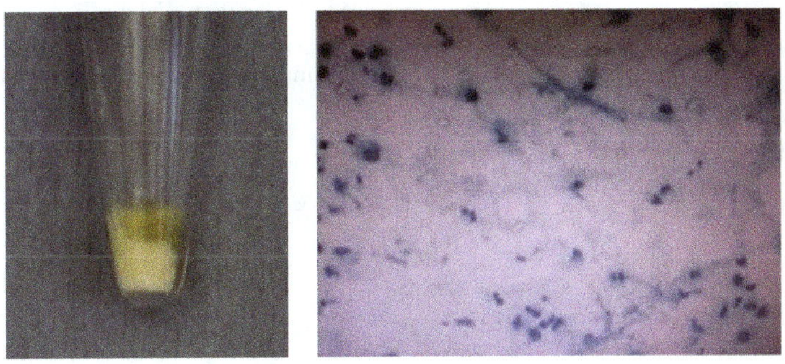

(a) (b)

FIGURE 5: (a) Aspiration of the L3-4 interspinous space yielded a murky, pus-like synovial effusion. (b) Multiple cultures of the synovial fluid tested negative for bacteria and fungi, whereas compensated polarized light microscopy revealed monocle or triclinic intracellular crystal with a positive birefringence.

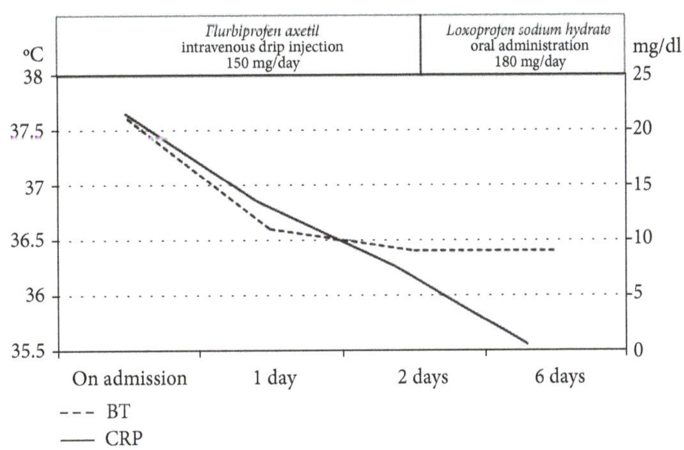

FIGURE 6: Flurbiprofen axetil was administered by intravenous drip injection for 3 days, and local and systemic inflammatory signs dramatically improved.

TABLE 1: The articles that describe about acute CPPD crystal arthritis of the lumbar spine.

Studies	Sex/age	Duration of symptoms	Precedent infection	Fever	Neurologic deficit	Level of involvement	Joint CPPD deposition	Treatment
Lee et al. [8]	M/59	2 days	Unknown	No	Yes	L4-5 disc	Unknown	Surgery
Fujishiro et al. [13]	F/71	2 days	Unknown	Yes	No	L4-5 facet	Yes	Aspiration
Our case	F/86	1 day	Yes	Yes	Yes	L3-4-5 LF, L4 lysis, L3-4 interspinous	Yes	NSAIDs

Lysis: spondylolysis.

Consent

The patient represented in this article was informed that the data would be deidentified and used in a journal publication.

References

[1] M. C. Hall and G. Selin, "Spinal involvement in Gout," *The Journal of Bone & Joint Surgery*, vol. 42, no. 2, pp. 341–343, 1960.

[2] K. J. Bridges, C. L. Bullis, A. Wanchu, and K. D. Than, "Pseudogout of the cervical and thoracic spine mimicking infection after lumbar fusion: case report," *Journal of Neurosurgery. Spine*, vol. 27, no. 2, pp. 145–149, 2017.

[3] H. Zhang, D. Jin, and E. Sun, "The early and late stages of crowned dens syndrome: two case reports," *The Spine Journal*, vol. 15, no. 10, pp. E65–E68, 2015.

[4] E. Y. Chang, W. Y. Lim, T. Wolfson et al., "Frequency of atlantoaxial calcium pyrophosphate dihydrate deposition at CT," *Radiology*, vol. 269, no. 2, pp. 519–524, 2013.

[5] G. Cacciotti, F. Novegno, and D. Fiume, "Calcium pyrophosphate dihydrate deposition disease of the filum terminale," *European Spine Journal*, vol. 22, Supplement 3, pp. 501–505, 2013.

[6] S. Odate, J. Shikata, S. Fujibayashi, N. Hosaka, T. Soeda, and H. Kimura, "Progressive thoracic myelopathy caused by spinal calcium pyrophosphate crystal deposition because of proximal junctional vertebral compression fracture after lumbopelvic fusion," *European Spine Journal*, vol. 21, no. 12, pp. 2436–2442, 2012.

[7] M. R. B. M. Namazie and M. R. Fosbender, "Calcium pyrophosphate dihydrate crystal deposition of multiple lumbar facet joints: a case report," *Journal of Orthopaedic Surgery*, vol. 20, no. 2, pp. 254–256, 2012.

[8] J. Lee, K. T. Cho, and E. J. Kim, "Cauda equina syndrome caused by pseudogout involving the lumbar intervertebral disc," *Journal of Korean Medical Science*, vol. 27, no. 12, pp. 1591–1594, 2012.

[9] A. J. Fenoy, A. H. Menezes, K. A. Donovan, and S. F. Kralik, "Calcium pyrophosphate dihydrate crystal deposition in the craniovertebral junction," *Journal of Neurosurgery. Spine*, vol. 8, no. 1, pp. 22–29, 2008.

[10] H. Y. Lam, K. Y. Cheung, S. W. Law, and K. Y. Fung, "Crystal arthropathy of the lumbar spine: a report of 4 cases," *Journal of Orthopaedic Surgery*, vol. 15, no. 1, pp. 94–101, 2016.

[11] S. H. Lin, E. T. Hsieh, T. Y. Wu, and C. W. Chang, "Cervical myelopathy induced by pseudogout in ligamentum flavum and retro-odontoid mass: a case report," *Spinal Cord*, vol. 44, no. 11, pp. 692–694, 2006.

[12] T. Mahmud, D. Basu, and P. H. P. Dyson, "Crystal arthropathy of the lumbar spine," *Journal of Bone and Joint Surgery (British)*, vol. 87-B, no. 4, pp. 513–517, 2005.

[13] T. Fujishiro, Y. Nabeshima, S. Yasui, I. Fujita, S. Yoshiya, and H. Fujii, "Pseudogout attack of the lumbar facet joint: a case report," *Spine*, vol. 27, no. 17, pp. E396–E398, 2002.

[14] N. Magarelli, R. Amelia, N. Melillo, M. Nasuto, F. Cantatore, and G. Guglielmi, "Imaging of chondrocalcinosis: calcium pyrophosphate dihydrate (CPPD) crystal deposition disease – imaging of common sites of involvement," *Clinical and Experimental Rheumatology*, vol. 30, no. 1, pp. 118–125, 2012.

[15] J. L. Rosales-Alexander, J. Balsalobre Aznar, and C. Magro-Checa, "Calcium pyrophosphate crystal deposition disease: diagnosis and treatment," *Open access Rheumatology: Research and Reviews*, vol. 6, pp. 39–47, 2014.

[16] A. K. Rosenthal, L. M. Ryan, and D. J. McCarty, "Calcium pyrophosphate crystal deposition disease, pseudogout, and articular chondrocalcinosis," in *Arthritis and Allied Condition*, W. J. Koopman and L. W. Moreland, Eds., pp. 2373–2396, Lippincott Williams & Wilkins, Philadelphia, USA, 15th edition, 2005.

[17] A. K. Rosenthal, "Pseudogout: presentation, natural history, and associated conditions," in *Crystal-Induced Arthropathies: Gout, Pseudogout, and Apatite-Associated Syndromes*, R. L. Wortmann, H. R. Schumacher Jr., M. A. Becker, and L. M. Ryan, Eds., pp. 99–116, Taylor & Francis Group, New York, 2006.

[18] F. Martinon, V. Pétrilli, A. Mayor, A. Tardivel, and J. Tschopp, "Gout-associated uric acid crystals activate the NALP3 inflammasome," *Nature*, vol. 440, no. 7081, pp. 237–241, 2006.

41

Glossopharyngeal and Hypoglossal Nerve Paralysis Secondary to Prevertebral Phlegmon

Ryunosuke Fukushi, Izaya Ogon, Yoshinori Terashima, Hiroyuki Takashima, Tsutomu Oshigiri, Noriyuki Iesato, Mitsunori Yoshimoto, Makoto Emori, Atsushi Teramoto, and Toshihiko Yamashita

Department of Orthopedic Surgery, Sapporo Medical University School of Medicine, Sapporo, Japan

Correspondence should be addressed to Ryunosuke Fukushi; ryunosuke_fukushi_521@yahoo.co.jp

Academic Editor: Johannes Mayr

A 50-year-old man presented to the clinic with severe neck pain, fever, and difficulty breathing and was subsequently admitted to the local orthopedics department with possible retropharyngeal abscess and pyogenic spondylitis. Antibiotic therapy was initiated; however, due to poor oxygenation, he was referred and transferred to our department and admitted. Magnetic resonance imaging showed signal changes at the left C1/2 lateral atlantoaxial joint, posterior pharynx, longus colli muscle, carotid space, and medial deep cervical region, predominantly on the left side. In addition, despite lymph node enlargement from the posterior pharynx to the deep cervical region, there was no abscess formation. There were no signs of a space-occupying lesion or signal changes in the jugular foramen. One day postadmission, the patient's temperature had risen to 39.1°C and his SpO_2 had fallen. His neck pain had also worsened, and emergency surgery was decided. Preoperatively, we suspected retropharyngeal abscess and pyogenic spondylitis. On day 13 postadmission, the patient exhibited dysphagia, deviated tongue protrusion, and the curtain sign. Glossopharyngeal and hypoglossal nerve paralysis were diagnosed. The patient's swallowing functions recovered and he was discharged on day 36. We experienced a case of glossopharyngeal and hypoglossal nerve paralysis secondary to pyogenic cervical facet joint arthritis.

1. Introduction

Jugular foramen syndrome is a rare systematic cranial neuropathy that presents characteristic clinical symptoms due to the paralysis of jugular foramen cranial nerves. In addition, a lesion in the carotid space, which surrounds the common carotid and internal carotid arteries, can cause cranial neuropathy. Although both jugular foramen syndrome and carotid space lesions have been reported rarely in patients treated in otolaryngology, no cases have been reported in the orthopedic field. Here, we report a case of cranial neuropathy caused by prevertebral phlegmon.

2. Case Report

A 50-year-old man with severe neck pain, fever, and difficulty breathing and no initial cause was later diagnosed with cervical spondylosis deformans and prescribed analgesics. Neck pain worsened after 5 days, and he was examined for suspected meningitis, which was ruled out. He was admitted to the local orthopedics department to diagnose a possible retropharyngeal abscess with pyogenic spondylitis. Antibiotic therapy was initiated; however, due to poor oxygenation, he was transferred to our department the same day and admitted to the intensive care unit (ICU). Upon hospitalization, his body temperature was

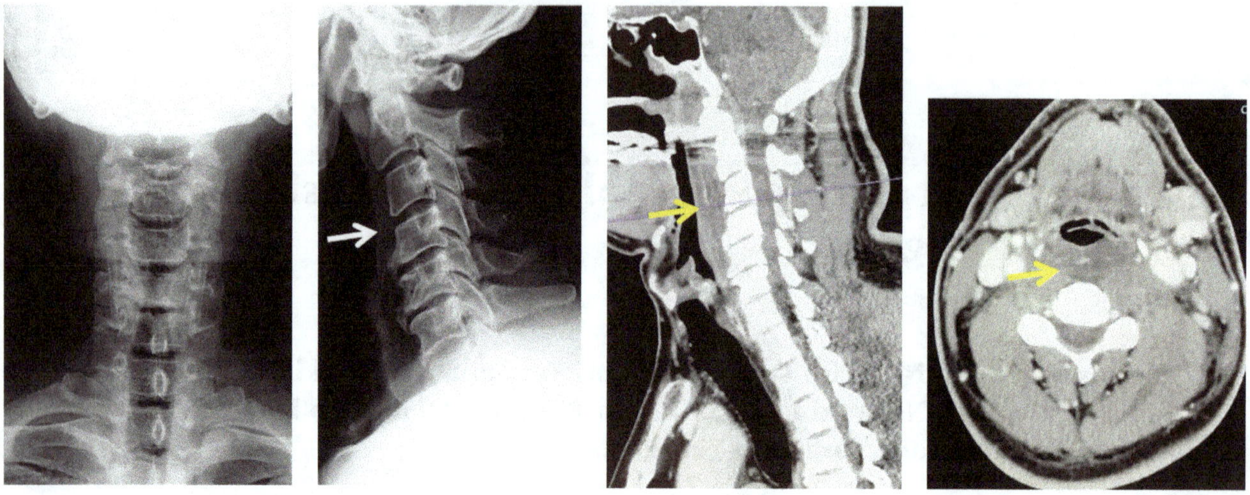

(a) (b) (c) (d)

Figure 1: Initial radiographic and computed tomography (CT) assessment of the cervical spine. Posteroanterior (a) and lateral plane (b) radiograms. A lateral plane radiogram showed soft tissue swelling anterior to the vertebral bodies (white arrow). Sagittal (c) and axial (d) CT indicated soft tissue swelling in the posterior pharynx (yellow arrows), but there were no clear signs of abscess formation.

38.7°C and SpO_2 was 92% (transnasal, 2 L). Physical findings included neck pain at rest and upon movement along with redness, swelling, feeling of warmth, and pressure around the entire neck. There were no signs of motor paralysis, sensory disturbances, abnormal deep tendon reflexes, or pathological reflexes. A blood test revealed leukocyte and C-reactive protein (CRP) levels of 20,900/μL and 25.25 mg/dL, respectively.

On X-ray examination at admission, soft tissue swelling was noted anterior to the vertebral bodies. Contrast-enhanced computed tomography revealed soft tissue swelling in the posterior pharynx without any clear signs of abscess formation (Figures 1(a)–1(d)). Magnetic resonance imaging (MRI) demonstrated signal changes at the left C1/2 lateral atlantoaxial joint, posterior pharynx, longus colli muscle, carotid space, and medial deep cervical region, predominantly on the left side. In addition, lymph node enlargement was observed from the posterior pharynx to the deep cervical region; however, no abscess formation was noted (Figures 2(a)–2(d)). In other image slices, there were no signs of space-occupying lesions or signal changes in the jugular foramen (Figures 3(a) and 3(b)).

Otorhinolaryngological examination revealed that the patient was able to converse and had no airway obstructions, stridor, or difficulty in swallowing. Examination using a fiberscope indicated swelling of the posterior oropharyngeal wall but revealed no abscess or other abnormal findings. The blood culture was positive for *Staphylococcus aureus*, but the results of other rapid tests were negative.

One day postadmission, the patient's temperature increased to 39.1°C and his SpO_2 decreased. Moreover, his physical symptoms deteriorated with worsening neck pain, increased blood CRP levels, and impaired respiratory status. Therefore, emergency surgery was performed. Imaging findings indicated that the likelihood of abscess formation was low; however, urgent, experimental surgery was performed to make a definitive diagnosis. Since the patient exhibited fever and a sharp rise in the inflammatory response, we also aimed to identify the bacteria responsible for the inflammation. An anterior cervical approach was selected for incision, drainage, and irrigation.

Intraoperative findings revealed no abscess formation in the posterior pharynx or vertebral bodies, or anterior to the intervertebral discs. Irrigation was performed with a large amount of physiological saline, and a drain was placed. The patient was then admitted to the ICU without being extubated and fitted with an Aspen® Cervical Collar.

Postoperatively, white blood cell (WBC) count and CRP levels exhibited a decreasing trend. On day 4 of hospitalization, he was extubated and released from the ICU, and the drain was removed on day 9. A catheter tip culture was positive for *S. epidermidis*; this result differed from that of the blood culture. This false positive was thought to be from contamination. The patient's previous physician had administered IPM/CS; however, based on the blood culture results of the previous physician, the patient's treatment regimen was changed to ABPC/CVA after being transferred to our hospital. Continued administration of antibiotics gradually decreased WBC count and CRP level. On day 13 of hospitalization, the patient had dysphagia, deviated tongue protrusion, and the curtain sign. Based on these findings, glossopharyngeal and hypoglossal nerve paralysis were diagnosed. Despite the presence of glossopharyngeal and hypoglossal nerve paralysis, WBC and CRP levels were negative and the patient was switched to antibiotic administration via a gastric tube.

The patient's swallowing functions recovered over the next month in the hospital, and he was discharged on day 36. An MRI was performed on postoperative day 68 while the patient was still hospitalized; signal change was observed in the facet joint, suggesting that swelling had subsided. At the 3-month follow-up, there was no recurrence, and radiographic images showed no abnormal findings.

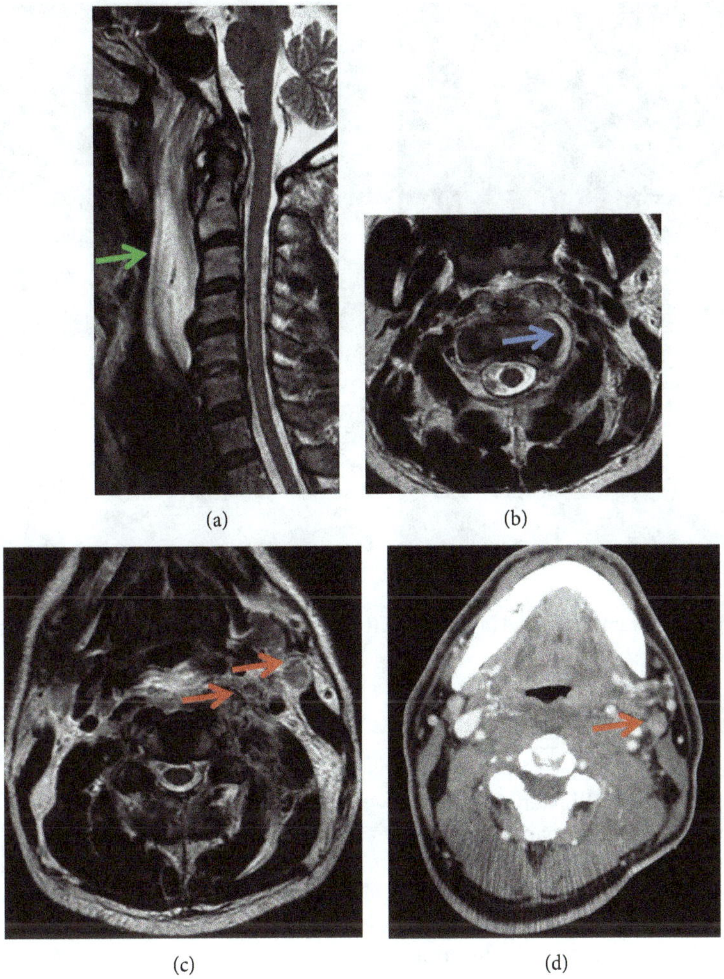

FIGURE 2: Initial magnetic resonance imaging (MRI) assessment of the cervical spine. Sagittal (a) and axial (b–d) MRI showed signal changes at the left C1/2 lateral atlantoaxial joint (blue arrow), posterior pharynx (green arrow), longus colli muscle, carotid space, and the medial deep cervical region, predominantly on the left side. Lymph node enlargement (red arrows) was observed from the posterior pharynx to the deep cervical region; there was no abscess formation.

3. Discussion

Until now, three studies have reported the incidence of glossopharyngeal and hypoglossal nerve paralysis caused by infection. Ohara et al. reported a case of glossopharyngeal, vagal, and hypoglossal nerve paralysis that recovered with antibiotics in a 1-year-old boy [1]. They reported that the paralysis was caused by pressure on the carotid space. Miyamoto et al. reported a 62-year-old woman with glossopharyngeal nerve paralysis, as well as vagal and accessory nerve paralysis [2]. The causative pathogen in the aforementioned case was *Mycobacterium tuberculosis*; although the patient was treated with antitubercular agents, some vocal cord paresis remained. Shiratsuchi et al. reported a 71-year-old man with glossopharyngeal and hypoglossal nerve paralysis [3]. In this case, the causative agent was a fungus and the patient's condition improved with the use of an antifungal agent. Miyamoto et al. and Shiratsuchi et al. reported that paralysis was caused by jugular foramen syndrome.

The jugular foramen is located on the inferior surface of the temple and acts as a pathway for the internal jugular vein and glossopharyngeal, vagal, and accessory nerves. If the jugular foramen is damaged by infection, trauma, cerebrovascular accident, and polyangiitis or is occupied by tumor, dysfunction of the glossopharyngeal, vagal, or accessory nerves can result [3, 4]. The carotid space is present in the region of the common carotid artery and internal carotid artery. Moreover, its height extends from the jugular foramen to the aortic arch, cervicofacial area, and superior mediastinum. The carotid space is anteriorly, laterally, medially, and posteriorly surrounded by the pharyngeal space, parotid gland, retropharyngeal space, and anterior vertebrae, respectively [5, 6]. In addition, glossopharyngeal and hypoglossal nerve dysfunction can result from pressure arising from lymph node enlargement due to infection, tumors, or other pathologies [5].

Jugular foramen syndrome does not generally involve damage to the hypoglossal nerve [7–11]; however, pressure exerted on the carotid space may lead to hypoglossal nerve dysfunction. In the present case, the patient had hypoglossal nerve paralysis, which made us believe that the pathogenesis was due to pressure on the carotid space.

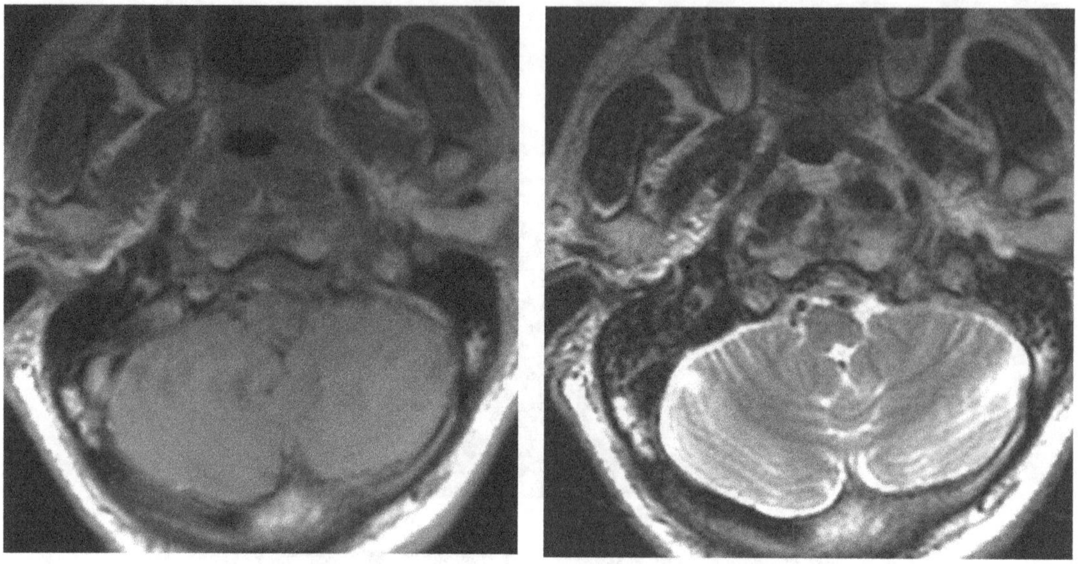

(a) (b)

FIGURE 3: MRI assessment of the jugular foramen. Sagittal (a) and axial (b) MRI showed no signs of a space-occupying lesion or signal changes in the jugular foramen.

The lateral retropharyngeal lymph nodes (LRPLNs) are present on the medial side of the carotid space, which contains the glossopharyngeal and hypoglossal nerves [5]. Ohara et al. demonstrated that infection led to LRPLN enlargement, which resulted in pressure on the carotid space from the medial to lateral side, causing glossopharyngeal and hypoglossal nerve paralysis. The lack of symptoms associated with the accessory, vagal, and sympathetic nerves, which also pass through the carotid space, may be explained by the location of these tissues' pathways. They are on the dorsal side of the space and are thus less likely to be affected by pressure from an abscess [1]. We believe that the pathogenesis in the present case was through the same mechanism.

Further enlargement of LRPLN may have caused symptoms involving the accessory, vagal, and sympathetic nerves. To our knowledge, this is the first study to report a case of cranial neuropathy caused by prevertebral phlegmon in orthopedics.

The current case report had several limitations. We did not perform direct suctioning from the facet joint, or gadolinium in MRI. One significant limitation of this study is that we were unable to confirm the actual location of the compression. However, we surmised the pathological diagnosis of this case based on several findings including the absence of abscesses and the presence of lymphadenopathy near the carotid space on images, and by citing previous literature.

4. Conclusions

We report a case of glossopharyngeal and hypoglossal nerve paralysis that occurred secondary to prevertebral phlegmon. Although the presence of an abscess was not confirmed in the images or intraoperative findings, the patient's symptoms improved with antibiotic administration. We believe lymph node enlargement due to inflammation resulted in pressure on the carotid space, which affected the functioning of the glossopharyngeal and hypoglossal nerves passing through this space.

Consent

Written informed consent was obtained from all patients prior to their participation in the study.

References

[1] T. Ohara, T. Okamoto, H. Naganuma, A. Maki, T. Nasuno, and M. Okamoto, "A pediatric case of retropharyngeal abscess causing multiple instances of cranial nerve palsy," *Nippon Jibiinkoka Gakkai Kaiho*, vol. 118, no. 5, pp. 657–661, 2015.

[2] S. Miyamoto, T. Okamoto, and M. Nakayama, "A case of tuberculous jugular foramen syndrome and hypertrophic pachymeningitis," *Koutou (THE LARYNX JAPAN)*, vol. 27, no. 2, pp. 108–113, 2015.

[3] H. Shiratsuchi, T. Yamamoto, T. Nakashima, N. Hirakawa, T. Mihara, and S. Komune, "A case of Collet et Sicard syndrome due to a probably epipharyngeal fungal infection induced by the long term use of steroids," *The Oto-Rhino- and Laryngological Clinic Practica Otologica Kyoto*, vol. 51, no. 3, pp. 183–188, 2005.

[4] M. J. Streitmann and A. Sismanis, "Metastatic carcinoma of the temporal bone," *The American Journal of Otology*, vol. 17, no. 5, pp. 780–783, 1996.

[5] K. Ichimura and H. Tojima, "The carotid space; its clinical implication," *Practica Oto-Rhino-Laryngologica*, vol. 92, no. 1, pp. 1–11, 1999.

[6] A. Gervasio, G. D'Orta, I. Mujahed, and A. Biasio, "Sonographic anatomy of the neck: the suprahyoid region," *Journal of Ultrasound*, vol. 14, no. 3, pp. 130–135, 2011.

[7] F. Graus and N. E. Slatkin, "Papilledema in the metastatic jugular foramen syndrome," *Archives of Neurology*, vol. 40, no. 13, pp. 816–818, 1983.

[8] K. T. Robbins and R. S. Fenton, "Jugular foramen syndrome," *The Journal of Otolaryngology*, vol. 9, no. 6, pp. 505–516, 1980.

[9] J. Biller, P. W. Brazis, and J. C. Masdeu, *Localization in Clinical Neurology*, Lippincott Williams & Wilkins, Hagerstown, MD, 2011.

[10] N. P. Shine and P. O'Sullivan, "Collet-Sicard syndrome: a rare presentation of metastatic prostate adenocarcinoma," *Auris Nasus Larynx*, vol. 32, no. 3, pp. 315–318, 2005.

[11] A. Agarwal, N. Baisakhiya, A. Kakani, A. Bhake, M. Nagrale, and S. Reddy, "Metastatic lung cancer presenting with jugular foramen syndrome in a case of von Recklinghausens disease," *Journal of Cancer Research and Therapeutics*, vol. 6, no. 3, pp. 391–393, 2010.

42

Baseball Related Injuries: A Case Report on Acute Compartment Syndrome of the Forearm

Charles B. Pasque and Christopher Hendrix

Department of Orthopaedic Surgery and Rehabilitation, University of Oklahoma College of Medicine, Oklahoma City, Oklahoma, USA

Correspondence should be addressed to Charles B. Pasque; charles-pasque@ouhsc.edu

Academic Editor: Federico Canavese

Acute compartment syndrome is a difficult diagnosis to make due to its wide range of clinical presentations. Delay or misdiagnosis can cause devastating consequences such as Volkmann's ischemic contracture, permanent nerve damage, amputation, and death. Lower extremity compartment syndrome is more common than upper extremity compartment syndrome, with the forearm being the most common location for upper extremity compartment syndrome. Acute compartment syndrome is most caused by acute fracture trauma but can also be due to soft tissue crush injuries or vascular problems. We report a unique case of a male umpire being struck on the forearm by a baseball with subsequent progression to an acute compartment syndrome that required emergent fasciotomies. The patient made a full recovery with no known long-term sequelae.

1. Introduction

Acute compartment syndrome of the extremity occurs when the interstitial pressure of the tissues exceeds the capillary perfusion pressure either from bleeding or edema in the compartment [1]. This can result from external pressure on the compartment or decreased arterial inflow [2]. The majority of compartment syndromes occur as a result of high-energy trauma with an accompanying fracture. Around one-fourth of forearm compartment syndromes occur because of soft tissue injury alone, and in 10 percent of these cases, the patient has an underlying coagulopathy or known bleeding disorder [3]. Acute compartment syndrome is largely a clinical diagnosis, and it is vitally important that the health-care provider recognizes it within the appropriate period. Acute compartment syndrome is typically diagnosed by using somof the five "P's," which includes pain, paresthesia, paralysis, pallor, and pulselessness. The outcome of any acute compartment syndrome significantly hinges on the time elapsed from the onset of pathology to the diagnosis and subsequent compartmental release. In general, irreversible damage occurs after eight hours has elapsed from the onset of ischemia [4–7]. We present a case of acute volar and dorsal compartment syndrome of the forearm after an impact injury during a baseball game. To our knowledge, this is the first case report in the literature of a compartment syndrome after being struck by a baseball.

2. Narrative

A 51-year-old right-hand dominant male and home plate baseball umpire was struck on the right proximal dorsal forearm approximately three hours prior to his presentation to the Emergency Department. The patient stated that he was struck during the first game of a double-header and continued to umpire while leaving his right arm in a dependent position. He subsequently developed progressive worsening pain and paresthesia in his right forearm and hand. The patient had no other medical problems and was taking no medications.

On the initial physical exam, the patient's right upper extremity had a swollen dorsal forearm over the mobile extensor muscle wad. The patient was able to flex and extend his fingers with a painless passive arc of motion. His sensation was slightly decreased in the sensory radial nerve distribution but fully intact in the median and ulnar nerve distribution. The patient was sent for X-ray, which was negative for fracture. On return from X-ray, his repeat exam revealed tense compartments, pain with passive stretch causing nausea, absent sensation in the radial nerve distribution, and decreased sensation in the median nerve distribution. The dorsal forearm compartment pressures were measured in the emergency department using the Quick Pressure Monitor System (Stryker Instruments, Kalamazoo, MI, U.S.A.). The dorsal compartment measured 45 mmHg and the volar compartment measured 30 mmHg. The patient's coagulation studies were normal.

The patient was taken to the operating room for immediate forearm fasciotomies. Under general anesthesia, a dorsal compartment release was performed through a midline dorsal incision. The dorsal mobile extensor muscle wad was released. The muscles appeared very swollen without necrosis evident. The volar fasciotomy was performed with decompression of the superficial and deep volar compartments. The muscles were minimally swollen and there was a small hematoma within the deep volar compartment. The fasciotomy incisions were left open after the initial surgery. The patient required two more trips to the operating room over the following seven days for repeat irrigation and debridement to allow the swelling to improve for delayed primary closure of his incisions. The median nerve sensation returned to normal after the initial fasciotomy surgery.

On discharge, the patient was placed in a soft dressing and started on range of motion exercises. At four weeks postoperatively, the patient had no pain and the paresthesia in the sensory radial nerve had resolved. At three months, the patient had regained full range of motion and strength in his forearm without any pain.

3. Discussion

Compartment syndrome is one of the true orthopedic emergencies and occurs due to bleeding or edema within a closed osteofascial compartment. This leads to compression of the veins and a decreased arteriovenous pressure gradient, ultimately resulting in ischemia [1, 2, 4, 6]. Tissue fascia is avascular and nonelastic, making it resistant to acute stretching and resulting in fixed spaces [8]. If the period from the onset of ischemia to compartment release is within four hours, complete resolution is most often seen. Damage is variable between six to eight hours and irreversible damage can occur after eight hours [4]. Compartment syndrome remains largely a clinical diagnosis and is often difficult to recognize due to the variety of etiologies and injury patterns. Swollen and tense compartments are sometimes an obvious and important clinical finding. In addition, the five "P's" are historically used when making the diagnosis and include pain (out of proportion), paresthesia, paralysis, pallor, and pulselessness. Pain with passive stretching is often used as the sixth "P," and along with pain out of proportion, they are the first and most sensitive signs of acute compartment syndrome [1–4, 6, 8]. Pallor and pulselessness are not normally present on initial presentation and typically are a sign of late-stage compartment syndrome and probable irreversible damage [4, 9]. A critical analysis review found that risk factors for a delay in diagnosis included relying only on clinical signs, having an associated neurological injury, acute compartment syndrome in children or a patient with reduced or altered consciousness, regional or patient-controlled analgesia, and lack of experience of evaluating medical personnel [10].

As soon as the diagnosis of acute compartment syndrome is made, a fasciotomy should be performed to prevent the devastating complications of Volkmann's ischemic contracture, neurologic deficits, infection, amputation, or rarely death [6]. Volkmann's ischemic contracture is usually the chronic end stage and is the result of replacement of the compartment's muscle tissue with fibrotic tissue, causing contracture and nerve dysfunction [5]. The deep flexor muscles are more susceptible to compression and ischemic injury due to their fascial boundaries preventing expansion [4, 8]. The median nerve is the nerve most often injured in forearm compartment syndrome, lying between the flexor digitorum superficialis and the flexor digitorum profundus [8].

There have been many different recommendations over time regarding thresholds of tissue pressure indicating a need for fasciotomy. Normal resting tissue pressure is within 0-10 mmHg [6, 8]. The most widely accepted indication is a tissue pressure that is within 10-30 mmHg of the diastolic blood pressure, known as the delta pressure [2, 3, 5–11]. An absolute pressure greater than 30 mmHg is also an indication for fasciotomy, especially when other clinical signs are present [3, 5–8]. A concerning physical exam and an absolute pressure of greater than 20 mmHg are accepted as an indication to proceed to compartment release [3]. Diastolic pressure is often used as a guide due to hypotensive patients being more prone and hypertensive patients being less prone to compartment syndrome [4, 9]; thus, hypertension can be a protective factor and may be another reason older patients are less commonly affected [12].

A study published in 2019 found that the relative risk of morbidity and mortality is higher in those treated with fasciotomy than with a nonsurgical approach [13]. However, another recent study stated that a nonsurgical approach is not recommended, and patients successfully treated nonsurgically likely did not have true compartment syndrome after all [8]. Above all, the health-care provider must remember that these are only clinical guidelines and that the ultimate decision-making is up to the knowledge and experience of the health-care provider.

There are three different forms of compartment syndrome which are acute, chronic, and neonatal. Chronic is otherwise known as chronic exertional compartment syndrome and is characterized by recurring, transient increases in tissue pressure, usually during exercise, causing pain and neurologic symptoms that resolve with rest [5]. Neonatal is extremely rare and occurs within the first 24 hours of life. It is usually identified by swelling and discoloration of the limb and is caused by an unknown pathophysiology [14]. Acute compartment syndrome in adults most commonly affects males, with an incidence ten times greater when compared to females [15]. The higher incidence in males is thought to be due to their larger muscle mass within a fixed compartment, and that males are more likely involved in high-energy trauma [6, 12]. In adults and children, the most common location of acute compartment syndrome is the lower extremity and is usually due to a fracture. The most common location of fracture to cause acute compartment syndrome occurs in the tibia and distal radius [7]. In the upper extremity, it is estimated that 1.22 percent of all forearm fractures require fasciotomy [16]. Distal radius fractures are the most common cause of acute compartment syndrome of the forearm in adults, while supracondylar fractures are the most common cause in children. The second most common overall cause of acute compartment syndrome is soft tissue related, making up an estimated 23 percent of all cases [3, 8, 10]. Soft tissue injuries can be subdivided into crush injuries, burns, edema, intramuscular hematoma, snake bites, drug, or alcohol overuse induced stupor, with these causes being more common in patients with an underlying coagulopathy or known bleeding disorder [7, 15]. A relatively rare cause includes high-pressure injection injury to the upper extremity, such as by gunshot and pressurized gas and liquids, with the overwhelming majority occurring via occupational injury [17]. Other factors associated with forearm compartment syndrome secondary to soft tissue injury include increased age, medical comorbidities, and anticoagulation [10]. While 10 percent of soft tissue injuries resulting in compartment syndrome have a coagulopathy or known bleeding disorder [3], our patient in this case report's coagulation studies was normal.

Due to baseball's widespread popularity, it has one of the highest numbers of Emergency Department visits. The number of visits is likely underestimated because it does not include physician visits outside of the Emergency Department [18]. Baseball-related injuries have significantly declined over the last twenty years due to increased safety measures and precautions. The upper extremity is the second most common body part injured trailing only the face, with most being a soft tissue injury after being hit by a baseball [19]. This is one of two reports in the literature of an acute forearm compartment syndrome after being struck by a ball without a fracture. The other such report was published in 2006 of a man suffering from three separate acute compartment syndromes from minor trauma and without a fracture over a seven-year span [20]. The patient's coagulation studies were normal, except for one abnormal bleeding time after his first acute compartment syndrome case. The authors hypothesized that he may have had an underlying variant of Von Willebrand's disease.

The patient in our case report presented with elevated compartment pressures of 45 mmHg in the dorsal compartment and 30 mmHg in the volar compartment. The patient had volar and dorsal compartments that were tense, pain with passive motion of the fingers, paresthesia, and pain out of proportion to his injury. All these findings were consistent with an acute forearm compartment syndrome. The patient's volar, dorsal, and mobile wad compartments were all released, and the patient's symptoms improved gradually over the next four weeks.

4. Conclusion

This case report highlights that acute upper extremity compartment syndrome can develop after a major blow to the forearm soft tissues with high velocity objects, such as a baseball that may not result in bone fractures or obvious soft tissue damage on initial impact. This emphasizes the importance of complete and thorough serial physical examination, even after an initially benign-appearing injury. All healthcare providers at athletic events and Emergency Departments must be aware of the potential for compartment syndrome after blows from an object such as a baseball. In addition, maintaining a high level of clinical suspicion and diligence is important to make a timely diagnosis and treatment that will provide the patient with the best possible outcome. To our knowledge, this is the first case report of an acute forearm compartment syndrome during a sporting event due to a blow by a baseball.

Data Availability

No data are associated with this article.

Consent

This patient was lost to follow up.

References

[1] A. R. Hargens and S. J. Mubarak, "Current concepts in the pathophysiology, evaluation, and diagnosis of compartment syndrome," *Hand Clinics*, vol. 14, no. 3, pp. 371–383, 1998.

[2] P. Hosseinzadeh and C. B. Hayes, "Compartment syndrome in children," *The Orthopedic Clinics of North America*, vol. 47, no. 3, pp. 579–587, 2016.

[3] M. L. Prasarn and E. A. Ouellette, "Acute compartment syndrome of the upper extremity," *American Academy of Orthopaedic Surgeon.*, vol. 19, no. 1, pp. 49–58, 2011.

[4] T. E. Whitesides and M. M. Heckman, "Acute compartment syndrome: update on diagnosis and treatment," *The Journal of the American Academy of Orthopaedic Surgeons*, vol. 4, no. 4, pp. 209–218, 1996.

[5] F. J. Leversedge, T. J. Moore, B. C. Peterson, and J. G. Seiler, "Compartment syndrome of the upper extremity," *The Journal of Hand Surgery.*, vol. 36, no. 3, pp. 544–559, 2011.

[6] A. Hanandeh, V. R. Mani, P. Bauer, A. Ramcharan, and B. Donaldson, *Donaldson B*, Identification and surgical management of upper arm and forearm compartment syndrome, Cureus, 2019.

[7] S. Gourgiotis, C. Villias, S. Germanos, A. Foukas, and M. P. Ridolfini, "Acute limb compartment syndrome: a review," *Journal of Surgical Education*, vol. 64, no. 3, pp. 178–186, 2007.

[8] J. M. Kistler, A. M. Ilyas, and J. J. Thoder, "Forearm compartment syndrome: evaluation and management," *Hand Clinics*, vol. 34, no. 1, pp. 53–60, 2018.

[9] T. E. Whitesides, T. C. Haney, K. Morimoto, and H. Harada, "Tissue pressure measurements as a determinant for the need of fasciotomy," *Clinical Orthopaedics and Related Research*, vol. 113, no. 113, pp. 43–51, 1975.

[10] A. D. Duckworth and M. M. McQueen, "The diagnosis of acute compartment syndrome," *JBJS Reviews.*, vol. 5, no. 12, article e1, 2017.

[11] J. M. Clayton, A. C. Hayes, and R. W. Barnes, "Tissue pressure and perfusion in the compartment syndrome," *The Journal of Surgical Research*, vol. 22, no. 4, pp. 333–339, 1977.

[12] M. M. McQueen, P. Gaston, and C. M. Court-Brown, "Acute compartment syndrome," *Journal of Bone and Joint Surgery. British Volume (London)*, vol. 82, no. 2, pp. 200–203, 2000.

[13] J. D. Oliver, "Acute traumatic compartment syndrome of the forearm: literature review and unfavorable outcomes risk analysis of fasciotomy treatment," *Plastic Surgical Nursing*, vol. 39, no. 1, pp. 10–13, 2019.

[14] B. Martin and L. Treharne, "Neonatal compartment syndrome," *The Annals of The Royal College of Surgeons of England.*, vol. 98, no. 7, pp. e111–e113, 2016.

[15] A. Jimenez and R. Marappa-Ganeshan, *Forearm compartment syndrome. Stat Pearls*, Stat Pearls Publishing Copyright © 2020, Stat Pearls Publishing LLC, Treasure Island (FL), 2020.

[16] A. M. Saiz, A. C. Wellman, D. Stwalley, P. Wolinsky, and A. N. Miller, "The incidence and risk factors associated with the need for fasciotomy in tibia and forearm fractures: an analysis of the National Trauma Data Bank," *Journal of Orthopaedic Trauma*, vol. 34, no. 5, pp. e154–e158, 2020.

[17] F. Yılmaz, Ö. Köse, and E. Erol, "High-pressure injection injuries to the hand: a case report," *The Annals of Clinical and Analytical Medicine*, vol. 11, no. 3, pp. 242–244, 2020.

[18] D. H. Janda, "The prevention of baseball and softball injuries," *Clinical Orthopaedics and Related Research*, vol. 409, pp. 20–28, 2003.

[19] B. R. Lawson, R. D. Comstock, and G. A. Smith, "Baseball-related injuries to children treated in hospital emergency departments in the United States, 1994-2006," *Pediatrics*, vol. 123, no. 6, pp. e1028–e1034, 2009.

[20] F. W. Ortmann and J. B. Carr, "Metachronous acute compartment syndromes," *Orthopedics*, vol. 29, no. 7, pp. 647–649, 2006.

Permissions

All chapters in this book were first published by Hindawi Publishing Corporation; hereby published with permission under the Creative Commons Attribution License or equivalent. Every chapter published in this book has been scrutinized by our experts. Their significance has been extensively debated. The topics covered herein carry significant findings which will fuel the growth of the discipline. They may even be implemented as practical applications or may be referred to as a beginning point for another development.

The contributors of this book come from diverse backgrounds, making this book a truly international effort. This book will bring forth new frontiers with its revolutionizing research information and detailed analysis of the nascent developments around the world.

We would like to thank all the contributing authors for lending their expertise to make the book truly unique. They have played a crucial role in the development of this book. Without their invaluable contributions this book wouldn't have been possible. They have made vital efforts to compile up to date information on the varied aspects of this subject to make this book a valuable addition to the collection of many professionals and students.

This book was conceptualized with the vision of imparting up-to-date information and advanced data in this field. To ensure the same, a matchless editorial board was set up. Every individual on the board went through rigorous rounds of assessment to prove their worth. After which they invested a large part of their time researching and compiling the most relevant data for our readers.

The editorial board has been involved in producing this book since its inception. They have spent rigorous hours researching and exploring the diverse topics which have resulted in the successful publishing of this book. They have passed on their knowledge of decades through this book. To expedite this challenging task, the publisher supported the team at every step. A small team of assistant editors was also appointed to further simplify the editing procedure and attain best results for the readers.

Apart from the editorial board, the designing team has also invested a significant amount of their time in understanding the subject and creating the most relevant covers. They scrutinized every image to scout for the most suitable representation of the subject and create an appropriate cover for the book.

The publishing team has been an ardent support to the editorial, designing and production team. Their endless efforts to recruit the best for this project, has resulted in the accomplishment of this book. They are a veteran in the field of academics and their pool of knowledge is as vast as their experience in printing. Their expertise and guidance has proved useful at every step. Their uncompromising quality standards have made this book an exceptional effort. Their encouragement from time to time has been an inspiration for everyone.

The publisher and the editorial board hope that this book will prove to be a valuable piece of knowledge for researchers, students, practitioners and scholars across the globe.

List of Contributors

Hamed Ghoddusi Johari
Thoracic and Vascular Surgery Research Center, Shiraz University of Medical Sciences, Shiraz, Iran
Trauma Research Center, General Surgery Department, Shiraz University of Medical Sciences, Shiraz, Iran

Mohammad-Ali Erfani and Mohammad-Mehdi Karami
Research Center for Bone and Joint Diseases, Department of Orthopedic Surgery, Chamran Hospital, Shiraz University of Medical Sciences, Shiraz, Iran

Amirhossein Erfani and Reza Shahriarirad
Thoracic and Vascular Surgery Research Center, Shiraz University of Medical Sciences, Shiraz, Iran
Student Research Committee, Shiraz University of Medical Sciences, Shiraz, Iran

John H. Cabot, Khang H. Dang and Anil K. Dutta
Department of Orthopaedics, UT Health San Antonio, San Antonio, TX 78229, USA

Tsuyoshi Yamada
Department of Orthopaedic Surgery, Saiseikai Kawaguchi General Hospital, Saitama 332-8558, Japan
Department of Orthopaedic Surgery, Graduate School, Tokyo Medical and Dental University, 1-5-45 Yushima, Bunkyo-ku, Tokyo 113-8510, Japan

Ichiro Torigoe, Kenichiro Sakai and Yoshiyasu Arai
Department of Orthopaedic Surgery, Saiseikai Kawaguchi General Hospital, Saitama 332-8558, Japan

Atsushi Okawa
Department of Orthopaedic Surgery, Graduate School, Tokyo Medical and Dental University, 1-5-45 Yushima, Bunkyo-ku, Tokyo 113-8510, Japan

Aurélien Traverso, Benjamin Tschopp, Tristan Mekdade, Barbara Kwiatkowski and Nicolas Lutz
Department of Pediatric and Adolescent Surgery, Lausanne University Hospital (CHUV) and University of Lausanne (UNIL), Lausanne, Switzerland

Ömer Serdar Hakyemez, Fatih Arslanoğlu, Murat Birinci, Mehmet Akif Çaçan and Adnan Kara
Medipol Mega University Hospital, Istanbul, Turkey

Aaron Seidman, Kelley Brossy and Alfred Faulkner
Department of Orthopedic Surgery, Beaumont Hospital, Farmington Hills, MI, USA

Jeffrey Taylor
Lake Erie College of Osteopathic Medicine, Erie, PA, USA

Maximiliano Barahona, Alvaro Zamorano, Cristian Barrientos, Yoshiro Sato and Jaime Hinzpeter
Orthopedic Department at Hospital Clinico Universidad de Chile, 999 Santos Dumont Street, Independencia, Santiago 8380456, Chile

Mauricio Guzmán
Radiology Department at Hospital Clinico Universidad de Chile, 999 Santos Dumont Street, Independencia, Santiago 8380456, Chile

C. Granier, E. Maury, B. Coulet, M. Delpont, J. Cottalorda, C. Sleth, R. Carré and D. Louahem
Department of Pediatric Orthopedic Surgery, Lapeyronie Hospital, University of Montpellier, 371 Avenue Doyen Gaston Giraud, 34090 Montpellier, France

Ryan Cheng, Jay Moran, Samantha Smith, Christopher A. Schneble, Shin Mei Chan and Elizabeth C. Gardner
Department of Orthopaedics and Rehabilitation, Yale University School of Medicine, New Haven, CT, USA

Don Li
Orthopedic Surgery, Hospital for Special Surgery-Weil-Cornell Medical School, New York, NY, USA

S. Craig Morris and Peter J. Wilton
Department of Orthopedic Surgery, Loma Linda University, Loma Linda, CA, USA
Department of Orthopedic Surgery, Arrowhead Regional Medical Center, Colton, CA, USA

Priyantha L. Wickramanayake and Jonathan L. Allen
Department of Orthopedic Surgery, Arrowhead Regional Medical Center, Colton, CA, USA

David C. Ebbott, Alexander J. Johnson and Christopher Haydel
Temple University, Department of Orthopaedics and Sports Medicine, 3401, N. Broad St. Zone B, 6th Floor, Philadelphia, PA 19140, USA

Desirae McKee and E. L. Domingo-Johnson
Department of Orthopaedic Surgery, Texas Tech University, 3601 4th Street, Mail Stop 9436, Lubbock, TX 79430-9436, USA

Mohamed F. Albana and Sean Z. Griffiths
Department of Orthopedic Surgery, Inspira Heath, 1505 W Sherman Ave, Vineland, NJ 08360, USA

Kris E. Radcliff
Department of Orthopedic Surgery, The Rothman Institute, 2500 English Creek Ave. Egg Harbor Township, NJ 08234, USA

Kentaro Mataki, Masao Koda, Yosuke Shibao, Hiroshi Kumagai, Katsuya Nagashima, Kousei Miura, Hiroshi Noguchi, Toru Funayama, Tetsuya Abe and Masashi Yamazaki
Department of Orthopedic Surgery, Faculty of Medicine, University of Tsukuba, 1-1-1 Tennodai, Tsukuba, Ibaraki 305-8575, Japan

Toru Morimoto, Masashi Izumi, Hiroaki Ueba and Masahiko Ikeuchi
Department of Orthopaedic Surgery, Kochi University, Kochi Medical School, Kohasu, Oko-cho, Nankoku 783-8505, Japan

Celeste Tavolaro, Hector Pulido, Richard Bransford and Carlo Bellabarba
Department of Orthopaedics & Sport Medicine, Harborview Medical Center, 325 Ninth Avenue Seattle, WA 98104, USA

Yohei Teramoto, Kensuke Fukushima, Tomohisa Koyama, Yoshihisa Ohashi, Katsufumi Uchiyama and Masashi Takaso
Department of Orthopaedic Surgery, Kitasato University School of Medicine, 1-15-1 Kitasato, Minami-ku, Sagamihara, Kanagawa 252-0374, Japan

Naonobu Takahira
Department of Rehabilitation, Kitasato University School of Allied Health Sciences, Japan

Hana Ueda, Shunpei Hama, Masataka Yasuda, Kenta Minato, Masahiro Miyashita and Kishik Shin
Department of Orthopaedic Surgery, Baba Memorial Hospital, 4-244 Nishiku Hamadera Funao-cho Higashi, Sakai, Osaka 592-8555, Japan

Paul A. Krebs
Premier Health, Department of Family Medicine, Wright State University Boonshoft School of Medicine, 2400 Miami Valley Drive Suite 160 Dayton, Ohio 45459, USA

James R. Borchers
The Ohio State University Wexner Medical Center Jameson Crane Sports Medicine Institute, 2835 Fred Taylor Drive, Columbus, Ohio 43202, USA

Patrick Brayfield
The Ohio State University, Athletic Training Staff, 615 Irving Schottenstein Dr., Columbus, OH 43210, USA

Karla Wyatt, Moustafa Zidane and Chyong-jy Joyce Liu
Department of Anesthesiology, Perioperative and Pain Management, Baylor College of Medicine/Texas Children's Hospital, Houston, TX, USA

Debora Schivo and Sébastien Durand
Department of Plastic, Reconstructive and Hand Surgery, University Hospital of Lausanne, CHUV, Lausanne, Switzerland

Ergys Gjika
Department of Hand Surgery, University Hospital of Geneva, HUG, Genève, Switzerland

Aurélien Traverso
Department of Orthopaedics and Traumatology, University Hospital of Lausanne, CHUV, Lausanne, Switzerland

Sachin M. Patil
Department of Medicine, Division of Pulmonary, Critical Care and Environmental Medicine, University of Missouri Hospital and Clinic, One Hospital Dr, Columbia, MO 65212, USA

Phillip Paul Beck, Taylor B. Nelson, Andres Bran Acevedo and William Roland
Department of Medicine, Division of Infectious Disease, University of Missouri Hospital and Clinic, One Hospital Dr, Columbia, MO 65212, USA

Devan Irving, Brent Geers and Bruce Lawrence
Ascension Genesys Hospital, 1 Genesys Parkway, Grand Blanc, MI. 48439, USA

Georgios Kalinterakis, Emmanouil Antonogiannakis, Arezoo Abdi, Georgios Demetriades, Alexandros Koulouktsis, Sotiria Vrouva, Anastasios Papagiavis and Miltiadis Ziogas
First Department of Orthopedics, 401 General Military Hospital of Athens, Athens 11525, Greece

Athanasios Syllaios and Antonios Koutras
First Department of Surgery, Laiko General Hospital, National and Kapodistrian University of Athens, Athens 11527, Greece

C. Passaplan, A. Simonin, G. Maestretti and E. Gautier
Orthopaedic Surgery, Cantonal Hospital of Fribourg (HFR), Chemin des Pensionnats 2, 1700 Fribourg, Switzerland

Juan M. Patiño and Juan M. Torres Moirano
Departamento de Ortopedia y Traumatologia, Servicio de Cirugía de Miembro Superior, Hospital Militar Central "Cosme Argerich", Buenos Aires., Argentina

Marco Odorizzi, Maurice FitzGerald, Jorge Gonzalez, Dario Giunchi, Flurim Hamitaga and Vincenzo De Rosa
Paediatric and Orthopaedic Surgical Department, Istituto Pediatrico della Svizzera Italiana (IPSI), Bellinzona and Valli Regional Hospital, Ticino, Switzerland

Ryutaro Iwasaki and Seiji Ohtori
Department of Orthopaedic Surgery, Graduate School of Medicine, Chiba University, Japan

Masaaki Sakamoto, Tomoyuki Rokkaku, Hitoshi Watanabe, Toshiyuki Yamada, Takeshi Yamaguchi and Yasushi Wako
Department of Orthopaedic Surgery, Chiba Municipal Aoba Hospital, Japan

Hitoshi Kubosawa
Department of Pathology, Chiba Municipal Aoba Hospital, Japan

Ali Wasel Almomen
King Fahad Specialist Hospital Dammam, Orthopedic Surgery, Saudi Arabia

Yaser Mansour Tawfeeq, Ahmed Khalid Almuhaisin and Abdulraheem Ayman Altalib
Imam Abdulrahman Bin Faisal University King Fahd Hospital of the University, Orthopedic Surgery, Saudi Arabia

Miguel Quesado, Ana Sofia Esteves, Nuno Vieira da Silva, Tiago Costa, Nuno Ferreira and Hélder Nogueira
Serviço de Ortopedia e Traumatologia, Centro Hospitalar do Tâmega e Sousa, Penafiel, Portugal

Ta-Li Hsu
Department of Orthopedic Surgery, Far Eastern Memorial Hospital, New Taipei City, Taiwan

Shang-Ming Lin
Department of Materials and Textiles, Oriental Institute of Technology, New Taipei City, Taiwan

Chih-Hung Chang
Department of Orthopedic Surgery, Far Eastern Memorial Hospital, New Taipei City, Taiwan
Yuan Ze University Graduate School of Biotechnology and Bioengineering, Taiwan

Tsung-Yu Lan
Department of Orthopedic Surgery, Far Eastern Memorial Hospital, New Taipei City, Taiwan
Department of Materials and Textiles, Oriental Institute of Technology, New Taipei City, Taiwan

Tadahiro Nakajima, Kaoru Tada, Mika Nakada, Masashi Matsuta and Hiroyuki Tsuchiya
Department of Orthopaedic Surgery, Graduate School of Medical Science, Kanazawa University, 13-1 Takaramachi, Kanazawa 920-1302, Japan

Dong Hu, Kai Xu and Songhua Xiao
Department of Orthopedic, Beijing Tsinghua Changgung Hospital, School of Medicine, Tsinghua University, Beijing, China

Rui Hirasawa, Takashi Itabashi, Tsuneji Kita and Chikato Mannoji
Department of Orthopedic Surgery, Japanese Red Cross Narita Hospital, 90-1, Iidacho, Narita-shi, Chiba 286-8523, Japan

Giovanni Bonaspetti, Giovanni Dib and Flavio Azzola
Department of Orthopaedics and Trauma Surgery, Clinical Institute S. Anna GSD, Via del Franzone 31 25127 Brescia, Italy

Shinya Ishizuka, Akinori Kobayakawa, Hideki Hiraiwa, Hiroki Oba, Takefumi Sakaguchi, Masaru Idota, Takahiro Haga, Takafumi Mizuno, Itaru Kawashima, Kanae Kuriyama and Shiro Imagama
Department of Orthopedic Surgery, Nagoya University Graduate School of Medicine, Nagoya, Japan

Emmanuel Gibon and Hari K. Parvataneni
Division of Adult Reconstruction, Department of Orthopedics and Rehabilitation, University of Florida College of Medicine, University of Florida, Gainesville, FL, USA

Jacquelyn A. Knapik
Department of Pathology, Immunology and Laboratory Medicine, University of Florida College of Medicine, University of Florida, Gainesville, FL, USA

Neven Starčević
Traumatology Department, University Hospital Sveti Duh, Sveti Duh, 64 Zagreb, Croatia

Andrija Karačić
Department of General Surgery, University Hospital Sveti Duh, Sveti Duh, 64 Zagreb, Croatia

F. M. Bombah
Department of Surgery, Faculty of Medicine and Pharmaceutical Sciences, University of Douala, Cameroon

M. Diawara and A. Mikiela
Orthopedic and Traumatologic Surgery Department, Army Instructional Hospital, Libreville, Gabon

B. Y. Ekani and T. Nana
Department of Surgery, Faculty of Medicine and Pharmaceutical Sciences, University of Buea, Cameroon

Hironari Kaneyama, Yuichiro Morishita, Osamu Kawano and Takeshi Maeda
Department of Orthopedic Surgery, Spinal Injuries Center, Iizuka, Japan

Takuaki Yamamoto
Department of Orthopedic Surgery, Fukuoka University, Fukuoka, Japan

Ryunosuke Fukushi, Izaya Ogon, Yoshinori Terashima, Hiroyuki Takashima, Tsutomu Oshigiri, Noriyuki Iesato, Mitsunori Yoshimoto, Makoto Emori, Atsushi Teramoto and Toshihiko Yamashita
Department of Orthopedic Surgery, Sapporo Medical University School of Medicine, Sapporo, Japan

Charles B. Pasque and Christopher Hendrix
Department of Orthopaedic Surgery and Rehabilitation, University of Oklahoma College of Medicine, Oklahoma City, Oklahoma, USA

Index

R

S

T

W

Z